TUMORS
OF THE HEAD AND NECK
IN CHILDREN

TUMORS
OF THE HEAD AND NECK
IN CHILDREN

CLINICOPATHOLOGIC PERSPECTIVES

Robert O. Greer Jr., D.D.S., Sc.D.

Gary W. Mierau, Ph.D.

Blaise E. Favara, M.D.

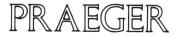

PRAEGER SPECIAL STUDIES • PRAEGER SCIENTIFIC

Library of Congress Cataloging in Publication Data

Greer, Robert O.
    Tumors of the head and neck in children.

    Includes index.
    1. Head—Tumors. 2. Neck—Tumors. 3. Tumors in
children. I. Mierau, Gary W. II. Favara, Blaise E.
III. Title. [DNLM: 1. Head and neck neoplasms—In
infancy and childhood. WE 707 G816t]
RC280.H4G73 1983   618.92'992   82-19114
ISBN 0-03-060093-6

Published in 1983 by Praeger Publishers
CBS Educational and Professional Publishing
a Division of CBS Inc.
521 Fifth Avenue, New York, New York 10175 U.S.A.

3456789   052   98765432

Printed in the United States of America

AUTHORS

Robert O. Greer, Jr., D.D.S., Sc.D.
Professor and Chairman
Division of Oral Pathology and Oncology
University of Colorado School of Dentistry
Denver, Colorado

Associate Professor of Pathology
University of Colorado School of Medicine
Denver, Colorado

Gary W. Mierau, Ph.D.
Electron Microscopist
Department of Pathology
The Children's Hospital
Denver, Colorado

Blaise E. Favara, M.D.
Chairman, Department of Pathology
The Children's Hospital
Denver, Colorado

CONTENTS

Chapter	Page

PREFACE

The problems attendant to accurate diagnosis and proper management of the child with a tumor of the head and neck represent a substantial challenge to the oncologist and pathologist. Lesions found in this location may herald the initial presentation of a more widespread disorder, such as a hematopoietic malignancy, or may represent the manifestations of a locally invasive and destructive process. Attention to cosmesis as it is affected by therapy and long-term complications of therapy are not inconsequential, but must be assessed in light of the potential lethality of many of these lesions.

This work presents a much needed description of the common lesions affecting the head and neck of children, and covers most of the important lesions to be encountered in that age group. It is comprehensive yet also represents the authors' personal experiences and is designed to be of assistance to the general pathologist who may encounter such lesions in his or her practice. The value of ultrastructural examination of the difficult lesion is to be emphasized and hopefully, the many illustrations will assist with proper classification of the numerous lesions manifesting in this area.

The work has been designed using a unique, easy-reference format that should allow quick resolution of statistical quandries related to the age, sex, site, and clinical presentation of a particular tumor. The pathogenesis of every lesion is also included. Chapters are presented with a central focus upon tissue type or specific disease entity rather than anatomic location.

A section on differential diagnosis is included for each neoplasm discussed. This section should be of interest not only to the pathologist, but to oral surgeons, pediatric general surgeons, otolaryngologists, and oncologists, as well. We believe this work will provide a useful document for those called upon to diagnose head and neck tumors as they affect the child.

It would be difficult to adequately acknowledge all the individuals who have contributed to the completion of this book in the short context of a preface; nonetheless, we are especially grateful to the following people:

Mrs. Patricia Yamashita had the arduous task of typing and editing the bulk of the original manuscript. Her dedication to detail and unselfish time commitment are gratefully acknowledged. We are also indebted to Ms. Wanda Valentine, Mrs. Paulette Newberry, and Ms. Pam Kanlet for their patience and diligence in this regard.

The bulk of the light microscopic photography represents the work of Dr. Todd Poulson who had the unenviable task of preparing much of the illustrative material while serving as a cancer fellow at the University of Colorado Health Sciences Center. His preparation of the hundreds of photomicrographs used to illustrate the diseases catalogued in this text deserves our sincere gratitude.

It would have been impossible to complete this undertaking without the support of our patient wives who offered encouragement during those periods when the challenge of completing this book seemed almost insurmountable.

Robert O. Greer, Jr.
Gary W. Mierau
Blaise E. Favara

TUMORS
OF THE HEAD AND NECK
IN CHILDREN

Chapter I

Clinicopathologic Approach to Head and Neck Tumors in the Child

APPROACH TO SURGICAL PATHOLOGY

The surgical pathology of tumors of the head and neck region in children is an exacting discipline because the pediatric oncologist depends on an accurate diagnosis and often a refined subclassification of that diagnosis in order to plan a multidisciplinary therapeutic program. Therapeutic modalities are potent and dangerous, thus an erroneously made malignant diagnosis of a benign process becomes a serious matter. The predominance of undifferentiated, embryonal tumors, which are often sarcomas, as compared to the rare occurrence of carcinomas in children, is in sharp contrast to the opposite experience in adults.

Best results of a pathological study follow pre-biopsy case discussions between pediatrician, oncologist, surgeon, and pathologist. Pre-biopsy evaluation should be thoughtful, thorough, and rapid. In the real and busy world of medicine, the pathologist too often learns of a case when previewing the operating schedule. A telephone call to the surgeon and/or attending physician will get the pathologist involved and thus benefit the patient. The pathologist should not hesitate to take the initiative!

If a malignant tumor is a strong pre-operative suspicion, a bone marrow examination should be done *before* surgery. A bone marrow aspirate and *biopsy* can be done under local anesthetic. The aspirate can be examined minutes after specimen procurement; and if a tumor is present, the type can often be diagnosed immediately thus sparing the child a general anesthetic and surgery. This point cannot be overemphasized!

Occasionally, a needle biopsy may result in diagnostic material, thus sparing the child a larger procedure.

The presence of elevated levels of serum lactate dehydrogenase in a patient suspected of having a malignant tumor when other (there are many) causes of that finding are absent, is strong evidence for malignancy and thus an indication for an approach to the malignancy.

That approach includes the following:

I. A thorough, pre-biopsy evaluation, such as chest x-ray, skeletal survey, abdominal films (supra-renal mass with mineralization is neuroblastoma until disproven), isotope scans, bone marrow study (some material should be processed for electron microscopy and immunological studies), body fluid studies for tumor makers, etc.

II. A pre-biopsy plan of surgery. How is the lesion approached: excision or incisional biopsy? Biopsy of draining lymph nodes? What is required for a proper operative staging of the disease? Will a frozen-section evaluation be useful? For diagnosis, which of the plans form an indication for additional "same-sitting" surgery? — Which of them determine adequacy of specimen for diagnosis? — and for determining extent of disease, when the extent dictates intra-operative management?

III. A specimen study. Tissue adequate for light microscopic, electron microscopic and immunopathological studies must be provided and processed immediately. The pathologist in the operating room can best advise on type of tissue to biopsy or excise; tissue can be promptly placed in glutaraldehyde, Zenker's, B-5, formalin, etc., touch imprints can be made, and material rapidly frozen. Cultures can be taken when findings suggest infection. The experienced pathologist can often "encourage" the surgeon to operate until the task at hand is accomplished, whether tumor resection or adequate biopsy.

If an adequate specimen is available, the tissue should be fixed in all four fixatives shown below, touch imprints made, and material frozen. If the tissue is inadequate for all fixatives, the priority or fixative choice is in the order shown below:

1. Zenker's, or B-5 (if lymphoma or leukemia is suspected).
2. Glutaraldehyde for electron microscopy.
3. 10% formalin.
4. Absolute alcohol (for PAS - glycogen studies).
5. Touch preparation - Wright's stain.
6. Material suitable for immunological studies.

When leukemia or lymphoma is suspected, B-5 fixative, touch imprints, immunological studies, and electron microscopy in that order of priority are indicated.

This ideal "team effort" is too often lacking but there is no question the patient benefits tremendously when it is operational.

Patients are spared needless surgery, pathologists make accurate diagnoses and therapists get better results.

The vast majority of tissue samples received from the oral cavity will represent one of the following: (1) excisional biopsy; (2) incisional biopsy; (3) bone biopsy; (4) aspiration biopsy; (5) punch biopsy; (6) exfoliative biopsy; (7) curettage biospy.

The punch biopsy is rarely encountered because of the nearly unlimited access, through use of the scalpel, that the clinician has to all oral sites. The aspiration or needle biopsy is typically used in the oral cavity to obtain fluid from a cavity of soft tissue or bone for chemical analysis.

Bone biopsies provide commonly encountered material from the oral cavity. The hard tissue requires decalcification prior to processing. The tissue sample sizes that the surgical pathologist must deal with are frequently rather small (less than 1 cm. in diameter). Commercial rapid decalcification solutions can be used; however, they tend to compromise cellular detail. Five percent nitric acid in neutral buffered formalin can be a reasonable alternative; decalcification, of course, takes longer, but cytologic detail is maintained. The tissue is considered properly decalcified when the decal solution that has been in contact with the hard tissue is mixed with both 5 ml. of ammonium hydroxide and 5 percent ammonium oxalate, and a clear solution results. A cloudy or milky solution indicates that further decalcification is necessary. Tissue submitted as curettings from a tooth socket often contain bone fragments. It is wise to decalcify this material to avoid sectioning difficulty.

Most soft tissue biopsies from the oral cavity are small, elliptical or wedge-shaped samples. If the tissue is received unfixed, it may be necessary to place thin, flat biopsies (e.g., floor of the mouth lesions) on a thin sheet of cardboard to prevent folding.

In suspected vesicular-bullous lesions, over aggressive handling of the delicate tissue can cause separation of epithelium from the underlying connective tissue, which of course impairs histopathologic interpretation.

Teeth are frequently only examined grossly, but each tooth must be adequately identified (i.e., first permanent maxillary second bicuspid). Often when teeth are submitted, the surgeon is interested in microscopic findings in soft tissue attachments to the root or crown of the tooth (e.g., dentigerous cyst, periapical cyst, odontogenic keratocyst). It is paramount to submit the attached soft tissue when such differential diagnoses are entertained by the submitting doctor.

Frozen sections are handled in much the same manner as tissue from elsewhere throughout the body. Automatically, considerable fatty tissue can be encountered in oral soft tissue specimens. These can be difficult samples on which to prepare frozen sections. The smaller the quantity of adipose tissue included, the simpler the sectioning process.

Very often the condition of artifact occurs as a result of the handling of oral tissues. Several types of artifact can be encountered including "crush artifact" which occurs most commonly in the manipulation of the tissue when it is removed using forceps or dull scalpel blades. This type of artifact is very dangerous in that it alters tissue morphology and squeezes the chromatin out of the cell nuclei. As inflammatory and tumor cells are the most susceptible to crush damage, this artifact can render an otherwise adequate specimen nondiagnostic. In order to prevent "crush artifact", tissue has to be handled very delicately, both at removal and at the surgical bench. A second very common condition of artifact seen in oral tissue specimens is "electrosurgery artifact". Electrosurgery, of course, provides adequate and prompt tissue hemostasis when a tissue sample is removed; however the cytological effect of electrosurgery on the tissue is to cauterize it, thereby precipitating protein and causing the resultant "cauterization artifact" which microscopically appears as coagulated, or shredded tissue. A third type of artifact seen in oral tissue samples is the artifact produced by the application of dyes, or medicaments to the tissues at the time of surgery.

Such medicaments can be introduced by the injection of a local anesthestic in or around the biopsy sites. A fourth kind of artifact is "dehydration artifact" caused by improper fixatives or air-drying of the specimen. Ten percent neutral buffered formalin remains the preferred fixative of choice for routine biopsy specimens. The last type of artifact that can inadvertently occur in oral tissue samples is "freezing artifact". This frequently occurs in the winter when outpatient biopsy specimens are mailed for evaluation. Ten percent formalin will freeze at -11° C, producing a "clefting artifact" that appears in the epithelium. "Freezing artifact" can be avoided by using Lillies AAF (acetic alcohol formalin). This fixative contains ten parts 40 percent formaldehyde, five parts glacial acetic acid, and five parts absolute ethyl alcohol. The solution will not freeze until it reaches -30° C.[1]

Electron microscopy may be an invaluable tool to the histopathologist and proper specimen handling is imperative if one is to utilize this technique to its fullest extent. Since the surgeon often cannot tell if such studies will be needed it is recommended that a 1 x 1 mm. sample of the fresh specimen be placed in 2 percent glutaraldehyde fixative as soon as possible after removal.

Thus the specimen is available for such study, —or may be discarded, if electron microscopy is not deemed necessary.

References

1. Bernstein, M.L. "Biospy technique: the pathological considerations." *J. Am. Dent. Assoc.* 96(1978): 438.

Chapter II

Papillary Lesions of the Oral Cavity, Nasosinus and Larynx

SQUAMOUS CELL PAPILLOMAS OF THE ORAL CAVITY AND SINUSES

Synonyms

1. Papilloma
2. Fibropapilloma
3. Squamous papilloma
4. Nasal papillomatosis
5. Squamous papillary epithelioma
6. Schneiderian papilloma

INCIDENCE

ORAL CAVITY:

The oral squamous cell papilloma is a very common benign epithelial neoplasm of children and young adults. The largest single survey of oral papillomas in the English literature was reported by Abbey and co-workers[1] in a review of 19,741 sequential surgical specimens from the oral cavity over a ten-year-period from 1968 to 1977. They defined papilloma as an exophytic arrangement of multiple papillary projections of stratified squamous epithelium arranged around a central fibrovascular connective tissue core. Four hundred and sixty-four lesions were considered histically acceptable as oral squamous papillomas.

Their series of 464 papillomas in 19,741 sequential specimens documents a 2.4 percent incidence. This figure is slightly higher than the 1.9 percent reported by Bhaskar,[2] and significantly lower than the 7.4 percent reported by Greer and Carpenter,[3] and the 3.0 percent reported by Thompson,[4] in similar evaluations of large numbers of sequential cases.

Abbey and associates[1] reported that 8.3 percent of their 464 oral papillomas occurred in patients less than ten-years-old. This figure correlates with the findings of Bhaskar[5] who reported the incidence of oral papillomas in children as 8 percent, and Jones[6] who reported a 7.5 percent incidence.

NASAL SINUS:

The squamous papilloma of the mucous membranes of the nasal cavity and paranasal sinuses is a relatively uncommon benign neoplasm. The reported incidence of nasal and paranasal sinus papillomas varies from 0.4 percent to 4.7 percent of all nasal and parasinus neoplasms.[7-10] Snyder and Perzin[11] reported that the lesion is four percent as frequent as the ordinary inflammatory nasal polyp.

Batsakis[12] reported four distinct histomorphological types of papillomas, and further categorizes them anatomically as: (1) papillary keratotic lesions arising from the squamous epithelial lining of the nasal vestibular mucosa; (2) inverted papillomas of the lateral nasal walls; (3) fungiform septal papillomas; and (4) the cylindrical cell papilloma of the maxillary sinus. Only the vestibular papilloma and the fungiform papilloma occur in significant numbers in children.[12;13]

Hyams[13] reported that the fungiform papilloma is the type most consistent with the common clinicopathological features of a papilloma. In a study of 315 papillomas of the nasal cavity and paranasal sinuses, Hyams was able to document only one fungiform papilloma arising in a child; however, he pointed out that, excluded from the study were classic nasal vestibular papillomas with clinical and histologic features and behavior patterns identical to papillomas arising from surfaces lined with squamous epithelium elsewhere in the body.[13]

Cummings and Goodman documented one inverted papilloma in a 12-year-old child out of a review of 29 inverted papillomas of the nose and paranasal sinus.[14] Two extensive reviews of inverted papillomas by Norris,[15] and Snyder and Perzin[11] failed to document a single inverted papilloma in a child.

AGE AND SEX

Eighteen to twenty-two percent of all oral squamous cell papillomas occur in childhood and adolescence.[1;3;5] Abbey and associates,[1] Greer and Carpenter,[3] and Greer and Goldman[16] all found the lesions to be somewhat more common in the second decade than in the first. Although the peak age of occurrence for oral papillomas has been reported to be the third through the fifth decades,[5;16;17] Abbey reported that 8.3 percent of his 464 cases were less than 10-years-old.

There are numerous conflicting accounts in the literature concerning the sexual predisposition in the incidence of the oral papilloma. Kohn and associates[18] reported that males outnumbered females three-to-one in their series; Greer and Goldman[16] documented a slight female predominance (1.25-to-1) in a review of 110 oral papillomas, and Waldron[17] noted equal numbers of males and females in a series of 125 lesions. Abbey and associates reported a slight predisposition towards males (1.04-to-1) in their review of 464 lesions.

The typical papilloma of the nasal vestibular mucosa shows no age specificity in childhood.

PATHOGENESIS

ORAL CAVITY:

Most investigators maintain that the oral papilloma is a true benign epithelial neoplasm.[19-21] Batsakis, however, questioned whether papillomas are not more accurately classified as a local reaction to injury rather than a true neoplasm.[12]

The viral etiology of oral papillomatous lesions in animals has been established;[22] but this etiology has never been substantiated with respect to human oral papillomas.[19;23] Without question, some lesions diagnosed as oral papillomas are one of the four varieties of virus-induced warts that can occur on the skin and mucous membranes.

Verruca vulgaris and condyloma acuminatum are the two most likely lesions to be more broadly diagnosed as "typical papillomas" on the oral mucosa. These two lesions are caused by the same Papova group virus, but show different clinical and pathologic manifestations according to their location.[24;25] It is very possible that the typical oral mucous membrane papilloma in many instances represents a manifestation of verruca vulgaris or condyloma acuminatum without histologic evidence of the atypical vacuolated cells seen in the stratum spinosum of these lesions when they are identified on the skin.

NASAL CAVITY AND PARANASAL SINUSES:

It is commonly suggested that papillomas of the nasal cavity and paranasal sinuses arise as a result of chronic inflammation of either allergic or bacterial origin. Hyams[13] discounts this postulate and reports that in a study of 315 nasosinus papillomas, there was no evidence to link the papillomas to local chronic inflammation or allergy. He also discounts the theory of neoplastic transformation of the inflammatory nasal polyp to a papilloma.

While a viral origin has been strongly suggested for nasal and paranasal sinus papillomas,[26;27] Hyams was unable to document intranuclear or cytoplasmic viral inclusion bodies in his survey. Gaito and associates reviewed the ultrastructure of the human nasal papilloma but were unable to identify virus-like particles.[28] It is commonly conceded that the paucity of reported papillomas of the nasal cavity and paranasal sinuses in the child tends to discredit a viral etiology because this younger age group would almost assuredly show increased involvement at these anatomic sites if a viral agent were active. So-called papillomas of the nose have been produced in hamsters using parenterally and topically applied carcinogens;[29] however, environmental carcinogenic agents have not been linked to human papillomas of the nasal sinuses.

CLINICAL FINDINGS

ORAL CAVITY:

Papillomas of the oral mucous membranes are most often perceived as broad based or pedunculated, raised, corrugated, oval swellings (Fig. 2-1). The vast majority are asymptomatic tumorfactions which rarely elicit from patients a "chief complaint". Abbey and associates[1] reported that the most common terms used by clinicians to describe papillomas are: sessile, pedunculated, cauliflower-like, and smooth. Most oral papillomas are white, pink, or red.

Lesions generally vary in size from less than 2-to-3 cm. in diameter.[1;16;30] Abbey and co-workers reported that in more than 50 percent of the lesions they reviewed, the lesions had existed from 2 to 11 months.[1]

These same investigators[1] reported that the palatal complex (hard palate, soft palate, uvula, tongue dorsum, and lips) were the most commonly affected oral anatomic locations, while Greer and Goldman[16] found that the tongue, palatal complex, and buccal mucosa were the most commonly affected areas.

NASAL SINUSES:

Childhood papillomas of the nasal vestibular mucosa are the most common of the four types of nasal and paranasal sinus papillomas to exhibit the typical raised, confluent cauliflower or verrucous excrescence which are consistent with the common visual concept of papilloma. Fungiform papillomas have a similar appearance.

Inverted papillomas are usually depicted as much more bulky and a great deal firmer than the vestibular papillomas common to the

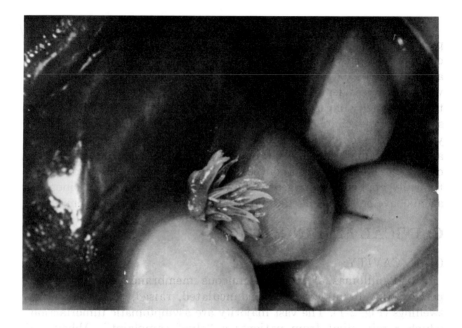

Fig. 2-1 Exophytic papilloma of the gingiva.

child.[13] Cylindrical cell papillomas are generally described as having a more ragged, beefy consistency than the typical papilloma of the nasal vestibule in children.

Nasal obstruction, epistaxis, pain, and allergic symptoms have all been reported as manifesting symptomatology for nasal and paranasal sinus papillomas.[13] None of these symptoms appear to be more common than others when viewed singularly in childhood.

LIGHT MICROSCOPY

ORAL PAPILLOMA:

The oral papilloma is classically an exophytic lesion demonstrating a complex pattern of multiple finger-like projections of stratified squamous epithelium surrounding a central vascular connective tissue core (Fig. 2-2). Hyperkeratosis is quite common. Superficial ulceration may be seen because nearly all oral lesions are subject to trauma during mastication. Regardless of whether the surface is intact or ulcerated, inflammatory cellular infiltration of the supporting connective tissue is an almost constant finding.

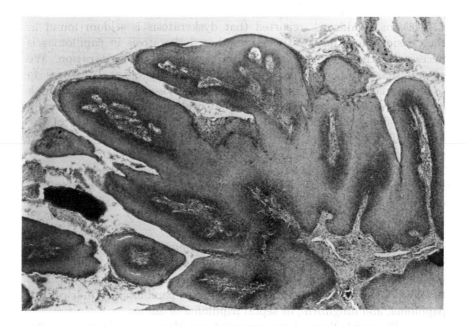

Fig. 2-2 Oral papilloma showing corrugated papillary fronds and thin connective tissue cores. (H&E x 250).

The literature contains varying accounts concerning the malignant potential of these lesions. Some reports have maintained that oral papillomas can display malignant alteration.[30-33] Shklar[34] stated that dyskeratosis and cellular atypia are found in a large number of papillomas, and he reported that carcinoma develops in large papillomas where the major portion of the lesion proves benign. Other investigators[11;16;19] considered the lesion unquestionably benign and found the biological behavior and histopathological appearance unassociated in any way with malignancy.

The biological relationship of dyskeratosis to malignancy in oral papillomas has received considerable attention in the literature. The question of whether the papilloma can represent a premalignant lesion has been somewhat unclear. Shklar[34] suggested that lesions having atypical epithelium have already undergone the early stages of malignant change, and he regarded papillomas with dyskeratotic changes as premalignant. The principal atypical feature documented in oral papillomas has been dyskeratosis, although Greer and Goldman[16] failed to encounter a single lesion exhibiting dyskeratotic change in a review of

110 lesions. Waldron[17] reported that dyskeratosis is seldom found in these lesions, and he questioned whether dyskeratosis in papillomas is necessarily the precursor of eventual carcinomatous alteration. We suspect that oral papillomas exhibiting atypical histological features do so in association with an intense inflammatory response or rapid growth rate; and we agree with Batsakis[12] that oral papillomas are uniformly benign lesions. Statements concerning the precancerous nature of the oral papilloma may have been due to confusion of this lesion with verrucous carcinoma.

Three acceptable cases of inverted papilloma of the oral cavity have been reported in the English literature.[35-37] None have occurred in children.

NASAL AND PARANASAL SINUS:

The histological features of the squamous papilloma of the nasal vestibular mucosa, the most frequent nasal sinus papilloma in childhood, are similar to those of the oral squamous papilloma (Fig. 2-3). This lesion must be distinguished from the inverted papilloma, cylindrical cell papilloma, and fungiform, or septal papilloma of adults.

The epithelium of the *inverted papilloma* invaginates into the supporting stroma and the exophytic papillary fronds of the more common vestibular papilloma of children are absent. Surface lining cells are usually squamous, but both Hyams and Batsakis[12;13] reported that ciliated columnar epithelium may also cover the inverted papilloma. Mucous-filled microcystic spaces are frequent throughout the epithelial portion of the tumor. There is no consistent inflammatory pattern within the edematous, myxomatous, or densely fibrous supporting stroma.

The *fungiform papilloma* has histological features that are quite comparable to those of the inverted papilloma, including microcyst formation. The connective tissue stroma may be a bit more reticular than in inverted papilloma, and a glandular component is generally absent. The principal feature of note that distinguishes the two lesions is the exophytic projection of squamous papillary frons in the fungiform papilloma.

The *cylindrical cell papilloma* is an exceedingly rare lesion. Hyams[13] was able to document only 10 such lesions in his review of 315 nasal sinus papillomas. He characterized the lesion as a papillary proliferation of multilayer, occasionally ciliated, column cells with eosinophilic cytoplasm, and round to oval, dark nuclei. Mucus cysts are frequently seen as epithelial inclusions.

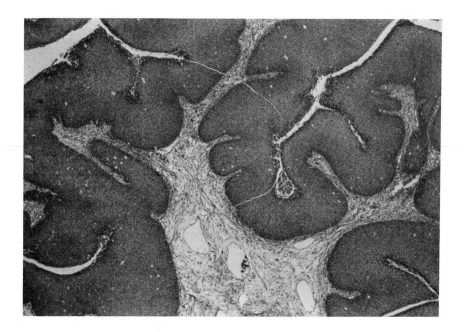

Fig. 2-3 Nasal papilloma. Note the loose, well-vascularized, connective tissue stroma that supports the seemingly inverted squamous papillary projections. (H&E x 220).

DIFFERENTIAL DIAGNOSIS

The solitary oral mucosal papilloma is usually easily recognizable clinically by virtue of its exophytic, corrugated surface. It may be indistinguishable from the common skin wart, *(verruca vulgaris)*, on the lips. Although clinically the lesions are quite similar, viral inclusion bodies are usually discernible in the upper spinous layer of verruca vulgaris.

Verruciform xanthoma of the oral mucosa is usually described clinically as a white, wart-like lesion resembling papilloma. Neville and Weathers reviewed a series of 21 of these lesions, and failed to document a single case in a child.[38] Histologically, the papilloma can be distinguished from the corrugated, rough-surfaced xanthoma as the latter lesion shows invaginating parakeratin crypts, elongated rete ridges, and foamy xanthoma cells in the lamina propria.

Condyloma acuminatum is a corrugated papillary lesion that may be, on clinical grounds, indistinguishable from the common oral papilloma. Condylomata are commonly referred to as *venereal warts*, and anatomically, they are predominately lesions of the anogenital region. Although oral condylomas are well-documented,[24] their occurrence in children is rare.

Eversole[39] pointed out that the clinical resemblance of condyloma acuminatum to the common oral papilloma is striking; however, he noted that the condyloma tends to appear more racemose, and also shows a tendency for multiplicity with clustering. Differentiation between the two can also normally be made clinically by a history of sexual transmission.

The most significant histological feature that separates condyloma from oral papilloma is the presence of vacuolated cells containing deeply hyperchromatic nuclei in the deeper portions of the epithelium.

Eversole and Sorenson reported a case of *florid oral papillomatosis* in a 13-year-old with Down's syndrome.[40] The lesions in the patient were identical clinically and histologically to diffuse confluent, cauliflower-appearing papillomas. The etiology of this generalized mucosal aberration is unknown. Multiple confluent papillomas of the lips and oral mucosa are a common feature of both *focal dermal hypoplasia syndrome (Goltz Syndrome)* and *nevus unius lateris.* The oral lesions are indistinguishable histologically from common oral papillomas.

Verrucous carcinoma of the oral mucosa may occasionally be confused with a large solitary papilloma. In the past, verrucous carcinoma was recognized as a disease of the elderly and it was rarely documented in children. The recent increased use of chewing tobacco by adolescents has accounted for our documentation of three pebbly, sessile, tobacco-associated verrucous lesions in patients less than 20 years of age at the University of Colorado School of Dentistry. Two of the three lesions were consistent microscopically with verrucous hyperkeratoses due to irritation; the third was verrucous carcinoma. Chewing tobacco is assumed to have been the etiologic agent since it had been applied locally to the site of all lesions for periods ranging from 6 months to 6 years.

NASAL SINUS:

It is of considerable importance to distinguish between papillomas of the nasal and paranasal sinuses as the biologic behavior of the four various types of papillomas are quite different.

Nasal polyps must be considered in the differential diagnosis of any suspected sinus papilloma in a child. Although the nasal polyp is primarily seen in adults, the well-documented association of nasal polyps with cystic fibrosis in children[41] must be remembered by both the clinician and the pathologist.

Prolonged symptoms, in a child, of nasal obstruction, recurrent epistaxis, and rhinorrhea are more foreboding than those commonly associated with the nasosinus papilloma. Angiofibroma, esthesioneuroblastoma, and extracranial meningioma are nasal lesions that may account for such symptomatology. These are discussed elsewhere in this text.

TREATMENT AND PROGNOSIS

Papillomas of the oral mucous membranes require complete local excision. Recurrence is uncommon. Abbey and associates reported a 4.1 percent recurrence rate in their review of 464 cases.[1] Twenty percent of the recurrent lesions recurred in the same year as excision. We agree with the findings of Goldman,[16] and Batsakis[12] that oral papillomas have no malignant potential. Batsakis reported that papillomas of the nasal vestibule (the typical papilloma of childhood) are probably, in truth, a collection of clinicopathologic lesions ranging from localized papillomatous keratosis to the keratinizing squamous papilloma that is identical to those found on other epithelial surfaces of the body. Their clinicopathologic behavior is benign and mimics that of similar lesions of skin. Complete local excision is the treatment of choice. Recurrence is uncommon.

When all four types of nasal and paranasal sinus papillomas are scrutinized for rates of recurrence, inverted and cylindrical cell papillomas show the highest recurrence rates.[11] Both types are almost nonexistent in children.

Malignant transformation in inverted papillomas has been reported to be as low as 2 percent,[42] and as high as 13 percent.[13] Such transformations appear limited to adults.

PAPILLOMAS OF THE LARYNX

Synonyms

1. Papilloma
2. Squamous cell papilloma
3. Juvenile papillomatosis
4. Juvenile papilloma
5. Juvenile laryngeal papilloma

INCIDENCE

The papilloma is the most common benign laryngeal neoplasm in children.[43-45] Only the subglottic hemangioma occurs with a frequency that remotely approaches the laryngeal papilloma.

AGE AND SEX

The onset of laryngeal papillomatosis is most frequent during the first seven years of life.[44] Majoros and associates[44] reviewed a series of 101 cases seen at the Mayo Clinic over a 46-year-period, and found that 37 percent of the children with laryngeal papillomas manifested symptoms, usually hoarseness, during the first two years of life. Halinger and co-workers[43] reviewed a series of 174 patients with papillomas of the larynx and found that 77 (44.3 percent) were in patients under 13 years of age. While some authors maintain that there is no sexual predisposition,[1;2] others report an inclination towards males.[44;46;47] Halinger suggested that the reason for such differences in sexual predominance relates to the fact that sexual distribution is equal in the prepubertal ages, but a male predominance is seen among the cases of immediately postpubertal children; a predominance that continues into adulthood. Blacks and whites appear to be affected equally.[43]

PATHOGENESIS

The association of chronic irritation and infection as etiological agents responsible for the growth, spread, and recurrence of the juvenile papilloma has been considered;[43;48] but, most evidence points to a viral etiology for juvenile papillomatosis.

The ultrastructural presence of virus-like particles in juvenile laryngeal papillomas has been documented throughout the literature in numerous reports.[49;50] Boyle and others have actually reported the occurrence of crystalline lattice assemblies characteristic of the Papova group virus in juvenile laryngeal papillomas. Quick and associates reported that there is a strong relationship between juvenile laryngeal papillomatosis and condylomata in the mother.[45]

Although a viral etiology remains the dominant acceptable causal factor for juvenile laryngeal papillomatosis, to date investigators have been unable to duplicate propogation of a laryngeal papilloma virus in cell culture by the establishment of culture lines from surgical specimens.[43]

Batsakis maintains that juvenile papillomas are not truly neoplastic lesions, but more than likely represent an abnormal tissue response to a viral stimulating factor.[12]

CLINICAL FINDINGS

Anatomically, the incidence of juvenile papillomas shows a predisposition of the true and false vocal cords, and the anterior commissure. Lesions can extend subglottically and may involve the trachea, bronchi, or epiglottis.[46] Kissane reported that approximately one percent of such cases originate in the trachea without evidence of laryngeal lesions.[51] Lynn and Takita[52] reviewed a series of tracheal papillomas and reported that 36 percent of tracheal lesions were associated with previous or present laryngeal papillomatosis. Esophageal juvenile papillomatosis is exceedingly rare,[53] as are juvenile papillomas of the pharynx and soft palate.

Hoarseness or a change in phonetics are the most commonly perceived symptoms. Majoros and co-workers[44] reported that hoarseness was the chief manifesting symptom in 91 of 101 cases in which they reviewed the clinicopathologic features of juvenile laryngeal papillomas. Respiratory difficulty is a rare manifesting symptom, and although it does occur, Majoros and associates reported only six instances of respiratory distress as the patient's chief complaint.

Juvenile papillomas appear as white, pink or red, corrugated, raspberry or cauliflower-like mucosal nodules (Fig. 2-4). They bleed quite readily and are frequently described as quite friable. Of the 101 cases reviewed by Majoros and co-workers,[44] 99 occurred as multiple lesions, and only 2 were solitary.

The disease may last five or more years and many reports document an average duration of more than 12 years.[44] Puberty has no effect on the course of the disease, and rarely do lesions regress spontaneously before the age of three.

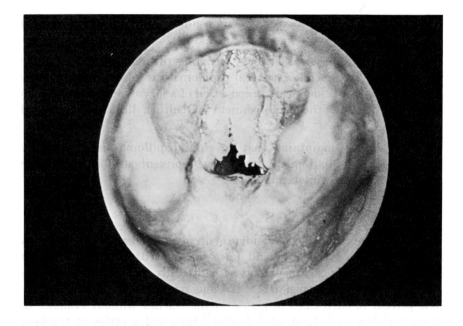

Fig. 2-4 Papilloma of the larynx in a child. Note the corrugated filliform character of the lesion. Courtesy of Dr. Bruce Jafek.

LIGHT MICROSCOPY

Both juvenile and adult papillomas have identical histological features; they are classically that of exophytic, papillary squamous epithelial frons, supported by a well-vascularized connective tissue core. Lesions may be sessile or pedunculated, and the squamous cells composing the lesion are generally well-differentiated without atypical features.

Quick and co-workers reviewed a series of 32 patients with laryngeal papillomatosis in childhood and adolescence in an attempt to better correlate histopathological features with clinical behavior.[45] These investigators identified three general clinical groups on the basis of recurrence rates and extent of papillomatosis. They found that the greatest frequency of recurrence was in those rare lesions with evidence of cytologic atypia.

Some of the lesions reviewed showed very disturbing atypical features including mitoses, cellular pleomorphism, and dyskeratosis. There was, however, no evidence of invasive carcinoma in any of their cases. The authors concluded that it was not possible to determine whether the atypia represented a response to rapid, benign cellular turnover, or neoplastic alteration. Based upon my own experience (ROG) with juvenile papillomatosis, histological evidence of cellular atypia is indeed a feature of note in a small percentage of cases, but the lesions as a whole have to be considered benign, and the atypia reactive, except for the rare, so-called invasive laryngeal papillomatosis described by Fechner and associates;[54] —although the lesion they describe bears a striking resemblance to verrucous carcinoma. The histological criteria for malignancy arising in a papilloma are identical to those used for diagnosing malignancy in other mucous membranes in the head and neck area. True papillary squamous cell carcinoma, although reported,[44;55] is a distinct rarity in the child and, as Batsakis[12] pointed out, unless induced by radiation or other means, the papillary squamous cell carcinoma does not pass through a benign papilloma phase. Altmann and others[56] suggested that when epithelial anaplasia is seen in papillomas of the adult larynx, repeated biopsies are mandatory; and while they made no reference to this necessity in laryngeal papillomatosis in childhood, they did suggest that the anaplastic changes in adult laryngeal papillomas are less alarming than those that arise in non-papillomatous epithelium of the larynx.

DIFFERENTIAL DIAGNOSIS

Although there are no apparent histological criteria that separate the juvenile papilloma from the adult papilloma, Halinger and co-workers maintained that there are clinical features quite unique for each of the lesions.[57] They reported the adult papilloma to be more friable than the childhood papilloma; but noted that the latter tends to be more penetrating, deep based, and firm. Otolaryngologists as a group agree with this observation.[58] Another clinical feature distinguishing the two lesions, is the much greater tendency for the laryngeal papilloma of the child to be multiple and confluent. The adult papilloma is characteristically solitary.

Atypical epithelial lesions showing transgression of the basement membrane are uniformly carcinomas. There is little difficulty in distinguishing these malignant lesions from the benign juvenile papilloma, even if they are papillary carcinomas. It should be noted that papillary squamous cell carcinoma tends to be a disease of adults and not children, and although the lesion is papillary in configuration, it has the cytologic hallmarks of malignancy. The papillary carcinoma is usually solitary and most often a lesion of the oropharynx or hypopharynx,[7] while juvenile papillomas occur chiefly on the true and false vocal cords, and the anterior commissure.

Great difficulty arises when lesions such as verrucous carcinoma and the so-called "invasive papilloma" described by Fechner[54] must be distinguished from a rapidly growing papilloma. We tend to agree with Quick and co-workers[45] who considered the "invasive papilloma" strikingly similar to verrucous carcinoma on both clinical and histological grounds.

As a last differential diagnostic consideration, it is paramount for the pathologist to remember that allowance must be made for the technical difficulties that are unavoidable in the preparation of histologic sections of laryngeal papillomas. The architecture of a papilloma produces many tangential sections which may be difficult to interpret. This difficulty is also compounded by the fact that a variation in the cytology of epithelial cells may occur from one part of the section to another. It is wise, therefore, to ask for input from the clinician, who may have a perspective about the nature of the growth of the specimen that makes the histological picture more or less tenable.

PROGNOSIS AND TREATMENT

The philosophy of treatment for multiple recurring papillomas of childhood should be along conservative management lines.[12] Halinger and co-workers[57] subscribed to a conservative treatment philosophy, and Szpunar,[59] and Batsakis[7] reported that the most successful management modality continues to be endoscopic excision of the lesions, often using microsurgical methods. Other forms of therapy have included cryotherapy, antibiotics, steroids, arsenicals, podophyllin, laser therapy, ultrasound, and radiation.[12]

Active spread of papillomas can occur as unexpectedly as their spontaneous regression. Szpunar[59] reported that even when the process seems to be completely cured, recurrence may be seen after a long symptom-free interval. This natural history dictates a follow-up period of no less than five years consisting of periodic, careful, and thoughtful re-examinations.

A 12-to-14 percent mortality rate has been expressed for the disease. This rather high mortality rate for a benign process is primarily related to therapeutic complications.

References

1. Abbey, L.M.; Page, R.G. and Sawyer, D.R. "The clinical and histopathological features of a series of 464 oral squamous cell papillomas." *Oral Surg.* 49(1980): 419-428.

2. Bhaskar, S.N. "Oral pathology in the dental office: Survey of 20,575 biopsy specimens." *J. Am. Dent. Assoc.* 76(1968): 761-766.

3. Greer, R.O. and Carpenter, M. "Surgical oral pathology at the University of Colorado School of Dentistry: A survey of 400 cases." *J. Colo. Dent. Assoc.* 54(1977): 13-16.

4. Thompson, C.C. "A six year regional report in the oral tumor registry and lesions diagnosed at the School of Dentistry biopsy service, University of Oregon Health Sciences Center." *J. Oral Med.* 36(1981): 11-15.

5. Bhaskar, S.N. "Oral tumors of infancy and childhood: A survey of 293 cases." *J. Pediatr.* 64(1963): 195-210.

6. Jones, J.H. "Non-odontogenic oral tumors in children." *Br. Dent. J.* 119(1965): 439-447.

7. Alford, T.C. and Winship, T. "Epithelial papillomas of the nose and paranasal sinus." *Am. J. Surg.* 106(1963): 764-767.

8. Lampertico, P.; Russell, W.D. and MacComb, W.S. "Squamous papilloma of upper respiratory epithelium." *Arch. Pathol.* 75(1963): 293-302.

9. Seydell, E.M. "Fibro-epithelial tumors of the nose (papillomata) and their relationship to carcinoma." *Ann. Otol. Rhinol. Laryngol.* 42(1933): 1081-1103.

10. Verner, J.L.; Maguda, T.A. and Young, J.M. "Epithelial papillomas of the nasal cavity and sinuses." *Arch. Otolaryngol.* 70(1959): 574-578.

11. Snyder, R.N. and Perzin, K.H. "Papillomatosis of nasal cavity and paranasal sinuses (inverted papilloma, squamous papilloma). A clinicopathologic study." *Cancer* 30(1972): 668-670.

12. Batsakis, J.G. *Tumors of the Head and Neck. Clinical and Pathologic Considerations.* 2nd ed. Baltimore: Williams and Wilkins, 1979.

13. Hyams, V.J. "Papillomas of the nasal cavity and paranasal sinuses. A clinico-pathological study of 315 cases." *Ann. Otol. Rhinol. Laryngol.* 80(1971): 192-206.

14. Cummings, C.W. and Goodman, M.C. "Inverted papillomas of the nose and paranasal sinuses." *Arch. Otolaryngol.* 92(1970): 445-449.

15. Norris, H.J. "Papillary lesions of the nasal cavity and paranasal sinuses. Part II: Inverting papilloma. A study of 29 cases." *Laryngoscope* 73(1963): 1-17.

16. Greer, R.O. and Goldman, H.M. "Oral papillomas. Clinicopathologic evaluation and retrospective examination for dyskeratosis in 110 lesions." *Oral Surg.* 38(1974): 435-440.

17. Waldron, C.A. "Oral Epithelial Tumors." In *Thoma's Oral Pathology*, edited by R.J. Gorlin and H.M. Goldman, pp. 801-802. St. Louis: C.V. Mosby, 1970.

18. Kohn, E.M.; Dahlin, D.C. and Erich, J.B. "Primary neoplasms of the hard and soft palates and uvula." *Proc. Staff Mtg. Mayo Clin.* 39(1963): 233-241.

19. Shafer, W.G.; Hine, M.K. and Levy, B.M. *A Textbook of Pathology*, 3rd ed. Philadelphia: W.B. Saunders, 1974.

20. Eversole, L.R. *Clinical Outline of Oral Pathology.* Philadelphia: Lea and Febiger, 1978.

21. Spouge, J.D. *Oral Pathology.* St. Louis: C.V. Mosby, 1973.

22. Gorlin, R.J.; Clark, J.J. and Chaudry, A.A. "The oral pathology of domesticated animals." *Oral Surg.* 11(1958): 500-535.

23. Frithof, L. and Wersall, J. "Virus-like particles in human oral papilloma." *Arch. Otolaryngol.* 64(1967): 263-266.

24. Shaffer, E.L., Jr.; Reimann, B.E.F. and Gysland, W.B. "Oral condyloma acuminatum. A care report with light microscopic and ultrastructural features." *J. Oral Pathol.* 9(1980): 163-173.

25. Praetarius-Clausen, F. "Rare and viral disorders (molluscum contagiosum localized keratoacontroma, verrucae, condyloma acuminatum and focal epithelial hyperplasia)." *Oral Surg.* 34(1972): 604-618.

26. Eggston, A.A. and Wolff, D. *Histopathology of Ear, Nose and Throat.* Baltimore: Williams and Wilkins, 1947.

27. Lehman, R.H. "Papillary sinusitis." *Ann. Otol. Rhinol. Laryngol.* 58(1949): 507-511.

28. Gaito, R.A.; Gaylord, W.H. and Hilding, D.A. "Ultrastructure of a human nasal papilloma." *Laryngoscope* 75(1965): 144-152.

29. Herrold, K.M. "Epithelial papillomas of the nasal cavity. Experimental induction in Syrian hamsters." *Arch. Pathol.* 78(1964): 189-195.

30. Lucas, R.B. *Pathology of Tumours of the Oral Tissues*, 3rd ed. London: Churchill Livingstone, 1976.

31. Archer, W.W. *Oral Surgery*, 4th ed. Philadelphia: W.B. Saunders, 1966.

32. Castiglian, S.G. "Oral Cancer." In *Oral Medicine*, 5th ed., edited by L.W. Burket, pg. 550. Philadelphia: J.B. Lippincott, 1965.

33. LaDow, C.S. "Surgical Aspects of Oral Tumors." In *Textbook of Oral Surgery*, 2nd ed., edited by G.O. Kruger, pg. 582. St. Louis: C.V.Mosby, 1964.

34. Shklar, G. "The precancereous oral lesions." *Oral Surg.* 20(1965): 58-70.

35. Moskow, R. and Moskow, B.S. "Inverted papilloma, report of a case." *Oral Surg.* 15(1966): 918-922.

36. Gettinger, R. "Atypical papilloma of the cheek: case report." *Archives of Clinical Oral Pathology* 3(1939): 62-82.

37. Greer. R.O. "Inverted oral papilloma." *Oral Surg.* 36(1973): 400-403.

38. Neville, B.W. and Weathers, D.R. "Verruciform xanthoma." *Oral Surg.* 49(1980): 429-434.

39. Eversole, L.R. *Clinical Outline of Oral Pathology. Diagnosis and Treatment.* London: Lea and Febiger, 1978.

40. Eversole, L.R. and Sorenson, H.W. "Oral florid papillomatosis in Down's syndrome." *Oral Surg.* 37(1974): 202-207.

41. Berman, J.M. and Colman, B.H. "Nasal aspects of cystic fibrosis in children." *J. Laryngol. Otol.* 91(1977): 133-139.

42. Osborn, D.A. "Nature and Behavior of transitional tumors in the upper respiratory tract." *Cancer* 25(1970): 50-60.

43. Halinger, P.H.; Schild, J.A. and Maurizi, D.G. "Laryngeal papilloma: Review of etiology and therapy." *Laryngoscope* 78(1968): 1462-1474.

44. Majoros, M.; Parkhill, E.M. and Devine, K.D. "Papilloma of the larynx in children: A clinicopathologic study." *Am. J. Surg.* 108(1964): 470-475.

45. Quick, C.A.; Foucar, E. and Dehner, L.P. "Frequency and significance of epithelial atypia in laryngeal papillomatosis." *Laryngoscope* 89(1979): 550-560.

46. Bjork, H. and Weber, C. "Papilloma of larynx." *Acta Otolaryngol.* 46(1956): 499-516.

47. del Villar et al. "Laryngeal papillomatosis. Its treatment at the Hospital Infantil de Mexico." *Arch. Otolaryngol.* 64(1956): 480-485.

48. Jenkins, J.C. "Preliminary report on the treatment of multiple juvenile laryngeal papillomata by ultrasound." *J. Laryngol. Otol.* 81(1967): 385-390.

49. Boyle et al. "Electron microscopic identification of papova virus in laryngeal papilloma." *Laryngoscope* 80(1973): 1102-1108.
50. Lundquist, P.G.; Frithiof, L. and Wersall, J. "Ultrastructural features of human juvenile laryngeal papillomas." *Acta Otolaryngol.* 80(1975): 137-149.
51. Kissane, J.M. *Pathology of Infancy and Childhood*, 2nd ed. St. Louis: C.V. Mosby, 1975.
52. Lynn, R.B. and Takita, H. "Tracheal papilloma." *Can. Med. Assoc. J.* 97(1967): 1354-1357.
53. Nuwayhid, N.S.; Ballard, E.T. and Cotton, R. "Esophageal papillomatosis. Case report." *Ann. Otol. Rhinol. Laryngol.* 86(1977): 623-625.
54. Fechner, R.E.; Gaepfert, H. and Alford, B.R. "Invasive laryngeal papillomatosis." *Arch. Otolaryngol.* 99(1974): 147-151.
55. Friedberg, S.A.; Stagman, R., and Hass, G.M. "Papillary lesions of the larynx in children. A clinicopathologic study." *Ann. Otol. Rhinol. Laryngol.* 80(1971): 683-693.
56. Altmann, F.; Basek, M. and Stout, A.P. "Papillomas of the larynx with intraepithelial anaplastic changes." *Arch. Otolaryngol.* 62(1955): 478-485.
57. Halinger, P.H.; Johnston, K.C. and Anison, G.C. "Papilloma of the larynx: a review of 109 cases with a preliminary report on aureomycin therapy." *Ann. Otol. Rhinol. Laryngol.* 59(1950): 547-564.
58. Jafek, B.W. Personal communication, 1981.
59. Szpunar, J. "Juvenile laryngeal papillomatosis." *Otolaryngol. Clin. North Am.* 10(1977): 67-70.

Chapter III

Cysts and Pseudocysts of the Soft Tissues

MUCOCELE

Synonyms

1. Mucous retention cyst
2. Mucous extravasation phenomenon
3. Mucous inclusion cyst
4. Ranula

INCIDENCE

The mucocele is the most commonly encountered of all lower lip swellings in children. After the lower lip, the most common sites in order of frequency in the head and neck area are the buccal mucosa, floor of the mouth, palate, tongue, upper lip, maxillary sinus, and retromolar areas.[1,2] Lesions involving the submandibular or sublingual glands and arising in the floor of the mouth are commonly termed ranulas. Ranulas and maxillary sinus mucoceles are discussed in Chapter VI under salivary gland tumors.

Greer and Carpenter[3] reviewed 400 surgical specimens seen during a one year period on the surgical oral pathology service at the University of Colorado School of Dentistry, and found that 5.7 percent represented mucoceles. Over half of the lesions they recorded were in children and young adults.

AGE AND SEX

Approximately one-third of all reported cases of mucoceles of the oral cavity have occurred in the first two decades of life. Greer and Carpenter[3] found that 35 percent of their cases were in patients between the ages of 1 and 19. Harrison[1] reported that 32 percent of salivary mucoceles he reviewed were in patients less than 20 years of age. Cohen[4] reviewed 356 mucoceles of the oral cavity and reported that nearly 50 percent occurred in patients less than 20 years of age. There was no sexual predisposition recorded in any of these studies.

PATHOGENESIS

Oral mucoceles develop in one of two manners. The most frequently encountered type arises (usually due to trauma) as a result of extravasation of mucus into adjacent tissues following rupture of the duct of a minor salivary gland. This rupture generally results in the formation of granulation tissue at the periphery of the lesion. These *extravasation type* mucoceles occur more frequently in children than adults.

Rarely, a second type of mucocele can be found in which a cavity lined by epithelium and filled with mucus is identified. This true mucous cyst (*retention mucocele*) usually results from obstruction of a salivary gland duct resulting in subsequent dilation.

CLINICAL FINDINGS

Mucoceles occur as painless, freely movable, smooth, dome-shaped, fluctuant swellings varying in size from a few millimeters to several centimeters (Fig. 3-1). They often have an intense blue color which may make them difficult to distinguish clinically from hemangioma. Mucoceles are frequently bitten by the patient, causing them to drain and heal. Following bite trauma, the swelling will usually recur, necessitating surgical management.

LIGHT MICROSCOPY

Most mucoceles are of the extravasation type and are considered to arise as a result of an extravasation of mucous from a torn main duct of a minor salivary gland. The consequences of such extravasation of mucous into the surrounding tissues is usually a peripheral inflammatory response and ultimately aggregation of granulation tissue. A fibrous capsular margin may encompass the entire accumulation of mucous and granulation tissue (Fig. 3-2). Minor salivary gland acinar and ductal elements are often prominent at the periphery of the extravasated mucous.

The retention-type mucocele usually consists of a channel of mucous limited either by a band of flattened fibroblasts, or rarely, by a true epithelial lining. A chronic inflammatory component usually infiltrates the surrounding connective tissue and residual salivary gland lobules.

DIFFERENTIAL DIAGNOSIS

Clinically, the mucocele may be confused with hemangioma while histologically, it can mimic low grade mucoepidermoid carcinoma

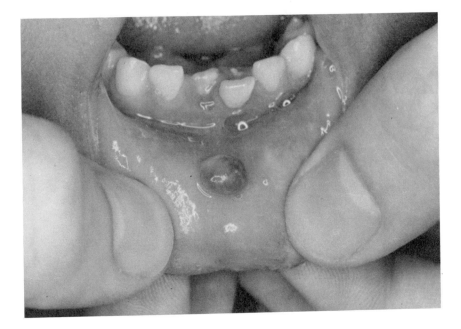

Fig. 3-1 Dome-shaped mucosal swelling characteristic of mucocele. Courtesy of Dr. Al Abrams.

or chronic sialadenitis. However, multiple entrapment cysts common to mucoepidermoid carcinoma are not common histologic features of mucocele.

TREATMENT AND PROGNOSIS

Mucoceles may regress spontaneously; however, the vast majority do not regress, necessitating surgical excision. Large mucoceles may have to be treated by marsupalization. If this surgical procedure is employed without extirpation of the associated gland responsible for pooling of the mucous, recurrence is quite likely.

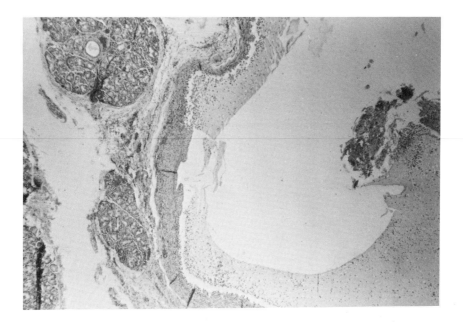

Fig. 3-2 Mucocele. A well-defined mucous pool is localized in the connective tissue. The pool is surrounded by a fibrous band, some granulation tissue, and minor salivary gland lobules. (H&E x 200).

LYMPHOEPITHELIAL CYST

Synonyms

1. Branchial cleft cyst
2. Bronchiogenic cyst

INCIDENCE

The lymphoepithelial cyst of the oral mucous membrane is a rare lesion that microscopically resembles the so-called branchial cleft cyst of the neck. They both are lined by stratified squamous epithelium and contain functioning lymphoid tissue. Giunta and Cataldo[5] reported a series of 21 cases of lymphoepithelial cysts and found that they represented only .09 percent of all the cases in the files of the Department of Oral Pathology at Tufts University School of Dental Medicine. In a review of 19,997 cases accessioned to the oral pathology service at the University of Colorado School of Dentistry, The Denver Children's Hospital surgical pathology service, and Western States Regional Oral Pathology Laboratory service during a five-and-one-half year period, Greer and Mierau recorded only 17 cases of lymphoepithelial cyst.[6]

AGE AND SEX

The lymphoepithelial cyst is usually noticed during late adolescence or early adulthood. Giunta and Cataldo[5] found age ranges from 7 to 65 years with a mean age of 32. Twenty percent of their cases occurred in patients less than 18. While there was no apparent predisposition of either sex in their study, Batsakis[7] has reported a male predisposition for this lesion.

PATHOGENESIS

The origin of the intraoral lymphoepithelial cyst is not known, but several theories have been postulated concerning its histogenesis.[8;9] Knappe[10;11] suggested that crypts of heterotopic oral lymphoid tissue become occluded, resulting in cystic proliferation of epithelium with lymphoid aggregations. Bhaskar[8] proposed that during embryogenesis, epithelium of glandular or ductal origin becomes included within lymphoid tissue, and subsequently, this epithelium undergoes cystic proliferation.

CLINICAL FINDINGS

Clinically, lymphoepithelial cysts are found as asymptomatic submucosal masses which are present prior to discovery for periods ranging from a few months to several years. They appear as freely movable nodular masses, varying in size from a few millimeters to two centimeters. The vast majority are seen in the floor of the mouth and the postero-lateral portion of the tongue. Usually the color of the cyst is yellow or yellow-white.

LIGHT MICROSCOPY

Histologically, a cystic cavity, lined by a thin flattened layer of stratified squamous epithelium, is seen subjacent to normal oral epithelium. The lumen usually contains acute and chronic inflammatory cells and amorphous eosinophilic coagulum. Immediately adjacent to the lining epithelium, there is well-organized lymphoid tissue, usually encompassing the entire cyst. The lymphoid tissue usually has a classic follicular arrangement often with germinal centers. The loose connective tissue adjacent to lymphoid aggregates may contain scattered inflammatory cells.

DIFFERENTIAL DIAGNOSIS

The most common lesions to clinically resemble lymphoepithelial cysts are mucocele, lipoma, and dermoid cysts. The histological features of these three lesions are so distinctly unique as to obviate confusion with lymphoepithelial cysts on histological grounds.

TREATMENT AND PROGNOSIS

The treatment of choice for the lymphoepithelial cyst is conservative surgical excision. None of the 21 cases reviewed by Giunta and Cataldo[5] or the 17 cases recorded by Greer and Mierau[6] recurred.

DERMOID CYST

Synonyms

1. Epidermoid cyst
2. Epithelial inclusion cyst
3. Teratoid cyst
4. Epidermal cyst

INCIDENCE

The term dermoid cyst has been defined by Meyer[12] to include three separate and distinct entities in the head and neck area. These three cystic entities include the epidermoid cyst, the dermoid cyst, and the teratoid cyst. *Dermoid* cyst is merely the clinical term used for all three types of cysts.

Head and neck dermoid cysts, regardless of subtype, account for approximately seven percent of dermoid cysts seen in all anatomic locations.[13]

Eighty percent of all dermoid cysts seen in the head and neck occur in the orbital area, the floor of the mouth, including the submandibular and submental areas, and the nasal region.[7] The remaining anatomic sites include the neck, lower lip, palate, and frontal or occipital midline.

Taylor and Erich,[13] in a review of dermoid cysts of the nose, found that lesions in this area accounted for just over 7.5 percent of all *dermoids* in the head and neck.

Dermoid cysts of the oral cavity account for about 25 percent of all dermoids in the head and neck region but represent less than 2 percent of dermoid cysts when all anatomic locations are considered.[14]

AGE AND SEX

The dermoid cyst is rarely seen at birth or in infancy. The majority occur in children, adolescents and young adults, and usually before the age of 35.[13] Yoshimura and associates[15] reviewed the world literature from 1949 to 1967 and found only eight reported cases of dermoid cyst in the sublingual region in infants and children. Taylor reviewed the literature concerning dermoid cysts of the nose and found an age range from 3 months to 59 years. The average age at the time of diagnosis and treatment in Taylor's review was between 12 and 13 years.

Meyer[12] suggested that development of dermoid cysts in the orbital region and the oral cavity are coincidental with the period of development of epithelial tissue derivatives including sweat glands, hair, and sebaceous glands. Most of the lesions in these two locations, therefore, become evident between the ages of 15 and 30 years.

A male predominance has been reported for the occurrence of dermoid cysts of the nose.[13] A similar sexual predisposition has not been noted for dermoid cysts in other head and neck regions.

PATHOGENESIS

Most dermoid cysts are derived from epithelial debris, or rests enclaved in tissue during embryonic closure or from traumatic implantation.[15] Dermoid cysts of the floor of the mouth may be caused by the ectodermal differentiation of multipotential cells that were probably pinched off at the time of closure of the anterior neuropore.[16] Congenital epidermoid cysts and teratomas have also been explained based upon this embryological enclavement phenomenon.[17;18] A very small percentage of dermoid cysts probably represent choristomas.[7]

CLINICAL FINDINGS

Dermoid cysts of the *nose* rarely result in dramatic clinical findings. The first clinical signs may be a small depression or pit on the bridge of the nose. Hairs may extend from the depression. Larger lesions often result in a freely movable, rubbery, subcutaneous mass. Cysts which are located deeply may result in nasal obstruction.

Dermoid cysts of the *oral cavity* most often affect the floor of the mouth (Fig. 3-3). These lesions generally range in size from a few millimeters to 12 centimeters in diameter[19] (Fig. 3-4). They have a rubbery or doughy consistency and are often filled with yellowish, cheese-like material derived from the cyst wall. Symptoms usually include a slowly enlarging swelling in the floor of the mouth and difficulty with speech or swallowing. Extraoral swelling, if present, is characterized by the gradual development of a "double chin" appearance. Dermoid cysts in the floor of the mouth have been described anatomically as sublingual, genioglossal, geniohyoid, or lateral. The lesions are invariably in the midline and pain is seldom a primary feature.

Dermoid cysts in a child's *orbital* region usually begin as small swellings along lines of embryonic closure. They have a doughy texture and may be multiple.

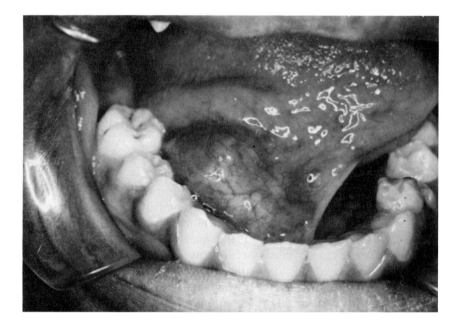

Fig. 3-3 Dermoid cyst arising above the mylohyoid muscle. Courtesy of Dr. Al Abrams.

LIGHT MICROSCOPY

The *dermoid cyst* is an epithelial-lined cavity containing an admixture of dermal appendages such as sebaceous glands, sweat glands, hair, and hair follicles in its supporting connective tissue wall (Fig. 3-5). The cyst lumen is often filled with cheesy, coagulated, proteinaceous debris or keratin.

The *epidermoid cyst* is generally lined by a thin, often corrugated layer of squamous epithelium which is supported by a connective tissue wall, devoid of adnexal structures. The contents of the cyst lumen are similar to those of the dermoid cyst.

The *teratoid cyst* is an epithelial-lined cavity usually filled with cheesy material. The cavity may be lined by stratified squamous or respiratory-type epithelium. Muscle, bone, fibers, and other mesodermal or endodermal structures, as well as dermal appendages, can be found in the supporting stroma.

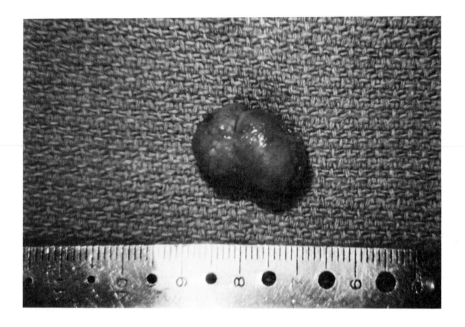

Fig. 3-4 Gross appearance of well-encapsulated dermoid cyst of the oral cavity. Courtesy of Dr. Bruce Jafek.

DIFFERENTIAL DIAGNOSIS

True *teratomas* of the head and neck are most frequently encountered in the neck and nasopharynx. A few are located in the orbit. Most teratomas arise at birth. Those in the nasopharynx affect females more frequently than males, and signs and symptoms depend upon the site and size of the teratomatous mass.

True teratoid tumors differ from the more common dermoid cyst because of their histologic inclusion of ectodermal, mesodermal, and endodermal derivatives and their frequent association with deformities of the skull. Teratocarcinomas are rarely seen in the head and neck region of children.

Several other pathological entities have to be distinguished from dermoid cyst. Many, including ranula, lymphoepithelial cyst, thyroglossal duct cyst, lipoma, cystic hygroma, and salivary and skin appendage tumors may have clinical features similar to dermoid cysts, but distinguishing histologically between them is not difficult.

Perhaps the most important differential diagnosis is that of encephalocele in the region of the nose. A thorough radiographic

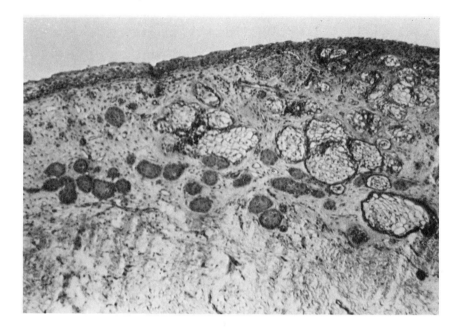

Fig. 3-5 Dermoid cyst showing sebaceous glands in wall of cyst. (H&E x 180).

examination of the skull and facial bones is mandatory when the possibility of encephalocele exists.[7]

TREATMENT AND PROGNOSIS

The treatment for dermoid cyst in the sublingual region of the oral cavity is complete surgical removal. The prognosis is excellent as the dermoid cyst, in this area, lends itself to simple surgical dissection.[20]

Dermoid cysts of the nose are also treated by complete surgical removal, but unlike their oral counterparts, 25 to 50 percent of them recur and require a second attempt at surgical correction.[13] Primary surgical failure is probably related to the fact that nearly half of the nasal dermoids extend deeply into nasal bones. Batsakis and colleagues suggested that recurrences in this location are less likely if the cystic lining is destroyed by electrocoagulation.[21] Orbital and occipital-frontal dermoid cysts in the midface are also treated by complete surgical removal. They recur less frequently than nasal dermoids but more often than dermoid cysts of the oral cavity.

LESIONS OF EMBRYONIC REMNANTS

Synonyms

1. Thyroglossal duct cyst
2. Branchiogenous cyst
3. Enterogenous cyst
4. Teratoma

INCIDENCE

Thyroglossal duct lesions are, in our experience, relatively common cystic masses of the head and neck region of children, as are branchiogenous cysts, while enterogenous cysts and teratomas are relatively rare (Table 3-1).

TABLE 3-1

LESIONS OF EMBRYONIC REMNANTS

— The Children's Hospital, Denver, Colorado —

Lesion	Annual Incidence
	Cases/1000 Surgical Specimens
Thyroglossal Duct Cyst	3.6
Branchiogenous Remnant	1.9
Enterogenous Cyst	0.04
Teratoma	0.04

AGE AND SEX

Most thyroglossal duct lesions are diagnosed between 2 and 7 years of age. Branchiogenous cysts and remnants are seen in infants but most are also diagnosed between 2 and 7 years of age. Enterogenous cysts of the neck manifest themselves in the first 2-to-3 years of life,[22] while teratomas are most often congenital.[23] No sexual predisposition is documented for the acquisition of any of these lesions.

PATHOGENESIS

Incomplete closure of the tract from foramen cecum at the base of the tongue to the normal pre-laryngeal site of the thyroid gland results in thyroglossal duct lesions, the most common being a mid-line cyst just cephalad to the thyroid gland.

The failure of normal morphogenesis of the first and second branchial systems results in the presence of a remnant lesion in the soft tissues along the anterior aspect of the sternocleido-mastoid muscle. This most often takes the form of a cartilaginous rest but may be a cyst, a sinus, or a combination of these elements.

Enterogenous cysts of the upper esophagus or tongue are the result of maldevelopment of that portion of the alimentary tract. Hypotheses related to:(1) aberrant luminal canalization seem plausible for such lesions in the duodenal area; (2) failure of diverticular involution may pertain to lesions of the cecal region; (3) aberrant notochordal closure seem relevant to such lesions when associated with vertebral defects, and (4) vascular insults may be operational in some mesenteric associated lesions.[22] Upper esophageal and lingual lesions are of unexplained pathogenesis.

Teratomas are neoplasms and/or malformations composed of varying types and amounts of tissue representing all three embryonal germ cell layers. The rare occurrence of such tumors in the head and neck is unexplained and the relationship to anomalous twinning is poorly documented.

CLINICAL FINDINGS

Lesions in this category most often manifest as masses, as painful masses, or with signs and symptoms of obstruction when the mass is initially inapparent. Infection and sterile inflammation are common in cystic lesions other than teratomas.

Thyroglossal duct lesions are nearly always cysts with inapparent tracts. Most are inflamed at the time of operation and have a midline pre-laryngeal, suprathyroid location in the neck (Fig. 3-6). Lesions are rarely cephalad to the hyoid bone but may be encountered at the base of the tongue. The cyst is usually not obvious at birth and can, particularly in the very young individual, cause airway obstruction by mass effect.

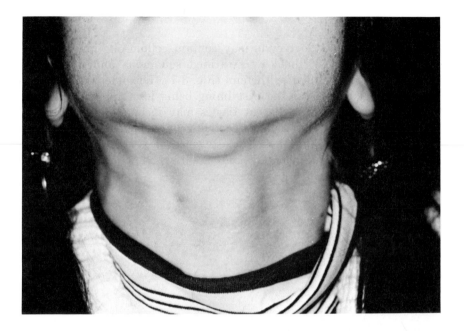

Fig. 3-6 Thyroglossal duct cyst in midline submental location.

Radiological studies uniformly fail to reveal calcified elements in the cyst or cyst wall.

Branchiogenous lesions usually appear as unilateral cystic masses of the pre-sternocleido-mastoid cervical region and are, in our experience, significantly inflamed in over 75 percent of the instances. Mature cartilaginous rests are the most common manifestation of branchial remnants in our cases and these are rarely associated with inflammation. Cystic lesions are commonly associated with inflammatory change and these occur as painful swellings.

Enterogenous cysts of the esophagus and posterior tongue are usually detected because of difficulty swallowing or because of upper airway obstruction.

Teratomas of the head and neck region may become manifest as huge masses in the neonate. When a nasopharyngeal tumor protrudes through a mid-facial defect, it is referred to as an epignathus. Smaller teratomas occur most often in the nasopharynx and thyroid region. Teratomas in these sites are rarely malignant.

Radiological examination of these teratomas often reveals osseous or dental elements within the mass.

PATHOLOGY

Thyroglossal duct cysts may contain colloid-like material and are, when preserved, lined by stratified squamous and/or ciliated pseudostratified columnar epithelium (Fig. 3-7). The older the child the greater the likelihood of the cyst lining being lost and inflammatory changes predominating. Adjacent tissues may include thyroid follicles but commonly show fibrosis and reactive cellular elements due to cyst rupture and/or inflammation. The existence of a tract from cyst to hyoid bone may be commonly demonstrated.

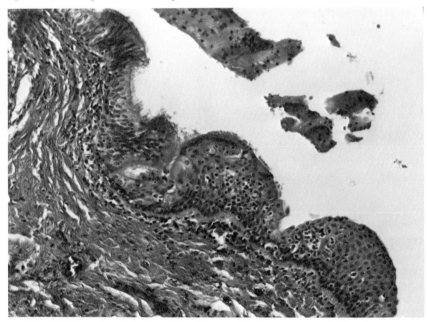

Fig. 3-7 Thyroglossal duct cyst lined by stratified squamous and ciliated pseudostratified columnar epithelium. Inflammatory changes are present. (H&E x 100).

Branchiogenous cysts (Fig. 3-8) are lined by stratified squamous and ciliated columnar epithelium unless the epithelium has been destroyed by inflammation. The latter is a very common event and, often, the presence of adjacent cartilage provides the only clue to derivation of this lesion. In well-preserved specimens, lymphoid tissue is often seen beneath the epithelium and may form well-developed follicles (Fig. 3-9).

Enterogenous cysts are recognized only when preservation of the cyst wall, mimicking some level of the gastrointestinal tract, has

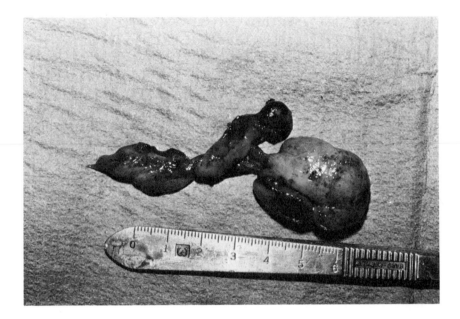

Fig. 3-8 Completely resected branchiogenous cyst and associated tract.

occurred. It may include mucosa, submucosa, and muscularis. The type of gastrointestinal mucosa is not necessarily related to the site of the lesion.

Teratomas of the head and neck region are usually solid masses which may have small cysts within them. They resemble teratomas in other sites, but, they usually contain large amounts of central nervous system tissue and/or embryonic neural tissue. This latter finding is not to be looked upon as a sign of malignancy. Generally, malignant elements in teratomas are epithelial embryonal carcinoma. Such malignant histology is found to be exceedingly rare in lesions of the head and neck, although the tumor can be lethal by position and extent of involvement.

DIFFERENTIAL DIAGNOSIS

Various cystic lesions of the head and neck can be difficult to distinguish histologically, particularly when destructive changes of inflammation are prominent. The major differential lesions include

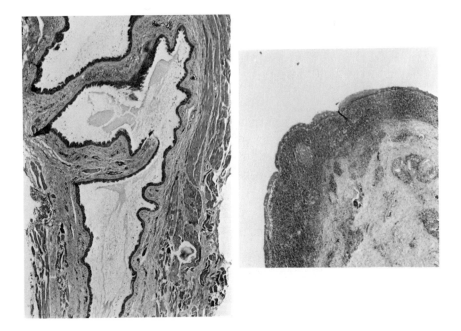

Fig. 3-9 (A) Branchiogenous sinus tract with intact pseudostratified column epithelium. (H&E x 25). (B) Same sinus tract with focal area of lymphoid tissue. (H&E x 25).

dermoid cyst, epidermal inclusion cyst, mucocele, and lymphangioma-tous lesions. All are benign and the difference, in general, bears little other than academic significance.

Encephalocele and nasal glial hamartoma (nasal glioma) are usually solid masses, the neural nature of which is inapparent until histologic sections are examined. The absence of entodermal and mesodermal elements distinguishes these lesions from teratomas with prominent neural components.

Encephaloceles (more correctly meningoencephaloceles) communicate with subarachnoid or ventricular spaces, are associated with bony defects, and occur anteriorly only rarely.[24]

The nasal bridge, lateral aspect of the nose, or intranasal location may be the site of neuroglial tissue associated with corrective tissue bands. These lesions, nearly universally referred to as nasal gliomas, are not neoplasms but may attach to the meninges through a small and subtle portal; these must be attacked with care by the surgeon.

TREATMENT AND PROGNOSIS

Surgical extirpation of these lesions is generally curative, but the presence of extensive inflammatory changes with or without infection can, on occasion, make surgical resection difficult.

Thyroglossal duct cysts must be removed en bloc with the midportion of hyoid bone since the tract usually extends to that level. Failure to execute this maneuver results in a high incidence of recurrence.

Large teratomas can be difficult to manage due to location and extent of involvement. There is no effective chemotherapy or radiotherapy for their treatment.

References

1. Harrison, J.D. "Salivary mucoceles." *Oral Surg.* 39(1975): 268-278.
2. Cataldo, E. and Mosadomi, A. "Mucoceles of the oral mucous membrane." *Arch. Otolaryngol.* 91(1970): 360-365.
3. Greer, R.O. and Carpenter, M. "Surgical oral pathology at the University of Colorado School of Dentistry: a survey of 400 cases." *J. Colo. Dent. Assoc.* 54(1976): 13-16.
4. Cohen, L. "Mucoceles of the oral cavity." *Oral Surg.* 19(1965): 365-372.
5. Giunta, J. and Cataldo, E. "Lymphoepithelial cysts of the oral mucosa." *Oral Surg.* 35(1973): 77-84.
6. Greer, R.O. and Mierau, G. *Tumors of the Oral Mucosa and Jaws in Infants and Children.* Denver: University of Colorado Medical Center Press, 1980.
7. Batsakis, J.G. *Tumors of the Head and Neck. Clinical and Pathological Considerations,* 2nd ed. Baltimore: Williams and Wilkins, 1979.
8. Bhaskar, S.N. "Lymphoepithelial cysts of the oral cavity. Report of twenty-four cases." *Oral Surg.* 21(1966): 120-128.
9. Doyle, J.L.; Weisinger, E. and Manhold, J.H. "Benign lymphoid lesions of the oral mucosa. Preliminary classification." *Oral Surg.* 29(1970): 31-37
10. Knappe, M.J. "Pathology of oral tonsils." *Oral Surg.* 29(1970): 295-304.
11. Knappe, M.J. "Oral tonsils: Locations, distribution and histology." *Oral Surg.* 29(1970): 155-161.
12. Meyer, I. "Dermoid cysts of the floor of the mouth." *Oral Surg.* 8(1959): 1149-1164.
13. Taylor, B.W. and Erich, J.B. "Dermoid cysts of the nose." *Mayo Clin. Proc.* 42(1967): 488-494.
14. Seward, G.R. "Dermoid cysts of the floor of the mouth". *Br. J. Oral Surg.* 3(1965): 36-47.
15. Yoshimura et al. "Congenital cyst of the sublingual region: report of case." *J. Oral Surg.* 23(1970): 366-370.

16. Katz, A.D. and Passy, V. "Sublingual dermoid tumors." *California Medicine* 111(1969): 96-98.
17. Quinn, J.H. "Congenital epidermoid cyst of anterior half of tongue." *Oral Surg.* 13(1960): 1283-1287.
18. Miller, A.P. and Owens, J.B., Jr. "Teratoma of the tongue." *Cancer* 19(1966): 1583-1586.
19. Figi, F.A. and Dix, C.R. "Dermoid cysts of the floor of the mouth. Report of a case." *Proc. Staff Mtg. Mayo Clin.* 14(1931): 289-291.
20. Korchin, L. "Dermoid cyst of the floor of the mouth." *U.S. Armed Forces Med. J.* 2(1951): 289-292.
21. Batsakis, J.G. and Farber, E.R. "Teratomas of the head and neck." *Eye, Ear, Nose and Throat Monthly* 30(1968): 67.
22. Favara, B.E.; Franciosi, R.A. and Akers, D.R. "Enteric Duplications." *Am. J. Dis. Child.* 122(1971): 501-506.
23. Potter, E.L. and Craig, T.M. In *Pathology of the Fetus and the Infant*, 3rd ed., pp.188-192, Chicago: Yearbook Medical Publisher, 1975.
24. Nakamura, T.; Grant, J.A. and Hubbard, R.E. "Nasoethmoidal Meningoencephalocele," *Arch. Otolaryngol.* 100(1974): 62-68.

Chapter IV

Odontogenic Tumors and Cysts
INTRODUCTION

Odontogenic tumors and cysts are lesions that arise in association with or directly from the precursors or remnants of the tooth germ. To understand the pathology of tumors arising from the tooth germ apparatus, it is necessary to understand the development of the tooth. The tooth germ originates as an invagination of a tubular epithelial extension of basal cells from the stomadeal ectoderm overlying the developing alveolar ridges. This tubular extension is composed of cuboidal epithelial cells enveloped by a basal lamina.

The dynamic relationships observed between tissues of the developing odontogenic apparatus are markedly influenced by epithelio-mesenchymal interactions. As the dental lamina progressively invades the underlying connective tissue, differentiation at the terminal end ensues. The lamina degenerates to form the inner enamel epithelium, outer enamel epithelium, and a central zone encased by these two epithelial layers. The central region is composed of an aggregate of stellate cells termed the stellate reticulum. The inner enamel epithelium differentiates further to become a layer of tall columnar cells with oval nuclei polarized away from the basal lamina. This characteristic cell, an ameloblast, is a hallmark of enamel epithelium. In juxtaposition to this ameloblastic layer and interposed between the ameloblasts and stellate reticulum is an intermediate layer of cuboidal cells termed the stratum intermedium.[1]

As the epithelial element differentiates in this fashion, the underlying connective tissue assumes a unique quality. Subjacent to the epithelial cap of the tooth germ is a condensation of mesenchyme that will become the vital tooth pulp. The cells are spindle-shaped and the fibrous element is delicate. At this stage, a layer of connective tissue cells begins to differentiate in juxtaposition to the ameloblastic layer. These cells are derivatives of the neural crest and are referred to as ectomesoderm. At the interface, the ectomesodermal cells (odontoblasts) become elongated and begin to elaborate an eosinophilic matrix that will become dentin, the principal calcified substance of the tooth. Subsequent to the elaboration of a predentin layer by odontoblasts, the ameloblasts begin to synthesize a keratin matrix that will eventually calcify as enamel, the surface structure of the tooth. The integrated efforts of the odontoblastic and ameloblastic layers eventually generate the crown of the tooth.[1]

The radicular (root) region is formed in a similar manner, whereby tubular extensions from the enamel epithelium progressively grow deeper into the developing alveolar bone, accompanied by continued differentiation of odontoblasts. After dentin is synthesized along this lattice, the epithelial component degenerates.[1] The connective tissue adjacent to the developing root region buttrices the dentin layer that was previously shielded by an epithelial layer; these mesenchymal cells differentiate into cementoblasts and generate a layer of cementum which coats the radicular dentin. Sharpey's fibers become inserted into the cemental tissues and pass through the adjacent fibrous tissue, interlacing with fibers inserted into the developing alveolar osseous tissue to create the periodontal ligament of the tooth. As root development proceeds, an eruptive force is created, pushing the tooth toward the surface epithelium until it erupts into the oral cavity.

As tooth development proceeds, remnants of progenitor cells remain entrapped within the jaws. Three primary sources for oncogenic change remain:[1]

1. Remnants of dental lamina residing in the mature adult gingiva (rests of Serres)
2. Remnants of the radicular epithelial projections of the tooth germ residing throughout the periodontal ligament (rests of Malassez)
3. Remnants of the ameloblastic layer overlying the crown of a tooth that failed to erupt (reduced enamel epithelium surrounding the crown of impacted teeth).

All these odontogenic epithelial rests can undergo neoplastic transformation. It is theorized that during odontogenic oncogenesis, the epithelial component alone may proliferate; the epithelial component may influence surrounding connective tissue to differentiate and to proliferate in the absence of the epithelium itself; or the neoplasm may recapitulate tooth formation by neoplastic proliferation of both epithelial and mesenchymal tissues. These three possibilities account for classifying odontogenic tumors as epithelial, mesenchymal, or mixed neoplasms, respectively. Tables 4-1, 4-2, and 4-3 delineate the proposed histogenesis and treatment of odontogenic neoplasms.

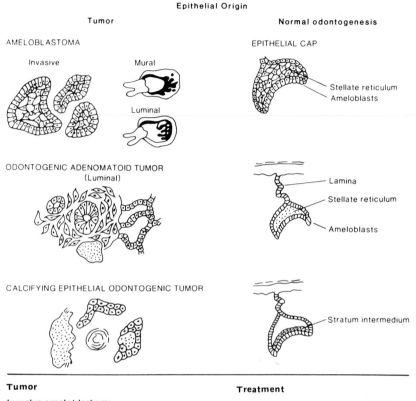

Epithelial Origin

Tumor   Normal odontogenesis

AMELOBLASTOMA   EPITHELIAL CAP

Invasive   Mural
                                                          Stellate reticulum
                                                          Ameloblasts
                Luminal

ODONTOGENIC ADENOMATOID TUMOR
          (Luminal)
                                                          Lamina

                                                          Stellate reticulum

                                                          Ameloblasts

CALCIFYING EPITHELIAL ODONTOGENIC TUMOR

                                                          Stratum intermedium

Tumor	Treatment
Invasive ameloblastoma	Resection (marginal or complete)
Mural and luminal ameloblastoma	Enucleation/curettage with saucerization
Odontogenic adenomatoid tumor	Enucleation
Calcifying epithelial odontogenic tumor	Resection

Table 4-1 Schematic diagram showing the histogenesis of epithelial odontogenic tumors. (Modified from: Greer, R.O. "The Oral Cavity." In *Pathology*, edited by S.G. Silverberg. New York: Wiley and Sons, 1982.)

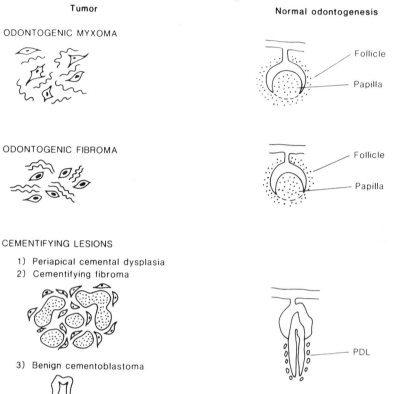

Mesenchymal Origin

Tumor   Normal odontogenesis

ODONTOGENIC MYXOMA

                                                                    Follicle

                                                                    Papilla

ODONTOGENIC FIBROMA

                                                                    Follicle

                                                                    Papilla

CEMENTIFYING LESIONS

   1) Periapical cemental dysplasia
   2) Cementifying fibroma

                                                                    PDL

   3) Benign cementoblastoma

Tumor	Treatment
Myxoma	Resection
Odontogenic fibroma	Enucleation
Periapical cemental dysplasia	None
Cementifying fibroma	Enucleation with saucerization
Benign cementoblastoma	Extraction with encleation

Table 4-2 Schematic diagram showing the histogenesis of mesenchymal odontogenic tumors. (Modified from: Greer, R.O. "The Oral Cavity." In *Pathology*, edited by S.G. Silverberg. New York: Wiley and Sons, 1982.)

Dual (Mixed) Origin

Tumor   Normal odontogenesis

AMELOBLASTOMA FIBROMA

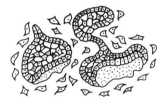

— Lamina

— Cap

— Papilla

AMELOBLASTIC FIBRO-DENTINOMA

— Lamina

— Cap

— Dentin

— Odontoblasts

— Papilla

ODONTOMA

— Epithelium

— Enamel

— Dentin

— Pulp

— Cementum

AMELOBLASTIC FIBRO-ODONTOMA
(Odontoma + Ameloblastic fibroma)

Tumor	Treatment
Ameloblastic fibroma	Enucleation; with saucerization
Ameloblastic fibro-dentinoma	if recurrent, resection
Odontoma	Enucleation; if gingival, excision
Ameloblastic fibro-odontoma	Enucleation
	Enucleation

Table 4-3 Schematic diagram showing the histogenesis of mixed odontogenic tumors. (Modified from: Greer. R.O. "The Oral Cavity." In *Pathology*, edited by S.G. Silverberg. New York: Wiley and Sons, 1982.)

AMELOBLASTOMA

Synonyms

1. Adamantinoma
2. Admantoblastoma

INCIDENCE

In an exhaustive review of 54,534 biopsy specimens submitted to the Department of Oral Pathology over a 41-year-period, Regezi and associates documented 706 tumors of odontogenic origin.[2] Seventy-eight (11 percent) of these odontogenic tumors and cysts were ameloblastomas. A mean age of 45 was recorded for the 78 ameloblastoma patients. These authors were able to document only seven tumors in patients less than 20 years of age. Young and Robinson,[3] Lewin,[4] and Dresser and Segal[5] have also reported cases of infrequent ameloblastoma in children.

AGE AND SEX

Most children having ameloblastomas are within 10 years of age. Small and Waldron[6] reviewed a series of 1,036 ameloblastomas occurring in all age groups and found that 24 patients (4 percent) were between birth and 9 years of age at the time their tumors were discovered. Young and Robinson[3] reviewed seven additional cases in children and found that all their patients were between the ages of 2 months and 7 years of age. There is no apparent sexual predisposition in the occurrence of this tumor in children, unlike the stronger tendency for occurrence in males among adults.

PATHOGENESIS

The etiology of ameloblastoma is unknown. Some authorities believe that the lesion arises in association with the difficult eruption of a third molar in association with a previous infection or cyst. Hertz[7] and Forsberg[8] suggested that trauma or inflammation are common etiologic agents. Tumors that appear to be histologically compatible with ameloblastoma in humans have been produced in mice by the injection of polyoma virus extracts.

Most investigators agree that the ameloblastoma is derived from odontogenic epithelium or certain derivatives or residua thereof. The histomorphological structure is reminiscent of the dental lamina as it penetrates the ectomesenchyme of the forming fetal jaw and differentiates into the epithelial enamel organ.[9] The dental lamina thus remains the most likely parent tissue.[10] The most convincing support for dental lamina origin of the ameloblastoma centers around the fact that the biologic and physiologic characteristics of the tumor remarkably parallel those of the dental lamina, —a structure that continues to grow from surface oral epithelium, pushing out columns of epithelial cells in an orderly fashion into the supporting connective tissue until the site of ultimate tooth germ formation is reached within bone.

Other sources have been suggested as potential tissues of origin for the ameloblastoma. They include surface oral epithelium, odontogenic cyst epithelium, epithelial rests of Malassez, and the enamel organ.[10] All of these, except the enamel organ origin, remain reasonable.[10] Perhaps the most convincing factor against direct enamel organ origin is the fact that enamel deposition is conspicuously absent from the histopathologic features of the ameloblastoma.

Young and Robinson[3] reported that the ameloblastoma in the child has quite a different genesis that its adult counterpart. Ameloblastomas in children most frequently arise in the walls of dentigerous cysts. Stanley[11] has documented that the epithelial lining associated with dentigerous cysts or the epithelium around impacted or unerupted teeth, especially third molars and cuspids, retains the columnar palisaded pattern common to reduced enamel epithelium up to age 22, when the tissue maturates to stratified squamous epithelium. This phenomenon may explain why the ameloblastoma is commonly found in association with impacted or unerupted teeth before the age of 33. Interestingly, Small and Waldron[6] reported that 33 is the average age for clinical identification of ameloblastomas after all ages are considered.

Two special types of ameloblastoma occur with great frequency in the child or young adult. These subtypes are referred to as mural and intraluminal ameloblastoma, —neoplastic variants that have a lesser degree of biologic aggressiveness than their central osseous counterparts.

CLINICAL FINDINGS

Shehdev and associates[12] have compiled the most complete recent review of the clinical statistics of ameloblastoma. In their review of 92 lesions, the vast majority occurred in the mandible. Maxillary ameloblastomas accounted for slightly less than 20 percent of their reported cases, consistent with findings in other large series in the literature.[13]

Painless swelling is the most common early symptom of ameloblastoma in either jaw. Shehdev and associates[12] found that in 14 of 20 patients with maxillary ameloblastoma, the duration of symptoms was less than one year. Nasal obstruction and epistaxis occurred late in the course of the disease. In mandibular ameloblastomas, the typical lesion appears as a slowly expanding swelling that usually causes thin-walled, bulging cortical plates.

Radiologically, the majority of ameloblastomas become manifest as intraosseous multilocular or "soap-bubble" type radiolucencies which may communicate with the oral cavity via destruction of the cortical plates (Fig. 4-1). The common cyst associated with ameloblastoma of childhood is a well-delineated, unilocular radiolucency most often surrounding the crown of a tooth that may be displaced superiorly in the maxilla or posteriorly in the mandible. When establishing a differential diagnosis for ameloblastoma on the basis of radiological information, it is important to remember that lesions such as central giant cell granuloma, aneurysmal bone cyst, odontogenic myxoma, and odontogenic keratocyst may all have similar radiological appearances.

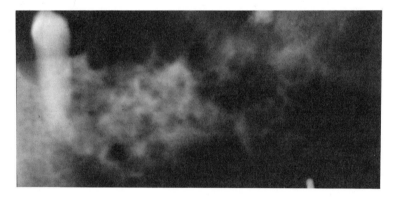

Fig. 4-1 Expansive multilocular radiolucency characteristics of ameloblastoma.

GROSS AND LIGHT MICROSCOPIC FINDINGS

The typical ameloblastoma surgical specimen is a solid gray-white tumor mass with a margin of peripheral bone. Resection may include the teeth at the periphery of the resected specimen. The tumor mass cuts readily, although there may be a gritty consistency to the tissue. Ameloblastomas do not contain a calcified product, and therefore hard tissue structures of the tooth will not be identified histologically. Frequently in children, the surgical specimen is a cyst. In such instances, one may find a sac-like lining with elevated white nodular areas in the cyst wall or lumen; the white nodular areas often represent *mural* or *intraluminal* ameloblastoma proliferation. It is important for the pathologist to examine all of the tissue sample in order that neoplastic proliferation in the wall of a cyst does not go unrecognized.

Classically, five histologic patterns have been described for ameloblastoma. The "follicular" variant is composed of tumor epithelium arranged in islands or sheets with a central area of polyhedral cells that resemble primitive stellate reticulum (Fig. 4-2). The plexiform or reticular pattern consists of irregular strands of epithelium bordered by columnar cells that surround an admixture of cells resembling stellate reticulum. The basal cell, granular cell, and acanthomatous variants contain central cells that have a basaloid, granular, or squamous or keratinaceous character respectively.

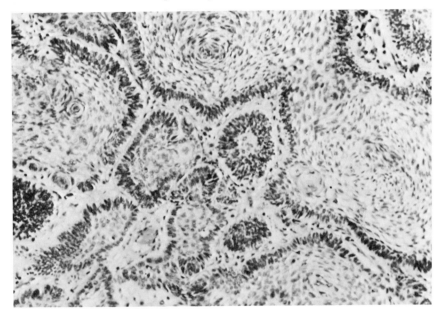

Fig. 4-2 Follicular ameloblastoma, showing islands of odontogenic epithelium with central stellate cells. (H&E x 320).

Cystic degeneration is not uncommon within the central portion of the epithelial component of ameloblastomas (Fig. 4-3). Of the five major histologic types of ameloblastoma, the follicular and plexiform patterns appear to be the most frequently encountered upon microscopic inspection. Quite frequently, a tumor displays one or more patterns throughout multiple sections of the tumor mass as it proliferates as

either sheets, nests, cords, or anastomosing strands of neoplastic epithelium into a well vascularized connective tissue stroma. Cells that rim
individual tumor islands are usually columnar or cuboidal cells resembling preameloblasts (Fig. 4-4). Individual tumor cells usually have oval
to vesicular nuclei which are polarized toward the central portion of the
follicular tumor nests. The cytoplasm ranges from granular to homogeneous; it is usually eosinophilic. Mitotic activity is minimal.

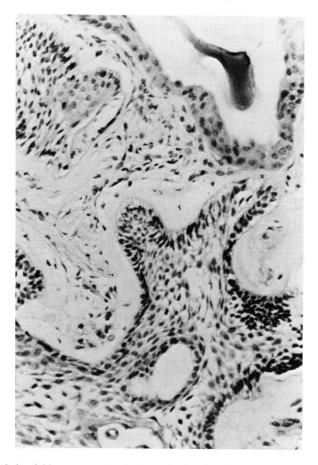

Fig. 4-3 Ameloblastoma arising in the wall of a dentigerous cyst in a child. Tumor
islands directly abut the overlying epithelial lining of the cyst. (H&E x 380).

Gardner[14] recently described a *plexiform unicystic ameloblastoma.* This variant clinically and grossly resembles a dentigerous cyst.

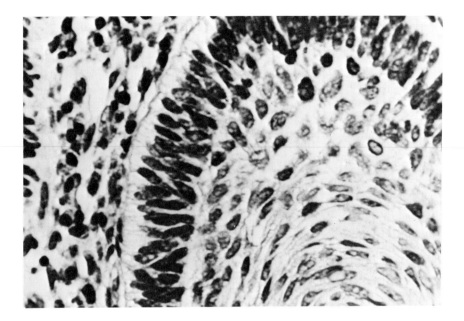

Fig. 4-4 Note tall columnar "preameloblasts" lining ameloblastoma tumor nests. (H&E x 500).

The classic microscopic finding is one displaying a unique histological pattern of anastomosing plexiform epithelial proliferations with hyperchromatic palisaded vacuolated basal cells that have their nuclei polarized away from the basement membrane.

This variant of ameloblastoma occurs primarily during the second and third decades of life, generally in the mandible. While Gardner[14] reported that enucleation, accompanied by good follow-up examination, is probably sufficient for tumors which have proliferated into the cystic lumen, more extensive surgery is indicated for those tumors involving the periphery of the fibrous connective tissue wall of the cyst.

ELECTRON MICROSCOPY

Ultrastructural studies of ameloblastoma are sparse.[15] Electron microscopic findings generally reveal a biphasic neoplasm; individual tumor islands are composed of peripheral columnar cells surrounding a central area of stellate cells. A continuous basement membrane surrounds the tumor islands. Peripheral columnar cells have parallel cellular membranes with little interdigitation of cell processes. Cell membranes are usually in close apposition, but occasionally separate focally, forming intercellular lacunae. Plasma membranes of adjacent tumor cells are intimately connected by desmosomes (Fig. 4-5). Cell nuclei remain oval or elliptical, and apically situated in the cells. One to two nucleoli are generally present. The cytoplasm of peripheral cells often contains abundant glycogen granules, frequently mitochondria, and rarely, lysosomes and rough endoplasmic reticulum. Clear cytoplasmic vesicles, slightly larger than mitochondria and bounded by a single membrane, may be prominent. Poorly-developed Golgi complexes can occasionally be seen adjacent to the nucleus at the pole pointing to the center of the lesion. Tonofilaments tend to be widely distributed in long, curved, and arching bundles around nuclei and adjacent to the plasma membranes (Fig. 4-6).

DIFFERENTIAL DIAGNOSIS

Ameloblastoma is frequently confused histologically with ameloblastic fibroma. Considerable care should be taken to differentiate the two entities, because the ameloblastic fibroma behaves in a much less aggressive manner than ameloblastoma, and management is correspondingly more conservative. The ameloblastic fibroma is composed of both epithelial and mesenchymal tooth germ components. Like the ameloblastoma, it produces no calcified dental structures. Histologically, ameloblastic fibroma consists of islands and cords of odontogenic epithelium resembling the dental lamina of early tooth development. The stroma is generally composed of fibromyxoid embryonic connective tissue that closely resembles the dental papilla of a developing tooth germ. Both the epithelial and mesenchymal components of the lesion are considered neoplastic. A useful histological feature distinguishing ameloblastic fibroma from ameloblastoma is the fact that the supporting stroma of the former remains primitive and quite cellular, whereas the connective tissue stroma of the ameloblastoma more closely resembles mature collagen. Ameloblastic fibroma also occurs in a much younger age group than ameloblastoma, with an average age of 15.5 years.[16] The mean age of patients with ameloblastoma is about two decades older.

The vast majority of ameloblastomas arise centrally within bone. Recently, a *peripheral (soft tissue) ameloblastoma* has become well-documented.[14,17] The peripheral ameloblastoma has all the histological characteristics of its medullary counterpart, but it occurs solely in soft tissues covering the tooth-bearing parts of the jaws. Extraosseous variants are rare in children.

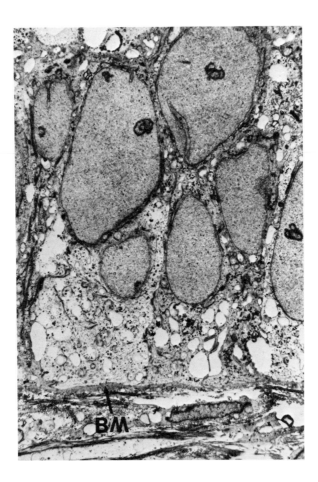

Fig. 4-5 Ultrastructural features of ameloblastoma. Peripheral columnar cells abut on continuous basement membrane (BM). Central polarization of nuclei is a consistent finding. (Orig. mag. x 7,850).

The *craniopharyngioma* is a rare lesion found in the bone beneath the sella turcica. It is histologically similar to ameloblastoma and is often referred to as a pituitary ameloblastoma. The origins of the two tumors are somewhat similar since Rathke's pouch does originate embryologically by invagination of oral epithelium. The histologic similarity between the ameloblastoma and the craniopharyngioma is a time-honored observation. Notable differences include the predominantly cystic nature of the craniopharyngioma and its striking tendency

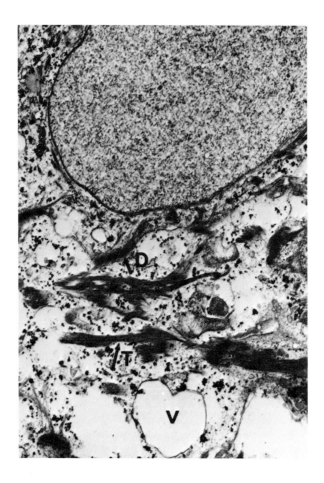

Fig. 4-6 Ameloblastoma. Cells in central stellate areas have prominent desmosomes (D) and tonofilaments (T). Cytoplastic vesicles (V) are prominent. (Orig. mag. x 26,800).

to form ghost keratin which undergoes dystrophic calcification. Although some tumors indeed reproduce solid proliferating islands histologically identical to ameloblastomas, the majority of these lesions more closely mirror the histology of the calcifying odontogenic cyst.

The so-called *adamantinoma of long bones* bears a superficial microscopic resemblance to ameloblastoma. It is doubtful whether any valid relationship between the two can be established.

TREATMENT AND PROGNOSIS

The standard form of therapy for central osseous ameloblastoma is wide en bloc excision to a border of normal tissue, uninvolved by tumor. For large aggressive lesions, hemimandibulectomy-maxillectomy or disarticulation of the mandible have been reported.

Tumors of childhood are usually managed much more conservatively by local excision with an adequate border of normal tissue, close postoperative observation, and a long-term follow-up. Although Mehlisch and associates[18] reported a 50 percent recurrence rate for ameloblastomas in adults where conservative removal of the lesion was reported, children do not seem to experience the same high recurrence rates following conservative surgery. Our own experience with five ameloblastomas arising in the walls of cysts has shown no recurrence with evaluations of up to five years. Conservative treatment was employed in all cases.

Becker and Perth[19] reported that patients who undergo radical forms of surgery for ameloblastoma, regardless of age, show a recurrence rate of 4.5 percent. The ameloblastoma of childhood is not considered to have a malignant potential.

ADENOMATOID ODONTOGENIC TUMOR

Synonyms

1. Adenoameloblastoma
2. Odontogenic adenomatoid tumor
3. Adenomatoid ameloblastoma
4. Ameloblastic adenomatoid tumor

INCIDENCE

The adenomatoid odontogenic tumor is a rare odontogenic neoplasm comprising 0.1 percent of all tumors and cysts of the jaws and approximately 1-to-3 percent of all odontogenic tumors.[2,20] This neoplasm, often characterized by formation of duct-like structures by the epithelial component of the tumor, is also known by the misleading name, adenoameloblastoma. Little more than 150 verifiable cases have been reported in the world literature.

AGE AND SEX

The adenomatoid odontogenic tumor is predominately a neoplasm of children, adolescents, and young adults. There exists a propensity for it in the second decade of life, although occasional cases have been reported in older patients. Courtney and Kerr[21] recently reported experience with 20 adenomatoid odontogenic tumors and found that 16 of their 20 patients were between the ages of 10 and 20. The mean age was 16.5. The oldest patient in their review was 37. Giansanti, in a review of 105 cases from the literature, found males to be affected twice as often as females.[22] Courtney and Kerr found that females outnumbered males in their series by a ratio of 4-to-1.[21]

PATHOGENESIS

From the time the adenomatoid odontogenic tumor was first recognized as a distinct clinicopathologic entity, there has been considerable controversy as to its histogenesis and cell of origin.

Most investigators now accede to its odontogenic source because it appears exclusively in the jaws, is also frequently found in association with dentigerous cysts or impacted teeth, and has characteristics in its cells which are similar to the various components of the enamel organ.

Since Stafne's report in 1948[23] of three cases of adenomatoid odontogenic tumor, which he called "epithelial tumors associated with developmental cysts", numerous cell origins have been proposed. Miles,[24] reporting a lesion he called a "cystic complex composite odontome", identified columnar ameloblast-like cells surrounding cyst-like spaces similar histologically to the adenomatoid odontogenic tumor. He believed the calcifications he saw were cementicles, and suggested an hamartomatous origin for what actually was an adenomatoid odontogenic tumor. There has been considerable support for the belief that the tumor is indeed a developmental overgrowth of odontogenic tissue.[24-33]

In 1955, Thoma[25] suggested that the adenomatoid odontogenic tumor arose from rests of Malassez which were thought to have the ability to differentiate along glandular lines. The following year, Oehlers[26] reported an adenomatoid odontogenic tumor he believed was an unusual pleomorphic salivary gland tumor arising in a dentigerous cyst. Subsequent study has largely discounted the likelihood of a salivary gland source.

Lucas[27] has observed that although the adenomatoid odontogenic tumor possesses a superficial resemblance to ameloblastoma, there are significant clinical and histologic differences between the two. He advocated the belief that the adenomatoid odontogenic tumor is a tumor of enamel organ epithelium, with the cells being derived from ameloblasts prior to their organizing stage. This theory of a pre-ameloblast derivation has had support from numerous investigators.[23;32;33]

Bhaskar[34] has suggested that the adenomatoid odontogenic tumor is simply a dentigerous cyst with proliferation of the lining epithelium within the cystic lumen. However, the lesion is, in many instances, a solid tumor occurring in anatomic sites in which dentigerous cysts are rarely seen. Shear[35] emphasized that the epithelial lining of a dentigerous cyst is reduced enamel epithelium "which differentiated, performed and completed its function" and is therefore unlikely to "redifferentiate and form a tumor". This same author suggests undifferentiated odontogenic epithelium as the source of the adenomatoid odontogenic tumor and proposes that the absence of the usual inductive relationships between epithelium and connective tissue results in incomplete differentiation of the tumor cells into ameloblasts.

CLINICAL FINDINGS

This biologically benign neoplasm generally occurs as a slow-growing, painless mass, involving the region of the anterior maxilla. The tumor is usually identified in the maxillary incisor, cuspid, or premolar area, although a few cases have been reported along the angle of the mandible. Sixty-five percent of the 105 cases described by Giansanti and

Waldron occurred in the maxilla.[22] In addition to the occasional cases reported in the mandible, a few instances of extraosseous expression of this tumor in the oral soft tissues have been reported.[36-38]

In nearly 75 percent of all cases, the tumor is associated with an unerupted tooth, most commonly the maxillary cuspid. This tendency for association with impacted teeth often results in a mistaken clinical impression of dentigerous cyst on roentgenographic examination.

Radiographically, the adenomatoid odontogenic tumor usually manifests as a solitary cystic-appearing lesion (Fig. 4-7). Calcification is sometimes seen in association with the tumor, and when present, produces a faintly detectable radiopacity. Lucas reports that most tumors are small, measuring in the range of 1-to-3 cm. in diameter at the time of discovery.[27] Our own experience with several of these tumors has been one in which all have been identified as masses greater than 5 cm. in diameter, at the time of their first clinical evaluation.

Cortical expansion is a common feature, but penetration of the cortical plates is unusual, and if present, should warrant consideration of a more aggressive tumor in the differential diagnosis.

GROSS AND LIGHT MICROSCOPIC FINDINGS

Grossly, these tumors are often encapsulated. Sectioning may reveal obvious areas of calcification, gritty, granular quality foci, or areas of cystic degeneration with mural excrescences. Solid tumor areas are generally gelatinous-to-firm and white-to-yellow.

The dominant histological feature of the tumor is one of a collection of sheets, nests and cords of epithelial cells which differentiate along columnar lines in numerous places to resemble ameloblasts. Frequently, the columnar cells form ducts or tubules with the central lumen ultimately encased by columnar cells (Fig. 4-8). The peripheral cells stain deeply and their nuclei are polarized away from the central portion of the neoplasm. In addition to the tubular and ductal structures, bands, sheets, and clusters of cells arranged in a spindle-like pattern may be identified. Occasionally these areas can take on a cartwheel or cribiform pattern reminiscent of salivary gland tumors, especially the mixed tumor (Fig. 4-9). Tumor nests are supported by a scant connective tissue stroma.

On occasion, tumor cells are arranged in a rosette pattern lined by cuboidal or columnar epithelium. Calcified material is common throughout the tumor. These calcifications develop primarily at junctions between aggregates of epithelial cells forming the tumor and the adjacent vascularized stromal tissues. The calcific foci have been shown

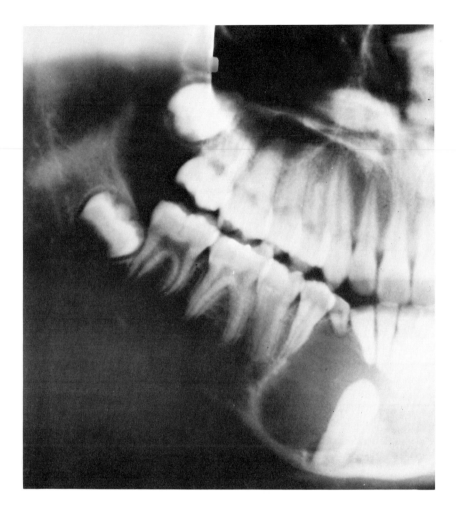

Fig. 4-7 Adenomatoid odontogenic tumor. This tumor, in an 11-year-old boy, greatly resembles a dentigerous cyst. A large unilocular radiolucency surrounds an impacted cuspid tooth. Courtesy of Dr. Robert Jones.

to resemble enamel, pre-enamel, or dentin morphologically and have similar staining and tinctorial qualities.

Other features of note may include the presence of an amorphous amyloid-like material filling the duct-spaces or occurring as intercellular droplets in areas with a more dense arrangement of tumor cells. This material gives a positive Periodic-Acid-Schiff reation and it is

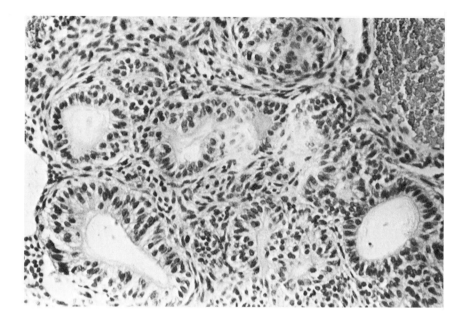

Fig. 4-8 Classic duct-like structures of adenomatoid odontogenic tumor. Note polarization of peripheral columnar cell nuclei away from the center of neoplastic islands. (H&E x 280).

metachromatically positive with toluidine blue, strongly suggesting that the material is of connective tissue orgin.

ELECTRON MICROSCOPY

Ultrastructural studies[39-42] have provided convincing support for the concept that the adenomatoid odontogenic tumor is of enamel organ origin. The cuboidal cells surrounding the duct-like spaces (Fig. 4-10) bear a striking resemblance to the cells of the inner enamel epithelium as they develop through the preameloblast stage.[43] That the duct-like spaces are not true ducts becomes immediately obvious upon electron microscopic examination, for they are found beneath the basal lamina upon which the epithelial cells rest. Surrounding and oriented perpendicular to the cuboidial epithelial cells is a population of spindle-shaped cells, containing prominent bundles of tonofilaments and desmosomes. These cells closely resemble and are believed to correspond to those of the stratum intermedium and stellate reticulum layers of the enamel organ.

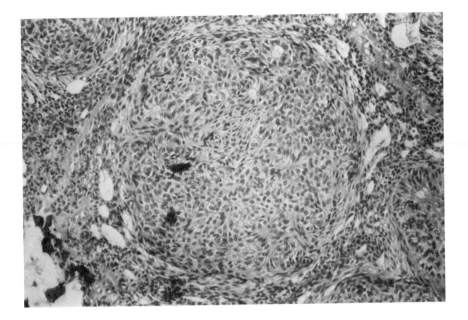

Fig. 4-9 Cartwheel clusters of cells and scattered calcified globules common to adenomatoid odontogenic tumor (H&E x 200).

DIFFERENTIAL DIAGNOSIS

The adenomatoid odontogenic tumor is most often confused with *ameloblastoma*; however, the two are distinctly different neoplasms with unique clinical, pathological, and behavior patterns.

The ameloblastoma is, classically, a tumor of the fourth decade, whereas the adenomatoid odontogenic tumor occurs predominately in the second decade. The occurrence of adenomatoid odontogenic tumor shows a marked female predominance, while the ameloblastoma is most commonly a tumor of males.

The adenomatoid odontogenic tumor is often associated with an impacted tooth, displays little biologic aggressiveness, and is easily enucleated with little chance for recurrence. Conversely, ameloblastomas are biologically aggressive tumors, at least locally, with a penchant for recurrence. They may require en bloc resection or extensive surgery, even in a child and certainly in adults.

Histologically the two tumors show distinct morphological patterns. The ameloblastoma almost consistently displays a follicular or stellate pattern, with tall columnar cells at the periphery of tumor

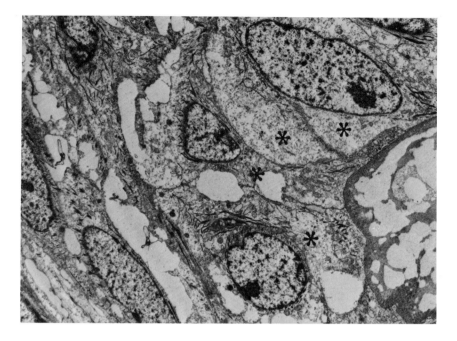

Fig. 4-10 As in the developing enamel organ, the spindle-shaped cells (far left) of adenomatoid odontogenic tumor surround a layer of cuboidal epithelial cells which, in turn, surround duct-like structures (lower right). (EM x 5,100).

islands and frequent epithelial metaplasia. The adenomatoid odontogenic tumor has a tubular or "ductal" pattern, with scant evidence of stellate areas of peripheral columnar cells resembling ameloblasts. Calcifications are common to the adenomatoid odontogenic tumor and frequently, there is elaboration of a hyalinized or eosinophilic product within epithelial tumor islands or the stroma. In the adenomatoid odontogenic tumor, the nuclei of the cells which line the duct-like spaces are polarized away from the lumen; in ameloblastoma, nuclei of epithelial islands are polarized toward the central stellate areas.

The *calcifying epithelial odontogenic tumor* may be misinterpreted as an adenomatoid odontogenic tumor, principally because both lesions frequently contain foci of amorphous, faintly eosinophilic cell product or small, round, or irregular calcified aggregates. However, the calcific foci in the calcifying epithelial odontogenic tumor generally becomes coalescent in a concentric ring phenomenon (Fig. 4-11), a feature that is rarely, if ever, present in the adenomatoid odontogenic tumor.

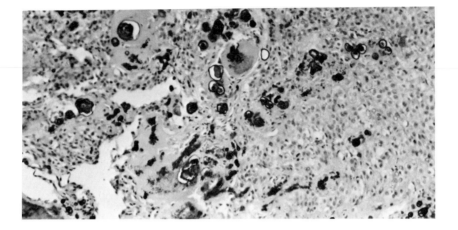

Fig. 4-11 Calcifying epithelial odontogenic tumor displaying coalescent concentric ring calcific foci. (H&E x 200).

The calcifying epithelial odontogenic tumor is a distinct rarity in children. The mean age of patients with this tumor is between 32 and 42,[44] and although Krolls has reported an occurrence in a 8-year-old child,[43] very few cases have been cited in patients under 20 years of age. Typically, the lesion appears as a radiolucent expansile lesion that is fairly well-delineated peripherally. A calcified central area is frequently identified. Half of the lesions reported in the world literature have been associated with an unerupted tooth.[45] Unlike the adenomatoid odontogenic tumor, the mandible appears to be affected more often than the maxilla, and the most frequent site of occurrence is the premolar/molar region.

The basic histological pattern of the calcifying epithelial odontogenic tumor is one of sheets and masses of polyhedral epithelial cells with deeply eosinophilic cytoplasm, supported by a well-vascularized connective tissue stroma. Intracellular bridging is an often noted characteristic, and there may be a moderate degree of pleomorphism, as well as considerable variance in chromaticity of individual cell nuclei.

Krolls and Pindborg[45] maintain that the treatment of choice for the calcifying epithelial odontogenic tumor is conservative surgical excision, but one must remember that calcifying epithelial odontogenic tumors with a classic histology have a potential for an aggressive infiltrative course, and unlike the adenomatoid odontogenic tumor, en bloc resection has been the management modality of choice in over 30 percent of all reported cases.

TREATMENT AND PROGNOSIS

The adenomatoid odontogenic tumor appears to grow very slowly and shows no tendency toward recurrence. When the lesion appears as a tumor mass, curettement or conservative surgical excision is usually employed. A large percentage of adenomatoid odontogenic tumors arise as proliferations within the walls of cysts, and these lesions are usually treated by enucleation. Abrams and co-workers have suggested that the behavior pattern of this lesion is so benign the lesion probably represents a hamartoma and not a true odontogenic tumor; they further report that recurrences have not been reported, even in cases that have been incompletely excised or enucleated.[38]

AMELOBLASTIC FIBROMA

Synonyms

1. Soft mixed odontogenic tumor
2. Soft mixed odontoma
3. Fibroadamantoblastoma

INCIDENCE

The ameloblastic fibroma is an odontogenic neoplasm derived from both epithelial (*ameloblastic*) and mesenchymal (*fibroma*) elements of the odontogenic apparatus. The tumor is uncommon even in childhood, and quite rare in adults. Greer and Mierau reviewed a series of 191 tumors of the oral mucosa and jaws in children seen at the University of Colorado Health Sciences Center over a five-and-one-half-year-period and recorded only three (1.5 percent) ameloblastic fibromas.[46] Regezi and Kerr,[2] in a review of 706 odontogenic tumors seen at the University of Michigan over a 41-year-period, reported that the oral pathology service catalogued only 15 as ameloblastic fibromas.

AGE AND SEX

Over 70 percent of patients diagnosed as having ameloblastic fibroma are under 20, with the average age being 15.[45] The youngest reported case, described by Huebsch and Stephenson in 1956, was in an 18-month-old boy.[47] The tumor is rarely seen in adults, and the oldest recorded instance that we could glean from the literature was in a 41-year-old man.[48] There is no predisposition in either sex nor does there appear to be a racial predisposition.

PATHOGENESIS

As previously noted, the ameloblastic fibroma is derived from both epithelial and connective tissue elements of the odontogenic apparatus. As these two cell types proliferate, they mimic normal odontogenesis in their differentiation patterns. The epithelial component represents numerous small, dental lamina extensions with foci of differentiation into epithelial tooth buds, with a zone of stellate reticulum.[49] The connective tissue element emulates the future tooth pulp or dental papilla, showing a myxoid or delicate collagenous background with a homogeneous distribution of plump fibroblasts. Differentiation in the ameloblastic fibroma is arrested prior to the synthesis of hard tissues. Thus, when dentin and enamel tissues are present within the tumor mass, the lesion represents an odontoma or one of the odontoma variants, and not an ameloblastic fibroma.[49]

CLINICAL FINDINGS

The classic clinical presentation is that of a painless swelling of the jaw. Eversole reported, however, that at least 20 percent of the tumors are discovered on routine dental radiographs without the patients being aware of any symptoms.[49] The three largest series of ameloblastic fibromas have been reported by Trodahl,[47] Gorlin,[50] and Regezi.[2] Their combination of cases exceeds 50. All three authors reported the predisposition of the posterior mandible (over 70 percent) as compared to the maxilla. Lesions ranged in size from 1-to-8.5 cm.

Radiographically, the tumor manifests as either a unilocular or multilocular radiolucency (Fig. 4-12). Large lesions generally show cortical expansion. Trodahl reported that 75 percent of the tumors reviewed in his series were associated with the crown of an impacted tooth, and that the majority of the tumors displayed a multilocular pattern.

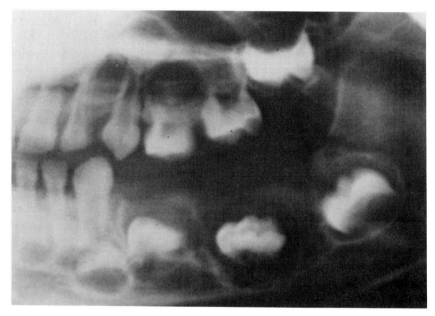

Fig. 4-12 Large loculated radiolucent ameloblastic fibroma of the posterior mandible in a two-and-one-half-year-old. Courtesy of Dr. Roy Eversole.

GROSS AND LIGHT MICROSCOPIC FINDINGS

Grossly, the ameloblastic fibroma has the consistency of a fibrous tumor. It may be rimmed by a definite peripheral collagenous capsule.

Ameloblastic fibromas represent odontogenic neoplasms in which both the epithelial component and the mesenchymal component are actively proliferating to produce a tumor mass.[49] The epithelial element is arranged in anastomosing cords of cuboidal back-to-back cells which rest against a well-defined basement membrane. These cords resemble the tooth germ primordial dental lamina (Fig. 4-13). In focal regions, these bilaminated epithelial cords manifest alveolar clusters whereby the double strands appear to open.[49] These saccular dilatations contain stellate and spindle-shaped epithelial cells, which emulate the stellate reticulum of the developing odontogenic apparatus (Fig. 4-14). The connective tissue element is the unique diagnostic feature of this neoplasm. Dense collagen fibers are lacking; while, the stroma assumes a somewhat myxoid character, being composed of delicate collagen fibers with a homogeneous distribution of plump, monomorphic, elongated fibroblasts.[49] In some areas of this neoplasm, an eosinophilic, nonstructured matrix material is interposed between the epithelial elements and the connective tissue in the region of the basement membrane. This matrix is believed to represent a collagenous product of the mesenchymal element, akin to predentin. On occasion, the central stellate reticulum may undergo cystic degeneration.

DIFFERENTIAL DIAGNOSIS

Ameloblastic fibroma is frequently confused with *ameloblastoma* at the time of microscopic examination. The most important histological feature distinguishing the two is that the ameloblastic fibroma has a supporting connective tissue composed of a loose proliferation of stellate connective tissue resembling that of the normal dental papilla. There is rarely any evidence of the dense collagen formation seen in the supporting stroma of ameloblastoma.

Ameloblastic fibroma can also be confused histologically with *calcifying epithelial odontogenic tumor, adenomatoid odontogenic tumor*, and *odontoma*. The calcifying epithelial odontogenic tumor is also composed of sheets and cords of neoplastic epithelial cells; however, these cells can be distinguished from the epithelial cells in ameloblastic fibroma because of their striking eosinophilic cytoplasm. Columnar ameloblasts with nuclear polarization are also absent in the calcifying epithelial odontogenic tumor. The calcifying epithelial odontogenic

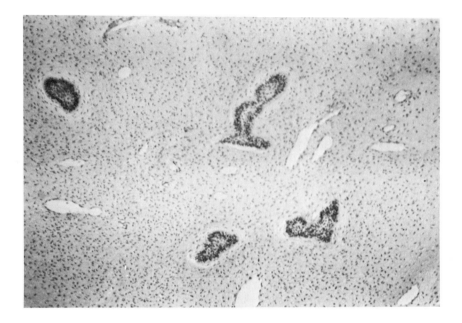

Fig. 4-13 Ameloblastic fibroma. Note that primitive connective tissue dominates the photomicrograph. Epithelial islands are arranged in isolated nests. (H&E x150).

tumor also has a mature collagenous stroma, as opposed to the immature mesenchymal stroma of ameloblastic fibroma.

Adenomatoid odontogenic tumor occurs in the same age group as the ameloblastic fibroma. It may also contain elongated and anastomosing cords of epithelium similar to that found in ameloblastic fibroma. A principal distinguishing feature between the two is the fact that the adenomatoid odontogenic tumor usually has a thick, fibrous capsule while such a capsule is usually not encountered in ameloblastic fibroma. The adenomatoid odontogenic tumor also often resembles a cyst with luminal epithelial proliferation, a feature not seen in ameloblastic fibroma. The stroma of the adenomatoid odontogenic tumor is extremely sparse and does not comprise a major portion of the neoplasm, whereas in ameloblastic fibroma, the loose, stellate connective tissue stroma is exceedingly prominent. Finally, although organoid rosettes, or ductal structures, are prominent features of the adenomatoid odontogenic tumor, they are not present in the ameloblastic fibroma.[51]

When dentin and enamel tissues are present in a suspected ameloblastic fibroma, the lesion more properly represents an *odontoma*

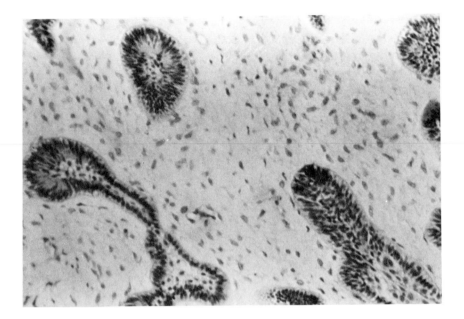

Fig. 4-14 Higher power photomicrograph showing epithelial islands and stroma, in ameloblastic fibroma. (H&E x 300).

or one of the odontoma variants, rather than ameloblastic fibroma, regardless of other histological features.

Ameloblastic sarcoma is considered the malignant counterpart of ameloblastic fibroma. The lesion is exceedingly rare and some authorities do not consider it to be true odontogenic malignancy, but rather a fibrosarcoma with fortuitous entrapment of active odontogenic epithelium, resembling that seen in ameloblastic fibroma.[46] The majority of these tumors have been reported in the mandible of patients who are significantly older than patients with ameloblastic fibroma.[46] The lesions are locally aggressive, but metastases are rare.

TREATMENT AND PROGNOSIS

Formerly, the ameloblastic fibroma was considered a nonaggressive, benign odontogenic tumor that could easily be enucleated and did not show a high recurrence rate. However, Trodahl has recently reported a recurrence rate of 43.5 percent.[47] Carr,[52] and Tanaka[53] have also documented high recurrence rates for this tumor. It appears that the lesion may be somewhat more aggressive than was originally thought and therefore, many authorities recommend that therapy include excision with adequate margins and not simply surgical curettage.

It has been postulated by some investigators that ameloblastic fibromas simply represent a unique step in the progression of mixed odontogenic tumors from immature to mature, ultimately resulting in an odontoma.

It has been suggested that some previously reported cases of *odontogenic fibroma*, were, in fact, mature ameloblastic fibromas which had gone undetected for many years. However, Eversole and co-workers[54] discounted, with reservation, the probability of such sequential differentiation resulting in a highly-differentiated odontogenic tumor (such as the odontoma) developing from an immature entity such as the ameloblastic fibroma.

Sawyer and associates[55] have reported a case of ameloblastic fibroma that developed over a span of 23 years. It was first noticed when the patient reached the age of 15. Throughout its course of more than two decades of growth, the tumor did not undergo transformation into an ameloblastoma, or any of the other mixed odontogenic neoplasms. The biologic behavior of this particular tumor gives strong credence to the view of Eversole and associates. [54]

MYXOMA

Synonyms

1. Odontogenic myxoma
2. Odontogenic fibromyxoma
3. Myxofibroma

INCIDENCE

Myxomas of bone are uncommon neoplasms of uncertain genesis with a potential for aggressive destruction of osseous tissues. Greer and Mierau found this tumor to account for 3.1 percent of 191 childhood tumors of the oral mucosa and jaws reviewed at the University of Colorado Health Sciences Center over a five-and-one-half-year period.[46] Myxomas accounted for 11.3 percent of 55 odontogenic tumors reviewed in the same series. In a review at the Mayo Clinic of 2,276 primary tumors of bone, Zimmerman and Dahlin documented only 26 myxomas; all were located in the jaws.[56] In 1975, Kangur and associates reported on 38 additional cases.[57]

Regezi and Kerr[2] reviewed 706 odontogenic tumors occurring within a 41-year-period and found that myxoma accounted for three percent of their total.

AGE AND SEX

In a recent review of the literature, Farman and associates reported 213 myxomas of the jaws.[58] They noted that 25 percent of the reported cases have occurred in patients under 20 years of age. What we believe to be the youngest patient affected by myxoma was reported by Ghosh and co-workers in the case of a five-month-old infant.[59]

The peak age of occurrence for myxoma appears to be the second and third decades. Appproximately 67 percent of patients are between 10 and 29 years of age.[56] Of the 20 tumors reported by Regezi and Kerr,[2] only five occurred in patients less than 20-years-old. Most of the cases reported by Greer and Mierau were in teenagers.

There is no sexual predisposition for the tumor in children; however, Farman[58] has reported a slight female predisposition in all age groups.

PATHOGENESIS

The myxoma is considered by most authorities to represent a tumor unique to the jaws that arises from the mesenchymal portion of the tooth germ apparatus. Gorlin,[60] however, suggested that perhaps two forms of myxoma exist; one, that has its genesis from primitive odontogenic tissue and the second, a far less common tumor, that arises from undifferentiated mesenchymal osseous precursors. Support for the second theory is based largely on the fact that myxomas have been reported not only in the non-tooth-bearing areas of the jaws (ascending ramus and condyles), but also in other bones.[61]

A few examples of myxomas as tumors of the oral soft tissue have been reported. Elzay and Duntz[62] believed that soft tissue myxomas are derived from early embryonic mesenchymal tissues. These investigators maintained that the neoplasms remain quiescent for long periods of time and have the ability to suddenly enlarge. The recommended therapy is surgical excision with adequate margins. The lesion is not thought to have the aggressive potential of its central osseous counterpart.

If one is to theorize the occurrence of true myxomas, then it becomes necessary to postulate the existence of a distinctive cell, perhaps a "myxoblast", that gives rise to the tumor, as suggested by Hodson and Prout.[63] But, in fact, most authorities who have evaluated the ultrastructure of myxomas support the theory that the lesion arises from fibroblasts and that the myxomatous appearance occurs because of the abundant amount of tumor intercellular mucin.[64]

CLINICAL FINDINGS

The vast majority of myxomas appear as slow-growing, expansile, nonpainful lesions that may cause jaw or facial deformity. The tumor may produce a myriad of symptoms, depending upon its site, ranging from tooth mobility to sinus obstruction if the maxilla is involved. The posterior mandible is the site of predisposition; the maxilla is less frequently affected.

The majority of lesions appear radiographically as multilocular radiolucencies (Fig. 4-15). They are generally described as "soap-bubble" or honeycombed in appearance. Occasional unilocular lesions have been described,[63] and some have resembled dentigerous cysts.[64] Fine trabecula of bone may rarely be seen at the periphery of the lesion, resulting in a "sunburst" pattern. Unlike the adenomatoid odontogenic tumor and ameloblastic fibroma, the myxoma shows no special tendency to be associated with impacted or partially erupted teeth.

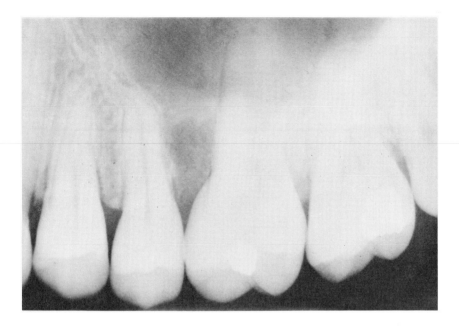

Fig. 4-15 Myxoma showing multilocular interproximal radiolucency.

GROSS AND LIGHT MICROSCOPIC FINDINGS

Upon gross examination, the myxoma can be a gray-white to yellow non-encapsulated fibrous mass that has a firm, glistening, cut surface that fails to bulge beyond surrounding tissues upon sectioning. Myxomas may also appear grossly as mucoid, slimy specimens with a semi-gelatinous consistency. In the latter instance, a capsule is not identified, and areas of bone are often present within the cut surface.

Microsopically, myxomas consist primarily of accumulations of triangular to stellate fibroblasts with rather lengthy anastomosing processes, and loose, mucoid intracellular material (Fig. 4-16). The cytoplasm of cells ranges from slightly basophilic to deeply eosinophilic, depending upon the degree of collagenization that has taken place. The supporting stroma is typically one of a mucopolysaccharide complex which may contain odontogenic epithelium (Fig. 4-17). Hasleton and colleagues[65] reported islands of odontogenic epithelium at all intervals throughout the cases they reported. Although odontogenic epithelium can be found in a high percentage of cases of central myxoma of bone involving the jaws, it may represent nothing more than a fetal remnant and is not necessarily important in the genesis of the tumor.

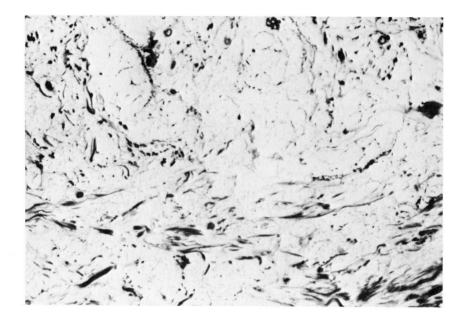

Fig. 4-16 Odontogenic myxoma. Note the delicate fibrillar cytoplasmic extensions, spindle-shaped nuclei, and loose myxoid stroma. (H&E x 380).

Regezi and Kerr[2] have evaluated myxomas for the presence of collagen and have graded the tumors on a scale of 1+ to 3+ by using polarized light. They found no correlation between the density of collagen and age of the patient. They found odontogenic rests in only 2 of 20 lesions.

ELECTRON MICROSCOPY

The ultrastructural features of odontogenic myxoma have shed some light on the cell of origin. The theory most commonly accepted today is that the tumor cell of origin closely resembles a fibroblast, a cell known to have an active secretory function. Goldblatt[66] has described two types of cells in odontogenic myxomas: a nonsecretory (Type I) and a secretory (Type II) cell (Figs. 4-18 and 4-19). Both of these cells appear to be of connective tissue origin. Redman, Greer, and Rutherford[67] have ultrastructurally identified cells resembling myofibroblasts with prominent microfilaments in odontogenic myxomas. This finding supports the theory that the cells of origin for the tumor may be periodontal ligament fibroblasts, which have also been shown to have

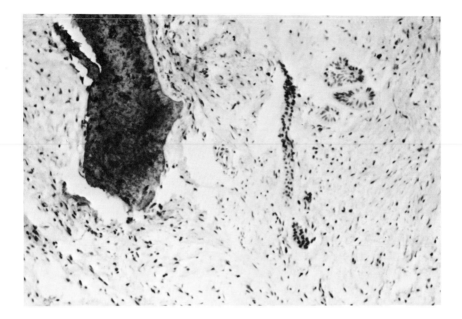

Fig. 4-17 Odontogenic myxoma. Note the delicate fibrillar stroma, odontogenic epithelial rests, and bony trabeculae. (H&E x 140).

such microfilament systems. The exact function of the myofibroblasts in the tumor is not known, although it has been postulated that their contractile mechanism is thought to be the device for allowing cell motility in the granulation tissue often associated with this tumor. Zimmerman and Dahlin[56] have attempted to define benign and malignant varieties of jaw myxomas, based largely upon the cytologic appearance of nuclei and anisocytosis. They have met with little success, and have been unable to distinquish between benign and malignant tumor variance. There is, however, some suggestion that the greater the mature fibrous component in the tumor, the less aggressive the biologic behavior.[46]

DIFFERENTIAL DIAGNOSIS

The principal lesions that most consistently resemble myxoma histologically are central odontogenic fibroma, dentinoma, and chondromyxoid fibroma. The *odontogenic fibroma* is an exceedingly rare tumor of odontogenic origin. Richardson[68] debated whether this is a true odontogenic tumor, although he has examples of a lesion showing

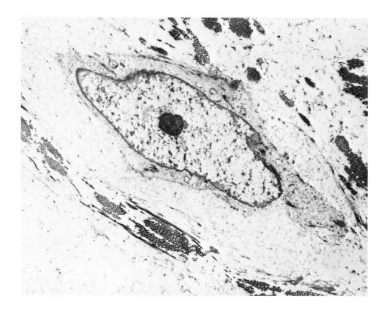

Fig. 4-18 Ultrastructural features of type I tumor cell in odontogenic myxoma illustrating elongated shape, prominent nucleolus, and microfilaments. (EM x 14,700).

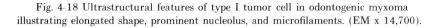

granular cell differentiation that is quite compatible with the so-called granular cell variant of ameloblastic fibroma. Many authorities feel that all lesions diagnosed as central odontogenic fibromas represent forms of central osseous nodular faciitis, non-ossifying fibroma, or juvenile fibromatosis; nonetheless, the lesion is recognized as a distinct entity by the World Health Organization.[69] Only a few adequately documented cases have been reported in the world literature. Wesley and others reported an age range of from 11-to-67 years in their studies.[70] The incidence of the lesions indicated no sexual predisposition. The mean age for all cases reported by Wesley and associates was 22 years. Odontogenic fibroma remains perhaps the most ill-defined and least understood of all odontogenic neoplasms. Wesley and colleagues gleaned only seven cases from the world literature; all tumors occurred clinically as slowly enlarging swellings. Most were multilocular radiolucencies, although unilocular lesions were identified.

There are reports in the literature which indicate that the tumor may contain radiographically visible calcified material.[71] All reported cases have occurred in the mandible.

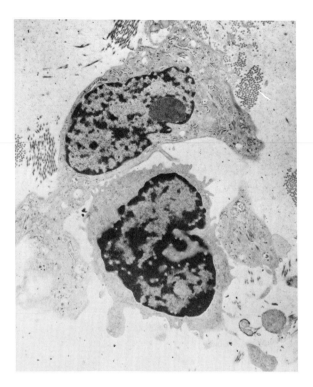

Fig. 4-19 Ultrastructural features of type II tumor cells in odontogenic myxoma illustrating prominent rough endoplasmic reticulum, indented nucleus, and absence of a prominent nucleolus. (EM x 14,700).

The odontogenic fibroma appears as an encapsulated neoplastic mass that has a homogeneous, white, cut surface that usually glistens. Typically, it is identified in association with an impacted tooth. Microscopically, one finds a moderately dense and relatively cellular proliferation of collagen, with a uniform distribution of fibroblasts (Fig. 4-20). The nuclei of the cells are usually round to oval and have finely dispersed chromatin and distinct small nucleoli. Occasionally, the nuclei can be spindle-shaped or vesicular. Cytoplasmic membranes are indistinct, and occasionally, amorphous calcifications can be identified in the tissue sample, but only in the supporting collagen. In some of the cases that have been reported, odontogenic epithelium has been identified. The presence of odontogenic epithelium should not negate a diagnosis of odontogenic fibroma. The greatest difference between the odontogenic fibroma and the lesion closely resembling it microscopically, odontogenic myxoma, is that, in the latter, the stroma exhibits only scant amounts of collagen and abundant ground substance, whereas in the odontogenic fibroma, the stroma is highly collagenous and much more cellular.

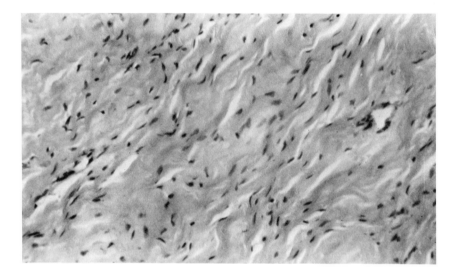

Fig 4-20 Odontogenic fibroma displaying a moderately dense, relatively cellular, proliferation of collagen with a uniform distribution of fibroblasts. (H&E x 150).

Ultrastructurally, the morphology of odontogenic fibroma is quite similar to that of odontogenic myxoma because cells in both neoplasms exhibit large amounts of endoplasmic reticulum. Two distinct cell types have not been identified in odontogenic fibroma as they have been in odontogenic myxoma. The odontogenic fibroma is benign and responds well to surgical enucleation with no tendency to recur or undergo malignant transformation.

Chemical and histochemical investigations by Borello and Gorlin[72] have demonstrated a high level of vanillylmandelic acid, a product of catecholamine metabolism in this tumor. Vanillylmandelic acid has also been identified in tumors of neural crest orgin, specifically, ganglioneuroblastoma, neuroblastoma, and retinoblastoma.

The *dentinoma* is an extremely rare, benign odontogenic tumor that consists of areas of "osteodentin" associated with odontogenic epithelium. The tumor has a stroma which resembles that of myxoma.[69]

Differentiation from myxoma depends upon finding areas of "osteodentin". Many investigators, including myself (ROG), doubt that this is a true neoplasm worthy of a separate classification.

Chondromyxoid fibroma may be confused with myxoma of the jaw. Grotepass and associates[73] found only five cases of chondromyxoid fibroma of the jaws when they reviewed the world literature, and added one new case. All six lesions occurred in the mandible. The histological appearance of this tumor differs from myxoma in that pseudolobules of myxomatous tissue are separated by septae of small, darkly-staining, hematoxyphilic cells. Dahlin[74] maintained that some of the lesions described in the literature as myxoma in bones other than the jaws may have been chondromyxoid fibromas.

Stout[75] has pointed out that fast-growing neoplasms may contain areas of myxomatous degeneration. Such areas are commonly found within fibrosarcoma, liposarcoma, and chondrosarcoma. In addition, mesenchymal chondrosarcoma contains large amounts of myxomatous tissue. Differentiation can only be made with certainty if adequate samples from various areas are viewed histologically. High mitotic activity is suggestive of malignancy.

TREATMENT AND PROGNOSIS

It is nearly impossible to differentiate between jaw myxomas that will behave aggressively and those that will have a totally benign biologic course. Farman, in his review of 213 myxomas, found no mortality related to the tumor.[58] I am aware, however, of three maxillary tumors in children that resulted in eventual orbital exenteration and maxillectomy. It appears that lesions of the maxilla spread rapidly throughout the surrounding cancellous bone and tend to have a more aggressive behavior than their mandibular counterparts.

Treatment has varied from curettage or enucleation to radical resection, with occasional cases being treated by radiotherapy, chemotherapy, chemical cautery or electrocautery.[58] Radiotherapy should be avoided as a management modality.

Wide surgical excision has generally resulted in lack of recurrence over periods of follow-up ranging from 9 months to 28 years.[55] This form of treatment and en bloc resection appear to be the most favored among surgeons. The rationale for such therapy, even with small lesions, is that the tumor has the potential to invade even the finest marrow spaces and probably extends beyond its apparent radiologic limits in most cases. The use of cautery has been advocated when wide excision is not anatomically possible.

Myxoma has a recurrence rate of at least 25 percent.[76] Our own experience has been that at least one-third of the 13 cases we have seen in all age groups in the past nine years have recurred. The same is true for our experience with six tumors seen over the past five years in children. Corio and associates[77] reported that recurrences have been noted as early as three months and as late as ten years following surgery. A two-to-three year interval between surgery and recurrences is seen most often.

CEMENTOBLASTOMA

Synonyms

1. True cementoma
2. Benign cementoblastoma
3. Attached cementoma

INCIDENCE, AGE AND SEX

Cementoblastoma is an uncommon, benign jaw neoplasm fused to the root of the involved tooth. Corio and others[77] recently reviewed a series of 24 cases of cementoblastoma presented in the world literature and added one of their own. They found that the lesion was not as uncommon as might be thought by its infrequent documentation in the world literature. Their investigations found an age range of 10-to-63 years; the mean age being 23.1 years. There appears to be a distinct male predisposition as over 60 percent of all recorded cases have occurred in males.

Although Abrams and associates[78] noted a similar sexual predisposition in an extensive review of cases in 1974, they reported a much narrower age distribution. All of their patients were between the ages of 15 and 22.

Greer and Mierau[46] reported only one cementoblastoma in an 11-year-old boy in their series of 191 tumors of the oral mucosa and jaws. Regezi and Kerr[2] reported a similar paucity of cases, recording only one cementoblastoma in their review of 706 odontogenic tumors recorded at the University of Michigan between 1934 and 1975. Abrams[78] suggested that the relative rarity of the lesion in the literature may be due to the fact that many authors fail to distinguish cementoblastoma (a true distinctive neoplasm) from periapical cemental dysplasia (a reactive process).

PATHOGENESIS

The cementoblastoma is a true neoplasm of functional cementoblasts.[79] The lesion is generally accepted to be a mesenchymal odontogenic tumor. The cementoblastoma's precise derivation has been alluded to as connective tissue from the periodontal ligament,[80] and/or the apical portion of the dental follicle.[81] Many authors have reported this lesion to be a response to irritation or to trauma, but careful consideration of such cases reveals most of them to be periapical cemental dysplasia.

CLINICAL FINDINGS

The cementoblastoma is usually located in the premolar or molar areas of the jaw with a rather equal distribution between the mandible and the maxilla. The lesion is classically attached to the apical half of the root surface of the tooth and undergoes enlargement as a spherical or lobulated mass that produces pain (Fig. 4-21).

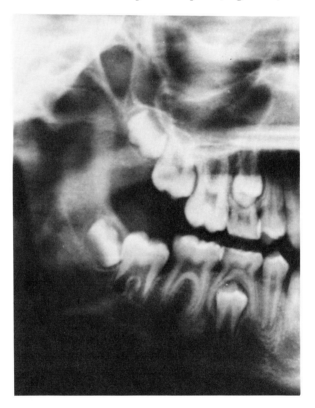

Fig. 4-21 Cementoblastoma. Note the attachment of radiopaque mass to mesial root of first mandibular molar tooth.

In most instances, pain is a significant feature of cementoblastoma. Well over half of all the cases documented by Corio featured pain as the primary manifesting symptom.[77] Associated teeth are vital, but may be nonresponsive to pulp tests, probably indicating disruption of normal neural impulse transmissions due to the fact that the tumor tends to encompass the root apex.

Radiographic features vary slightly from case to case, with the most constant feature being a central, generally dense, radiopacity, bordered by a well-demarcated, peripheral, radiolucent zone of variable width. Abrams and associates have reported a case in which the tumor involved the roots of two molar teeth,[78] and Eversole[82] has documented a rare instance in which the lesion was totally radiolucent. Evidence of root resorption of the affected tooth has also been reported.[78]

Pain and abnormal pulp tests, in association with the stated radiographic features, might suggest localized sclerosing osteomyelitis (condensing osteitis), but the consistent finding of a well-demarcated, radiolucent border in cementoblastoma is a clue to the true nature of the process. Radiographic features are occasionally misleading when excessive calcification obscures the sharp tumor border or when radiating trabeculae produce a "sunburst" effect. However, the so-called "sunburst" pattern is diagnostic of no specific entity and may be seen in a variety of benign conditions.

GROSS AND LIGHT MICROSCOPIC FINDINGS

Grossly, one can identify a sectioned tooth with an attached globular mass resembling hypercementosis if the specimen submitted is at least partially intact.

The microscopic appearance of cementoblastoma is fairly consistent. Histologically, there is a peripheral rim of radiating columns of cementum, lined by large pleomorphic (cemento) blastic cells (Fig. 4-22). In addition, at the peripheral border, islands of cementum and cementum-like substance can be seen set in a fibrous stroma. Frequently, the peripheral cementoblasts have quite hyperchromatic nuclei, marked pleomorphism, and appear to be packed on top of one another in a layer or lattice-like pattern. A portion of the tumor may show reactive cementum with tremendous reversal line activity. Giansanti[83] has demonstrated in his case studies a fine birefringence compatible with that of cementum and not bone.

However, Abrams and associates[78] have shown that trabeculae in active cellular areas of the tumor, examined under polarized light, show a birefringent pattern consisting of randomly arranged, intersecting groups of short, prominent, collagen fibers, typical of woven bone. Only the broad trabecular areas have a "quilt-like" pattern described by these authors as characteristic of cementum.

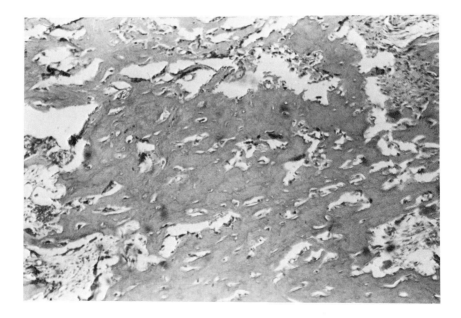

Fig. 4-22 Radiating columns of cementum, rimmed by cementoblasts are seen in this cementoblastoma from an 11-year-old-boy. (H&E x 180).

DIFFERENTIAL DIAGNOSIS

The histopathological similarities of *cementoblastoma, osteoid osteoma,* and *benign osteoblastoma* suggest a close relationship between the three conditions. Indeed, it has been stated by some investigators who have studied significant numbers of these tumor types that a histopathological separation of osteoid osteoma and benign osteoblastoma cannot be made and that these two entities can be distinguished only on the basis of clinical-radiological differences. [84]

Osteoid osteoma is generally described as a small, slow-growing lesion characterized by: (1) considerable pain; (2) frequent occurrence in patients less than 30 years of age; (3) origin in long tubular bones, and (4) a peripheral bone reaction that may be particularly prominent if much of the cortex is involved.

Benign osteoblastoma is usually regarded as a faster-growing, less painful tumor, principally involving flat bones, the vertebrae, and hands and feet of patients of about the same age as those afflicted with osteoid osteoma. Pain is less intense than with osteoid osteoma, and peripheral bone sclerosis is not a feature. [84]

Cementoblastoma also occurs primarily before the age of 30 years. It manifests pain of variable intensity, and shows, in at least some zones, active blastic proliferations with production of immature and irregularly mineralized trabeculae, focal resorption, and a well-vascularized, loose connective tissue stroma. These features are similar to those that characterize osteoid osteoma and, except for size, osteoblastoma. When examining the most cellular and active areas of cementoblastoma, it may not be possible to definitely distinguish its tumor histology from osteoid osteoma or osteoblastoma. However, broad trabecular regions with limited cellularity seem to be a feature prominent in and possibly unique to cementoblastoma. It may be that cementoblastoma is only a clinico-anatomic variant of osteoid osteoma and osteoblastoma.

In establishing a differential diagnosis for cementoid lesions, it is important to evaluate clinical, radiographic, and histological parameters. *Periapical cemental dysplasia, gigantiform cementoma,* and *cementifying fibroma* bear striking histological similarities to cementoblastoma.

Periapical cemental dysplasia is a lesion most commonly encountered in the anterior mandible and is frequently identified in middle-aged black females. This apparent ethnic propensity should be a prime consideration in any differential diagnosis which includes multiple blastic, lytic, or mixed radiographic lesions in the anterior mandible. *Cementifying fibroma (ossifying fibroma)* on the other hand, is typically present as a solitary lesion which may have a peripheral radiopaque rim around it; the lesion is usually identified in the mandibular posterior region and there is no sexual predisposition as with periapical cemental dysplasia. Except for the fact that the lesion contains cementum, it is identical to ossifying fibroma.

Another entity that should be considered in the differential diagnosis of cemental lesions is *gigantiform cementoma*. It is a lesion about which there is considerable confusion in the world literature. This diffuse lesion, most predominate in the mandible of middle-aged black females, appears radiographically as a large, dense, sclerotic, multifocal mass. Some authorities feel that there is a distinct histologic appearance to the lesion, while others, including myself (ROG), feel that the lesion represents a variant of ossifying fibroma, probably identical to the multiple endostoses that have been described by Bhaskar and Cutwright.[85]

TREATMENT AND PROGNOSIS

Cementoblastoma is thought to have a fairly unlimited growth potential, with a tendency toward expansion of the jaw, root resorption, and bone erosion. Although this growth potential has been demonstrated, a conservative surgical approach is the treatment of choice. Extraction of the associated tooth is indicated, regardless of whether or not one encounters a vital or nonvital pulp. Abrams, Kirby, and Melrose,[78] and Corio and others[77] have indicated that the tumor can easily be enucleated from adjacent bone. A malignant potential has not been documented for this lesion; therefore Abrams[78] indicated that the often-encountered term *benign* cementoblastoma is redundant. The lesion has little, if any, recurrence potential.

ODONTOMA

Synonyms

1. Complex odontoma
2. Compound odontoma
3. Odontome
4. Dilated odontome
5. Cystic odontoma

INCIDENCE

Odontomas are the most common of the odontogenic tumors; the majority are discovered in children and adolescents, upon routine radiographic examination of the jaws, as symptomless, calcified masses.

Odontoma accounted for 37 of the 191 lesions (19.3 percent) reviewed by Greer and Mierau in their study of consecutive lesions of the oral muscosa and jaws in children covering more than a five-and-one-half-year period at the University of Colorado School of Dentistry.[46]

Regezi and Kerr[2] found this lesion to be exceedingly common as well. In their review of 706 odontogenic tumors, 473 (67 percent) were odontomas. This strikingly large percentage of generally symptomless lesions lends some credence to the theory which states that the vast majority of the lesions may in fact be hamartomas and not true neoplasms.

AGE AND SEX

The most prevalent age for the diagnosis and treatment of odontomas is the second decade of life. Although most often found in this age group, these tumors can be discovered at any time throughout life. Budnick[86] reviewed a series of 149 odontomas seen in the Department of Pathology at the Emory University School of Dentistry and found that the mean age at detection was 14.8 years. Regezi and Kerr's[2] analysis of 473 lesions showed a mean age of occurrence of 19 years and Greer and Mierau[46] found a mean age of 16 years in their series. The youngest patient in these three studies was 2, the oldest 79. Regezi and Kerr[2] found nearly an equal distribution of tumors among males and females as did Greer and Mierau. Budnick[86] reported a slight male predominance.

PATHOGENESIS

Although odontomas are generally included in the classification of odontogenic tumors, most authorities will concede that these lesions are more properly considered to be malformations rather than true neoplasms.[46] A review of odontomas by Sprawson[87] in 1937 credits Paul Broca with the first use of the term *odontoma* in 1867. In 1887, Bland-Sutton proposed a classification based on the nature of the cell of the tooth germ from which the tumor originated.[88] Smith and associates suggested that the lesions originate from well-differentiated odontogenic epithelium, most likely reduced enamel epithelium.[88] Since Bland-Sutton's classification, a host of classifications have appeared in the literature. The most recent classification by the World Health Organization[69] included the following two distinct forms:

Complex odontoma — a malformation in which all the dental tissues are represented, individual tissues for the most part are well-formed but occur in a more or less disorderly pattern.

Compound odontoma — a malformation in which all the dental tissues are represented in a more orderly pattern than in the complex odontoma, so that the lesion consists of many tooth-like structures.

Tumors containing mature enamel and dentin, together with a neoplastic soft-tissue component, are properly classified as ameloblastic fibro-odontomas or odontoameloblastomas. These tumors should be distinguished from complex and compound odontomas and will be considered under the differential diagnosis heading in this chapter.

CLINICAL FINDINGS

The vast majority of odontomas occur as asymptomatic lesions identified on routine oral screening radiographs or in association with a retained or slowly erupting, deciduous or permanent, tooth. On occasion a slight expansion or swelling of the alveolar ridge may be noted. *Compound odontoma*, the most common variant, is characterized radiographically by a radiopaque accumulation of small denticle or tooth-like structures surrounded by a thin limiting radiolucent zone (Fig. 4-23). Compound odontomas are usually quite small, rarely attaining a size greater than 2 cm.

The anterior maxilla is the most common site for compound odontoma and although a female predisposition has been noted when all age groups are considered, no such predisposition has been noted in children.

In contrast to the compound odontoma, the *complex odontoma* is classically identified as a dense radiopaque mass, often associated with

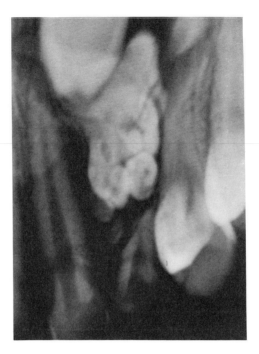

Fig. 4-23 Compound odontoma of the maxilla. Multiple opaque denticle-like structures are evident. Courtesy of Dr. Sidney Bronstein.

an impacted tooth, and surrounded by a well-demarcated radiolucent band. The occurrence of this variant indicates a predisposition of the posterior mandible and the lesion may attain a size that is somewhat greater than the compound odontoma.

LIGHT MICROSCOPY

The compound odontoma is characterized by a high degree of histodifferentiation and morphodifferentiation to the extent that the tumor is composed of an admixture of enamel, pulpal tissue, dentin, cementum, and connective tissue arranged into recognizable denticle or tooth-like structures. A peripheral fibrous connective tissue capsule often encapsulates individual denticles.

The complex odontoma is composed of a haphazard conglomerate of enamel, dentin, cementum, pulpal tissue, and connective tissue (Fig. 4-24). Morphodifferentiation is lacking or entirely absent, and normal tooth forms are not recongnizable.

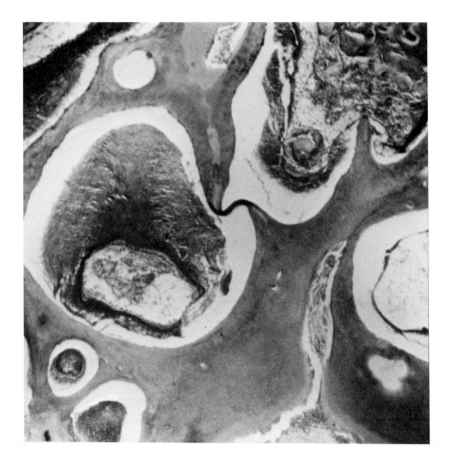

Fig. 4-24 Haphazard arrangement of dentin, pulpal tissue, poorly decalcified enamel, and periodontal ligament structures are evident in this complex odontoma. (H & E x 150).

In most odontomas, regardless of subtype, dentin forms the bulk of the tumor. Specimens that are examined during an active growth phase may show ameloblastic epithelium, odontogenic epithelial rests, epithelial ghost cells similar to those seen in the calcifying epithelial odontogenic tumor, and odontoblastic activity.

DIFFERENTIAL DIAGNOSIS

Odontoma must be distinguished from ameloblastic fibro-odontoma and ameloblastic odontoma, two lesions that have similar histological features, but not as limited a growth potential as odontoma.

Ameloblastic fibro-odontoma is a rare odontogenic tumor, histologically composed of features that are diagnostic of both ameloblastic fibroma and odontoma. Fewer than 25 cases of this tumor have been adequately documented in the world literature.[89-91] Regezi and associates[2] reported 11 lesions in their review of 706 odontogenic tumors.

The lesion has been principally identified in males in their early teens and indicates in its occurrence, a predisposition for the posterior mandible. It may be associated with unerupted teeth similar to ameloblastic fibroma. The lesion has been reported to be slow-growing, but expansile.[89-91]

The ameloblastic fibro-odontoma most commonly has a multilocular roentgenographic appearance with focal collections of calcified radiodense foci that resemble small denticles (Fig. 4-25). Histologically the ameloblastic fibro-odontoma has the microscopic features of a complex odontoma, but also contains a cellular soft tissue element similar to that of the ameloblastic fibroma[88] (Fig. 4-26).

Small foci of dentin and enamel are generally present, but these calcified components usually represent only a minor component of the lesion. It may be quite difficult to distinguish between ameloblastic fibro-odontoma and a developing complex odontoma. Regezi and associates[2] reported that complex odontomas have a greater amount of well-developed ameloblasts as well as more prominent stellate reticulum and odontoblasts than the ameloblastic fibro-odontoma. They also noted that hard tissue structures tend to be more evenly distributed throughout an odontoma.

The treatment of choice for ameloblastic fibro-odontoma is enucleation with adequate curettement. The tumor has little recurrence potential, —which is quite interesting, because ameloblastic fibroma, as a unique and separate tumor, appears to have a recurrence rate that approaches 40 percent.[47]

Odonto-ameloblastoma (ameloblastic odontoma) is defined by the World Health Organization[69] as an odontogenic neoplasm characterized by the presence of enamel, dentin, and odontogenic epithelium resembling that of an ameloblastoma in structure and behavior. The lesion is quite rare. There is a marked predisposition for the tumor in

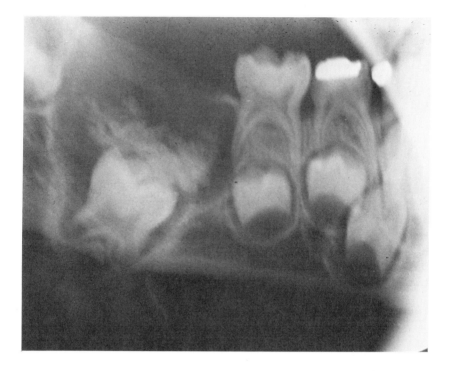

Fig. 4-25 Ameloblastic fibro-odontoma. Note the large radiolucency, totally encompassing the unerupted tooth and the calcified radiopaque area superior to the crown. Courtesy of Dr. Sidney Bronstein.

children and it is a far more common occurrence in males than females. Hooker.[91] reviewed a series of 26 cases from the Armed Forces Institute of Pathology and found a mean age of 11.5 years, with over 90 percent in patients under 15.

Most patients exhibit a slowly growing expansile mass arising centrally within bone and often delaying the eruption of teeth in the affected area. A multilocular or "soap-bubble" radiolucency is the dominant roentgenographic presentation. Within the radiolucency one finds irregular radiodense calcific foci that are, usually, rather easily identified as complex or compound odontomas (Fig. 4-27).

As noted previously, the tumor has microscopic features of both an odontoma and ameloblastoma. The differentiation of tumor hard tissues may be such that either tooth-like forms are produced or a haphazard arrangement of hard tissues may be present.[92] The stroma containing the ameloblastic tumor islands is composed of mature

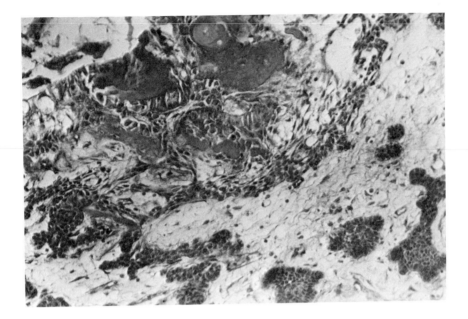

Fig. 4-26 Focal areas of dentin and cellular cementum, along with strands of odontogenic epithelium set in a primitive mesenchymal stroma, are characteristic of ameloblastic fibro-odontoma. (H&E x 220).

collagen unlike the myxoid or stellate stroma seen in ameloblastic fibro-odontoma.

There is no uniform agreement as to the treatment for this tumor. However, as the histopathological features undeniably substantiate ameloblastoma as a component of the tumor, Shafer [79] has suggested its treatment should be similar to that for ameloblastoma. Hooker [91] had obtained follow-up information on the clinical behavior of 16 out of the 26 tumors he reviewed, with follow-up ranging from 4-to-14 years. A single lesion recurred in one patient, three years after the initial surgical procedure. Four years after a second surgical intervention the patient was found to be free of disease.

TREATMENT AND PROGNOSIS

Odontomas are treated by conservative enucleation, excision, or curettage with preservation of associated permanent teeth if possible. Recurrence is exceedingly rare.

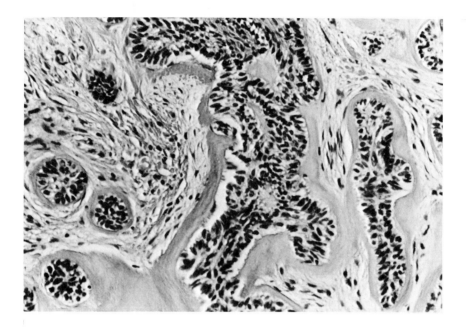

Fig. 4-27 A calcified product and ameloblastic epithelial islands are seen in this ameloblastic odontoma. Note that the connective tissue stroma is not as primitive as in ameloblastic fibro-odontoma. (H&E x 280).

ODONTONGENIC CYSTS, INTRODUCTION

The bulk of cysts that arise from odontogenic epithelium are classified as developmental cysts. In the broadest sense, a cyst occurring at the root apex of a nonvital tooth is also odontogenic in origin, but custom continues to dictate that such cysts be classified as inflammatory cysts. Odontogenic cysts can develop during any stage of odontogenesis, including development within the enamel organ, from reduced enamel epithelium, or in epithelial odontogenic remnants. The etiology of cyst formation is unknown. Table 4-4 is a schema of the various odontogenic cysts.

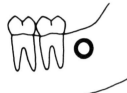

PRIMORDIAL CYST

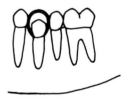

RADICULAR CYST (PERIAPICAL CYST)

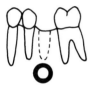
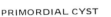

RESIDUAL CYST

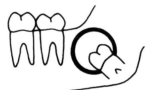

DENTIGEROUS CYST
(FOLLICULAR CYST)

ERUPTION CYST

GINGIVAL CYST

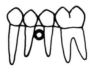

LATERAL PERIODONTAL CYST

Table 4-4 Cysts of odontogenic origin. (Modified from: Greer, R.O. "The Oral Cavity." In *Pathology*, edited by S.G. Silverberg. New York: Wiley and Sons, 1982.)

PRIMORDIAL CYST

Synonyms

1. Odontogenic keratocyst

INCIDENCE

The primordial cyst is typically a lesion of the child or young adult.[93] It is encountered less frequently in adults, but because the lesion grows slowly and usually asymptomatically, it may not be identified until late adulthood. Although Greer and Mierau[46] documented only two odontogenic keratocysts in the review of 191 tumors and cysts involving the oral mucosa and jaws of infants and children, the lesions are probably much more common.

AGE AND SEX

There is no apparent sexual predisposition for the primordial cyst, although a few reports in the world literature have documented a male predominance.[94;95] These reports presuppose all primordial cysts to be odontogenic keratocysts, an assumption that is not always valid.

PATHOGENESIS

The primordial cyst is thought to arise via cystic degeneration of the central stellate reticulum of the developing tooth germ before ameloblastic differentiation and the induction of a calcified product. After this cystic change has occurred, the development of a tooth is nullified, and the cyst takes the place of the tooth that would otherwise develop. It must be remembered that the primordial cyst can develop from any of the deciduous or permanent tooth germs, or it may arise from a supernumerary tooth germ. In addition, Gardner and Sapp,[96] and Soskalne and Shear[97] have documented the development of primordial cysts from remnants of the dental lamina. Most authorities now believe this derivation from the dental lamina is probably the most frequent mode of primordial cyst initiation.

CLINICAL FINDINGS

Primordial cysts are most commonly encountered in the mandible with well over two-thirds of the lesions located in the third molar area.[98] The roentgenographic manifestations of the primordial cyst can range from solitary well-circumscribed radiolucencies to large, expansile, multilocular lesions involving a large segment of the mandible or maxilla [99] (Fig. 4-28). As other cysts and tumors can have similar appearances, a clinical differential diagnosis of ameloblastoma, odontogenic myxoma, aneurysmal bone cyst, and hemangioma is often entertained.

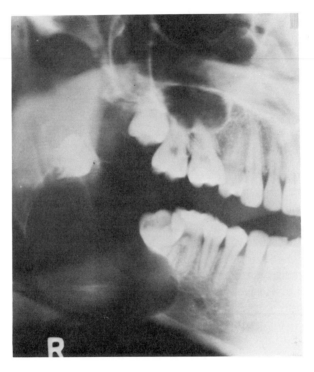

Fig. 4-28 Odontogenic keratocyst (dentigerous cyst type) occurring as a large, focally loculated cyst of the mandible, associated with an impacted third molar tooth. Courtesy of Dr. Sidney Bronstein.

LIGHT MICROSCOPY

The primordial cyst is typically a sac-like structure that is lined by a layer of statified squamous epithelium and supported by a dense relatively avascular connective tissue wall. When the lesion becomes secondarily infected, generally due to perforation of the cortical plates of bone, the epithelium may show rete ridge elongation.

Frequently, the primordial cyst will display the histological hallmarks of an odontogenic keratocyst. When such features are identified, it is paramount that the clinician and the pathologist understand the biological behavioral differences between the two lesions (see the following discussion under differential diagnosis).

DIFFERENTIAL DIAGNOSIS

So pervasive has the synonym, *odontogenic keratocyst*, become for primordial cyst, the World Health Organization uses the two terms interchangeably.[100] Unfortunately, this terminology functions under the supposition that only a cyst arising without association to a tooth can be a keratocyst. Although this may, in fact, be the general rule, exceptions certainly do occur, and there exist numerous well-documented reports in the literature supporting the fact that dentigerous cysts (those cysts associated with the crown of a tooth),[101] and even residual cysts (those remaining after previous extraction of a tooth or enucleation of a cyst),[102] can have histological features and a behavioral pattern consistent with those of the insidious odontogenic keratocyst.

Thus, critical facts for the surgical pathologist to remember are: the odontogenic keratocyst may be in direct association with a tooth; or, it may occur after tooth extraction. It need not always occur when there is a history of failure of a tooth to develop, as with the primordial variety.

Gardner and Sapp[96] suggested the use of the term *primordial* cyst be discontinued, and that this entity be viewed purely as a developmental concept. They further suggested that the term, *odontogenic keratocyst* be maintained to designate a specific entity with a characteristic microscopic appearance. The latter proposal appears to be a sound one; the former proposal is less acceptable, for despite their rarity, primordial cysts do occur. To further clarify this confusing issue, a simple and easily understandable sign-out diagnosis which the clinician can appreciate would be "odontogenic keratocyst: primordial, residual, dentigerous, or lateral periodontal type".

The term, odontogenic keratocyst, was first used by Philipsen[103] in 1956 to describe any odontogenic cyst displaying microscopic keratinization of the epithelial lining. The lesion has since been reported to account for within 8-to-10 percent of all jaw cysts.[104;105] The occurrence of these cystic lesions indicates a marked predisposition of the posterior body of the mandible and the most frequent incidence in the second and third decades of life. The lesion shows a variable radiologic pattern. Browne[105] described three distinct radiographic appearances in a series of 83 cases. He documented 56 percent as having a unilocular pattern, 20 percent as a solitary cavity with a locular periphery, and 23 percent as multilocular.

The odontogenic keratocyst tends to grow slowly and the patient is frequently symptomless. When a complaint is encountered, it is usually because the patient has noticed an expansion of the jaw, not pain.

The salient histological features of odontogenic keratocyst have been discussed by many authorities but probably are most succinctly described by Gardner and Sapp,[96] who have indicated that the following microscopic features are necessary to arrive at a diagnosis: (1) a thin, stratified squamous epithelial lining 6-to-8 cells thick, without rete ridge formation; (2) prominent or cuboidal basal cells with dense nuclear staining; (3) a corrugated surface layer of parakeratin, and (4) a thin connective tissue wall (Fig. 4-29).

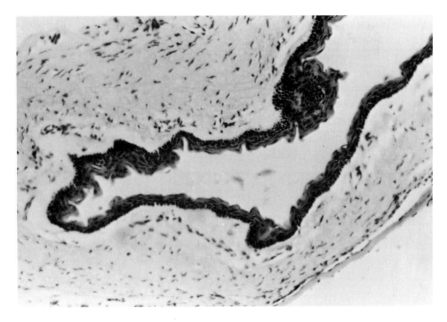

Fig. 4-29 Odontogenic keratocyst showing corrugated parakeratin surface and prominent basal epithelial layer without rete ridge formation. (H&E x 280).

The high rate of recurrence for this lesion may be related to the frequency of proliferation of daughter cysts in the wall, the penetration or budding of exceedingly thin epithelium into the connective tissue (often resulting in incomplete removal), or the reinitiated proliferation of cyst lining from remnants of the dental lamina.

A common histological feature associated with the odontogenic keratocyst has been the separation of the epithelial cyst lining from the supporting connective tissue capsule.[105] Wilson and Ross[106] examined this feature ultrastructurally as it had been hypothesized that the separation very likely accounted for the difficulty in surgical removal and a resultant high recurrence rate. These investigators found the basal lamina complex in odontogenic keratocyst to be ultrastructurally normal and could not fully explain the separation phenomenon except to hypothesize that there is somehow increased enzymatic collagen degradation.

Not all cysts displaying keratinization are odontogenic keratocyst. One cannot therefore render a diagnosis of odontogenic keratocyst simply because the cyst lumen is filled with keratin. If the salient features described by Gardner and Sapp[96] are not present, the lesion should not be designated an odontogenic keratocyst; it is probably some other form of odontogenic, fissural, or inflammatory jaw cyst.

It has been well documented that odontogenic keratocysts can be a component of the *basal cell nevus syndrome*, with its concomitant multiple cutaneous nevoid basal cell carcinomas and skeletal abnormalities. It is exceedingly important for the clinician and pathologist to consider the possibility of this syndrome in any patient with an established diagnosis of odontogenic keratocyst, especially when there have been multiple jaw cysts.

TREATMENT AND PROGNOSIS

The primordial cyst that is not an odontogenic keratocyst usually does not become very large or produce alarming symptoms. These lesions are generally treated by enucleation, with considerable care to remove the often fragile cyst lining by thorough curettement.

Treatments of odontogenic keratocyst have ranged from enucleation of unilocular lesions to resection of a considerable portion of the affected jaw in large multilocular, expanding, or erosive lesions.[107] The most striking clinical feature of the odontogenic keratocyst is its propensity for recurrence. The consistent recurrence rate documented in large reported series is about 25 percent, although reports in the literature range from 6-to-60 percent.[46]

DENTIGEROUS CYST

Synonyms

1. Follicular cyst

INCIDENCE

The dentigerous cyst is a relatively common odontogenic cyst that occurs in association with the crown of an unerupted tooth. It is the most common cyst of the jaws in childhood and adolescence. Greer and Carpenter, [108] in a review of 400 consecutively recorded cases seen on the surgical oral pathology service at the University of Colorado, found that 19.3 percent of their cases were dentigerous cysts.

AGE AND SEX

The average age in this study was 19 and no sexual predisposition was noted. The so-called *eruption cyst* is no more than a dentigerous cyst affecting infants (Fig. 4-30). This lesion is a self-limiting one.

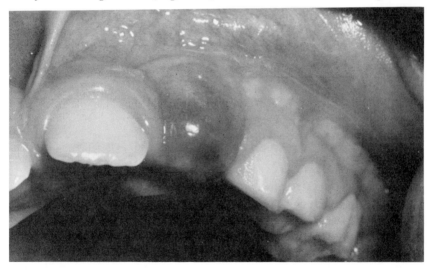

Fig. 4-30 Eruption cyst overlying a maxillary lateral incisor in a child. Courtesy of Dr. Al Abrams.

PATHOGENESIS

The dentigerous cyst develops when the enamel-forming apparatus (enamel organ) has been reduced to a few layers of epithelial cells surrounding the tooth crown. Fluid accumulates within the potential follicular space of the organ and a cyst eventuates. Typically, the crown of the tooth protrudes into the cystic cavity.

CLINICAL FINDINGS

The dentigerous cyst is most commonly found in association with impacted or partially impacted mandibular third molars, maxillary canine teeth (cuspid teeth), and maxillary third molars. Roentgenographically, the dentigerous cyst will manifest as a well-defined radiolucent area surrounding the crown of a tooth. The lesion may be displaced to one side of the tooth crown and need not always arise superficial to it.

The radiolucency may be unilocular or multilocular. The lesion has the potential to expand bone, and the cyst may cause extensive destruction of bone with almost complete replacement of the medullary portion of the ramus and body of the mandible by the cyst.[96] It is not always possible to definitively diagnose a dentigerous cyst radiographically, because odontogenic keratocysts and certain odontogenic tumors, such as ameloblastoma and odontogenic myxoma, may have similar appearances.

GROSS AND LIGHT MICROSCOPIC FINDINGS

Grossly, the lesion will appear as a sac, enveloping the tooth. The distinction between a dentigerous cyst and a hyperplastic dental follicle with cystic degeneration is often an arbitrary one because of the histological similarities between the two. The diagnosis of a dentigerous cyst is often based on the size of the gross specimen and the degree of radiographic involvement.

It is extremely important to examine the cyst wall for thickenings and outgrowths as there are well-documented instances of ameloblastoma and even squamous cell carcinoma arising in the walls of dentigerous cysts.

Histologically, the dentigerous cyst consists of a lining epithelium, supported by a fibrous connective tissue wall. The epithelium is generally of the stratified squamous variety and is only a few cell layers thick. Occasionally, the cyst may be lined by columnar or mucus-secreting cells.

The cyst wall may be diffusely inflamed or totally free of an inflammatory infiltrate. Frequently, the cyst wall contains extensive cholesterol clefting similar to that seen in a radicular or periapical cyst. When such features are noted microscopically, only the anatomic location of the lesion allows one to differentiate between a dentigerous cyst and a periapical cyst.

DIFFERENTIAL DIAGNOSIS

It is quite common to observe odontogenic epithelial rests in the wall of dentigerous cysts. There is considerable debate among pathologists as to whether these rests have the potential to develop along neoplastic lines. It is very important to relay to the clinician the presence of rest activity in the wall of all odontogenic cysts. All dentigerous cysts should be examined with multiple histologic sections for ameloblastoma.

Whether ameloblastomas arising in association with dentigerous cysts have their origin from cyst lining epithelium or from odontogenic rests in the connective tissue wall is still at issue. McMillan[109] offered an analysis of five cases, which he hoped would demonstrate that ameloblastoma arose by transformation of the epithelial lining of the cyst. In each one of the cases analyzed, the identification of the specimen as a dentigerous cyst was established first, and then the epithelium of the tumor was traced by serial sectioning to demonstrate that the lining epithelium was always continuous with that forming the ameloblastoma. Whether this process occurs in all instances cannot be determined by the evidence in these few cases, and the demonstration of one method of histogenesis does not rule out other possible methods. Our own experience indicates an apparent ability of ameloblastoma to arise either from cyst lining epithelium or from odontogenic rests within the cyst wall.[110]

Two of five cases reviewed by Poulson[110] showed ameloblastoma arising in the walls of odontogenic keratocysts. The majority of cyst-related ameloblastomas have been associated with dentigerous (follicular) cysts and not with other peculiar odontogenic cysts such as keratocysts.

Gingival cysts occur as two distinct entities; those of the newborn and those of the adult.[96] Gingival cysts of the newborn appear as a single or multiple small, white nodules along the crest of the alveolar ridge. These excrescences have been variously reported in the literature as microcysts of the gingiva,[111] Bohn's nodules, and Epsteins's pearls.[112] These outgrowths, in fact, represent cystic degeneration of remnants of the dental lamina. They are usually asymptomatic and exfoliated without consequence. Histologically, they appear as keratin-filled cysts, lined by stratified squamous epithelium.

Gingival cysts of the adult are quite common. They also are thought to originate from dental lamina remnants. Gardner and Sapp[96] point out that these lesions may also arise from traumatic implantation of surface epithelium from the oral cavity into the underlying connective tissue. The most frequent site for the gingival cyst of the adult is in the mandibular cuspid and premolar area; interestingly, this is a frequent site for supernumerary teeth as well. Gingival cysts usually occur clinically as painless swellings. Histologically, the gingival cyst of the adult mimics that of the newborn. Gingival cysts have little, if any, potential for recurrence and simple excision is curative.

TREATMENT AND PROGNOSIS

The dentigerous cyst can be adequately treated by complete surgical excision and curettage. Occasionally, lesions that show extensive bony involvement are managed by multiple surgical enucleation procedures. Recurrence is a possibility in all cysts that have odontogenic epithelial remnants within bone, following surgery.

CALCIFYING ODONTOGENIC CYST

Synonyms

1. Keratinizing and calcifying odontogenic cyst
2. Gorlin cyst

INCIDENCE

Although there is still controversy as to whether this lesion, first described by Gorlin in 1962,[113] should be regarded as a cyst or tumor, the World Health Organization contends that the lesion has gross and microscopic features most consistent with a tumor and, accordingly, prefers to classify it as such.[69]

In a recent review of 706 odontogenic tumors, Regezi and Kerr[2] documented that 115 (2 percent) of their lesions were calcifying odontogentic cysts.

AGE AND SEX

The calcifying odontogenic cyst is predominately a lesion of children and young adults. Freedman and associates[114] recently reviewed a series of 70 calcifying odontogenic cysts from the world literature and found that nearly 33 percent of all reported cases occurred in patients less than 20 years of age. The youngest acceptable case they were able to document occurred in a seven-year-old. Although both sexes appear to be equally affected, the lesion occurs more frequently in women before the fourth decade and more commonly in men after the fourth decade.

PATHOGENESIS

This curious lesion was first thoroughly described by Gorlin and associates, although they document that it was reported by Rywland much earlier.[113;115] There has been extended debate in the literature as to whether the calcifying odontogenic cyst represents a cyst or tumor, because the lesion can occur grossly as a cyst or as a solid tumor mass. The calcified structures identified roentgenographically can have the gross appearance of irregular hard tissue fragments or even small teeth or denticle-like structures.

Pindborg and Kramer[69] hold the view that the calcifying odontogenic cyst is non-neoplastic. Gorlin and colleagues[113] have actually demonstrated that the lesion can originate from the dental epithelium of a developing unerupted tooth. Lesions that develop in an extraosseous site most likely develop from remnants of odontogenic epithelium in the gingiva or alveolar muscosa. Smith and Turner[88] suggested that the intraosseous tumor arises from incompletely differentiated ameloblasts.

CLINICAL FINDINGS

The calcifying odontogenic cyst typically appears as a slow-growing, asymptomatic central osseous jaw lesion. Extraosseous examples have been documented in the literature, but they represent less than 25 percent of the reported lesions.[114;115] The mandible has a marked predisposition for this lesion. Regardless of a maxillary or mandibular occurrence, over 75 percent of the lesions reported in the series of Freedman and associates[114] occurred anterior to the first molar. Radiologically, the lesion most frequently appears as a unilocular or multilocular cystic, radiolucent area (Fig. 4-31). The margins may be well-defined or poorly-demarcated, and small, irregular calcified bodies of varying sizes have been reported in 29-to-37 percent of all reported cases.[116;117]

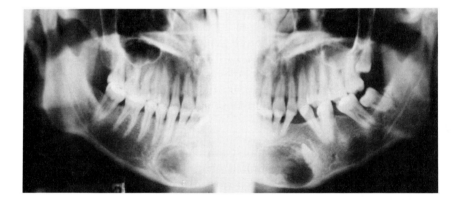

Fig. 4-31 Calcifying odontogenic cyst. Well-circumscribed, calcifying odontogenic cyst is present on split panographic film. Note the association with impacted tooth and the calcified areas within radiolucent zones. Courtesy of Dr. Don Biggs.

Calcifications may fill the cyst cavity entirely or they may be totally absent; therefore, the presence or absence of such calcifications is of questionable value in unequivocally establishing a radiologic diagnosis. Numerous odontogenic tumors can have radiographic features quite similar to the calcifying and keratinizing odontogenic cyst. Such lesions, including the calcifying epithelial odontogenic tumor, adenomatoid odontogenic tumor, ameloblastic odontoma, and the so-called cystic odontoma, should be included in the radiographic differential diagnosis.

LIGHT MICROSCOPY

Histologically, tissue sections reveal a cavity or potential cavity, lined by a prominent and well-defined basal layer of cuboidal or columnar cells having some resemblance to ameloblasts. These cells stain deeply-basophilic. Overlying the basal epithelial layer, loosely arranged epithelial cells that resemble the central stellate reticulum of the tooth germ can be identified. Distributed among these cells are large eosinophilic cells that have been termed "ghost cells" (Fig. 4-32). These cells are thought to have undergone aberrant keratinization, and occasionally, they flatten out in a manner similar to normal keratin. [98] The entire lumen of the cyst may be filled with aberrant keratin, and on occasion, foreign-body giant cell activity is prominent in the cyst wall and supporting capsular connective tissue wall.

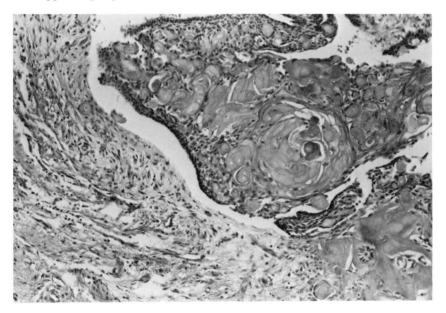

Fig. 4-32 A prominent basal epithelial layer is seen below loosely arranged epithelial and "ghost" cells of a calcifying odontogenic cyst. (H&E x 150).

Sauk[115] and Freedman and Lumerman[114] have documented that the basal epithelial layer can show prominent budding, and that odontogenic epithelium frequently penetrates deeply into the supporting collagenous wall. Dentin, enamel, and even melanin have been reported proliferating within the wall of calcifying odontogenic cysts.[113]

DIFFERENTIAL DIAGNOSIS

The calcifying odontogenic cyst is frequently confused with the odontogenic adenomatoid tumor. The characteristically prominent basal cell layer and "ghost cell" formation seen in the latter are the most definitive features that separate the two entities. Some authorities have observed that the calcifying odontogenic cyst has clinical and histological features closely resembling the first stage of the formation of a complex odontoma. However, Gorlin[113] reported that this is probably not the case, because extraosseous calcifying odontogenic cysts have been reported, whereas extraosseous odontomas have not.

TREATMENT AND PROGNOSIS

Recurrence of the calcifying odontogenic cyst is exceedingly rare. Even the most conservative form of enucleation appears to be curative. There appears to be little potential for the lesion to develop into an odontogenic tumor, and although there is a single report in the literature of the cyst occurring in association with an ameloblastic fibro-odontoma, there is doubt that the reported case represented a true calcifying odontogenic cyst.[118] The more likely sequence is that the lesion represented cystic change in an odontoma.

References

1. Greer, R.O "The Oral Cavity." In *Pathology*, edited by S. G. Silverberg pp. 1-48. New York: Wiley and Sons, 1982.
2. Regezi, J.A.; Kerr, D.A. and Courtney, R.M. "Odontogenic tumors: Analysis of 706 cases." *J. Oral Surg.* 36(1978): 771-779.
3. Young, D.R. and Robinson, M. "Ameloblastomas in children." *Oral Surg.* 15(1962): 1155-1162.
4. Lewin, M.L. "Non-malignant maxillofacial tumors in children." *Plast. Reconstr. Surg.* 38(1966): 186-196.
5. Dresser, W.J. and Segal, W. "Ameloblastoma associated with dentigerous cyst in a 6 year old child." *Oral Surg.* 24(1967): 388-391.
6. Small, I.A. and Waldron, C.A. "Ameloblastoma of the jaws." *Oral Surg.* 9(1955): 281-297.
7. Hertz, J. "Adamantinoma. Histopathologic and prognostic studies." *Acta Chir. Scand.* 102(1951): 405-432.

8. Forsberg, A. "A contribution to the knowledge of histology, histogenesis and etiology of adamantinoma." *Acta Odontol. Scand.* 12(1954): 39-64.
9. Greer, R.O. and Richardson, J.F. "Ameloblastoma of mucosal origin. A pathobiologic re-evaluation." *Arch. Otolaryngol.* 100(1974): 174-175.
10. Spouge, J.D. *Oral Pathology.* St Louis: C.V. Mosby, 1973.
11. Stanley, H.R. and Diehl, D.C. "Ameloblastoma potential of follicular cysts." *Oral Surg,* 20(1965): 260-268.
12. Shehdev et al. "Ameloblastoma of maxilla and mandible." *Cancer* 33(1974): 324-333.
13. Rockoff, W.M. "A statistical analysis of ameloblastoma." *Oral Surg.* 16(1963): 1100-1101.
14. Gardner, D.G. "Plexiform Unicystic Ameloblastoma: A Diagnostic Problem in Dentigerous Cysts." *Cancer* 47(1981): 1358-1363.
15. Greer, R.O. and Hammond, W.S. "Extraosseous ameloblastoma: light microscopic and ultrastructural observations." *J. Oral Surg.* 36(1978): 553-556.
16. Trodahl, J.N. "Ameloblastic fibroma: a survey of cases from the Armed Forces Institute of Pathology." *Oral Surg.* 3(1972): 547-558.
17. Gardner, D.G. "Peripheral ameloblastoma. A study of 21 cases including 5 reported as basal cell carcinoma of gingiva." *Cancer* 39(1972): 1625-1633.
18. Mehlisch, D.R.; Dahlin, D.C. and Mason, J.K. "Ameloblastoma: a clinicopathologic report." *J. Oral Surg.* 30(1972): 9-22.
19. Becker, R. and Perth, A. "Zur therapies des ameloblastomas." *Deutsch Zahn Mand. Kieferheilkd* 49(1967): 423-433.
20. Kahn et al. "Adenomatoid odontogenic tumor resembling a globulomaxillary cyst: light and electron microscopic studies." *J. Oral Surg.* 35(1977): 739-742.
21. Courtney, R.M. and Kerr, D.A. "The odontogenic adenomatoid tumor: a comprehensive study of twenty new cases." *Oral Surg.* 39(1975): 424-432.
22. Giansanti, J.S.; Someren, A. and Waldron, C.A. "Odontogenic adenomatoid tumor (adenoameloblastoma)." *Oral Surg.* 30(1970): 69-86.
23. Stafne, E.C. "Epithelial tumors associated with developmental cysts of the maxilla. A report of three cases." *Oral Surg.* 1(1948): 887-894.
24. Miles, A.E.W. "A cystic complex composite odontome." *Proc. R. Soc. Med.* 44(1951): 51-55.
25. Thoma, K.H. "Adenoameloblastoma." *Oral Surg.* 8(1955): 441-447.
26. Oehlers, F.A.C. "An unusual pleomorphic adenoma-like tumor in the wall of a dentigerous cyst. Report of a case." *Oral Surg.* 9(1945): 411-417.
27. Lucas, R.B. "Tumor of enamel organ epithelium." *Oral Surg.* 10(1957): 652-660.
28. Cina, M.T.; Dahlin, D.C. and Gores, R.J. "Ameloblastic adenomatoid tumors. A report of four new cases." *Am. J. Clin. Pathol.* 39(1963): 59-65.
29. Wee, L.K. "The so-called adenoameloblastoma. A radiological and histological study." *Malaysian Dent. Journal.* 5(1965): 8-30.
30. Spouge, J.D. "The adenoameloblastoma." *Oral Surg.* 23(1967): 470-482.
31. Abrams, A.M.; Melrose, R.J. and Howell, F.V. "Adenoameloblastoma: A clinical pathologic study of 10 new cases." *Cancer* 22(1968): 175-185.
32. Gorlin, R.J. and Chaudhry, A.P. "Adenoameloblastoma." *Oral Surg.* 11(1958): 762-768.
33. Oehlers, F.A.C. "The so-called adenoameloblastoma." *Oral Surg.* 14(1961); 712-725.

34. Bhaskar, S.N. "Adenoameloblastoma: its histogenesis and report of 15 new cases." *J. Oral Surg.* 22(1964): 218.

35. Shear, M. "The histogenesis of the 'Tumor of Enamel Organ Epithelium'." *Br. Dent. J.* 112(1962): 494-498.

36. Swinson, T.W. "An extra-osseous adenomatoid odontogenic tumor: a case report." *Br. J. Oral Surg.* 15(1978): 32-36.

37. Gorlin, R.J. and Chaudhry, A.P. "Adenoameloblastoma." *Oral Surg.* 11(1958): 762-768.

38. Abrams, A.M.; Melrose, R.J. and Howell, F.V. "Adenoameloblastoma: a clinical pathologic study of 10 new cases." *Cancer* 22(1968): 175-185.

39. Takagi, M. "Adenomatoid ameloblastoma. An analysis of nine case by histopathological and electron microscopic study." *Bull. Tokyo Med. Dent. Univ.* 14(1967): 487-506.

40. Hatakeyama, S. and Suzuki, A. "Ultrastructural study of adenomatoid odontogenic tumor." *J. Oral Pathol.* 7(1978): 295-310.

41. Smith et al. "Adenomatoid odontogenic tumor. Ultrastructural demonstration of two cell types and amyloid. *Cancer* 43(1979): 505-511.

42. Schlosnagle, D.C. and Someren, A. "The ultrastructure of the adenomatoid odontogenic tumor." *Oral Path.* 52(1981): 154-161.

43. Frank, R.M. and Nalbandian, J. "Ultrastructure of amelogenesis." In *Structure and Chemical Organization of Teeth*, edited by A.E.W. Miles, pp. 399-462. New York: Academic Press, 1967.

44. Saunders, B. *Pediatric Oral and Maxillofacial Surgery.* St Louis: C.V. Mosby, 1979.

45. Krolls, S. and Pindborg, J.J. "Calcifying epithelial odontogenic tumors. A survey of 23 cases and discussion of histomorphologic variants." *Arch. Pathol.* 98(1974)206-210.

46. Greer, R.O. and Mierau, G.W. *Tumors of the Oral Mucosa and Jaws.* Denver: University of Colorado Medical Center Press, 1980.

47. Trodahl, J.N. "Ameloblastic fibroma. A survey of cases from the Armed Forces Institute of Pathology." *Oral Surg.* 3(1972): 547-558.

48. Huebsch, R.F. and Stephenson, T.D. "Recurrent ameloblastic fibroma in a 3 year old boy." *Oral Surg.* 9(1956): 707-714.

49. Eversole, L.R. *Anatomic Pathology No. AP-59 Check Sample Series*, American Society of Clinical Pathology, n.l. (October 1978): 1-10.

50. Gorlin, R.J.; Chauhdry, A.P. and Pindborg, J.J. "Odontogenic tumors. Classification, histopathology and clinical behavior in man and domesticated animals. *Cancer* 14(1961): 73-101.

51. Shafer, W.G. "Ameloblastic fibroma." *J. Oral Surg.* 13(1955): 317-320.

52. Carr et al. "Recurrent ameloblastic fibroma." *Oral Surg.* 29(1970): 85-90.

53. Tanaka et al. "Recurrent ameloblastic fibroma. Report of a case." *Oral Surg.* 30(1972): 944-948.

54. Eversole, L.R.; Tomich, C.E. and Cherrick, H.M. "Histogenesis of odontogenic tumors." *Oral Surg.* 32(1971): 569-581.

55. Sawyer, D.R.; Nwoky, A.L. and Mosadomi, A. "Recurrent ameloblastic fibroma. Report of two cases." *Oral Surg.* 53(1982): 19-23.

56. Zimmerman, D.C. and Dahlin, D.C. "Myxomatous tumors of the jaws." *Oral Surg.* 11(1958): 1069-1080.

57. Kangur, T.T.; Dahlin, D.C. and Turlington, E.G. "Myxomatous tumors of the jaws." *J. Oral Surg.* 3(1975): 523-528.

58. Farman et al. "Myxofibroma of the jaws." *J. Oral Surg.* 15(1977): 3-18.

59. Ghosh et al. "Myxoma of the jawbones." *Cancer* 31(1973): 237-246.

60. Gorlin, R.J. "Odontogenic Tumors." In *Thoma's Oral Pathology*, 6th edition, edited by R.J. Gorlin and H.M. Goldman, pp. 481-415. St Louis: C.V. Mosby, 1970.

61. McClure, D.K. and Dahlin, D.C. "Myxoma of bone. Report of 3 cases." *Mayo Clin. Proc.* 52(1977)249-253.

62. Elzay, R.P. and Duntz, W. "Myxomas of the paraoral soft tissues." *Oral Surg.* 45(1978): 246-254.

63. Hodson, J.J. and Prout, R.E.S. "Chemical and histochemical characterization of mucopolysaccharides in jaw myxoma." *J. Clin. Pathol.* 21(1968): 582-589.

64. White et al. "Odontogenic myxoma." *Oral Surg.* 39(1975): 901-917.

65. Hasleton, P.S.; Simpson, W. and Craig, R.D.P. "Myxoma of the mandible a fibroblastic tumor." *Oral Surg.* 46(1978): 396-406.

66. Goldblatt, L.I. "Ultrastructural study of an odontogenic myxoma." *Oral Surg.* 42(1976): 206-220.

67. Redman, R.S.; Greer, R.O. and Rutherford, R.B. "Myofibroblasts in odontogenic myxoma." (Paper delivered at the Thirty-second Annual Meeting of the American Academy of Oral Pathology, Scientific Session, Fort Lauderdale, April 24, 1978), Abstract No. 12.

68. Richardson, J.F. Personal communiction, 1979.

69. Pindborg, J.J.; Kramer, I.R.M. and Torloni, H. *Histological Typing of Odontogenic Tumors, Jaw Cysts and Allied Lesions. International Classification of Tumors, No.5.* Geneva: World Health Organization, 1971.

70. Wesley, R.D.; Wysochi, G.P. and Mintz, S.M. "The central odontogenic fibroma. Clinical and morphologic studies." *Oral Surg.* 40(1975): 235-245.

71. Mallow et al. "Odontogenic fibroma with calcification." *Oral Surg.* 2(1964): 564-568.

72. Borello, E.D. and Gorlin, R.J. "Melanotic neuroectodermal tumor of infancy. A neoplasm of neural crest origin." *Cancer* 19(1966): 191-200.

73. Grotepass, F.W.; Farman, A.G. and Nortje, C. "Chondromyxoid fibroma of the mandible." *J. Oral Surg.* 34(1976): 988-994.

74. Dahlin, D.C. *Bone Tumors: General Aspects and Data on 6,221 Cases*, 3rd ed. Springfield: Charles C. Thomas, 1978.

75. Stout, A.P. "Myxoma, the tumor of primitive mesenchyme." *Ann. Surg.* 127(1948): 706-719.

76. Fu, Y.S. and Perzin, K.H. "Nonepithelial tumors of the nasal cavity, paranasal sinuses and nasopharynx. A clinicopathologic study. VII. Myxomas." *Cancer* 39(1977): 195-203.

77. Corio, R.L.; Crawford, B.E. and Schaberg, S.J. "Benign cementoblastoma." *Oral Surg.* 41(1976): 524-530.

78. Abrams, A.M.; Kirby, J.W. and Melrose, R.J. "Cementoblastoma." *Oral Surg.* 38(1974): 394-407.

79. Shafer, W.G.; Hine, M.K. and Levy, B.M. *A Textbook of Oral Pathology*, 3rd edition. Philadelphia: W.B. Saunders, 1974.

80. Hammer, J.E.; Scofield, H.H. and Cornyn, J. "Benign fibro-osseous jaw lesions of periodontal membrane origin. An analysis of 249 cases." *Cancer* 27(1968): 861-878.
81. Kline et al. "Large cementoma of the mandible. Report of a case." *Oral Surg.* 14(1961): 1421-1426.
82. Eversole, L.R.; Sabes, W.R. and Dauchess, V.G. "Benign cementoblastoma." *Oral Surg.* 36(1973): 824-830.
83. Giansanti, J.J. "The pattern and width of collagen bundles in bone and cementum." *Oral Surg.* 30(1970): 508-514.
84. Schajowicz, F. and Lemons, C. "Osteoid osteoma and osteoblastoma, closely related entites of osteoblastic derivation." *Acta Orthop. Scand.* 41(1971): 272-291.
85. Bhaskar, S.N. and Cutwright, D.E. "Multiple enostosis. Report of 16 cases. *J. Oral Surg.* 26(1968): 321-325.
86. Budnick, S.D. "Compound and complex odontomas." *Oral Surg.* 42(1976): 501-506.
87. Sprawson, E. "Odontomes." *Br. Dent. J.* 62(1937): 177-201.
88. Smith, R.M.; Turner, J.E. and Robbins, M.L. *Atlas of Oral Pathology.* St. Louis: C.V. Mosby, 1981.
89. Sanders, D.W.; Kolodny, S.C. and Jacoby, J.K. "Ameloblastic fibro-odontoma: report of a case." *J. Oral Surg.* 32(1974): 281-285.
90. Hanna, R.J.; Regezi, J.A. and Hayward, J.R. "Ameloblastic fibro-odontoma." *J. Oral Surg.* 34(1976)820-825.
91. Hooker, S.P. "Ameloblastic odontoma: an analysis of twenty-six cases." *Oral Path.* 24(1967): 375-376.
92. Miller et al. "Ameloblastic fibro-odontoma." *Oral Surg.* 41(1976): 354-365.
93. Shear, M. Singh "Age standardized incidence rates of primordial cyst (keratocyst) on the witwaterstrand." *Community Dent. Oral Epidemial.* 6(1978): 296-299.
94. Panders, A.K. and Hadders, H.M. "Solitary keratocysts of the jaws." *J. Oral Surg.* 27(1969): 931-938.
95. Radden, B.G. and Reade, P.C. "Odontogenic keratocysts." *Pathology* 5(1973): 325-334.
96. Gardner, D.G. and Sapp, J.P. "Odontogenic and fissural cysts of the jaws." *Pathol. Ann.* 13(1978): 177-200.
97. Soskalne, W.A. and Shear, M. "Observations on the pathogenesis of primordial cysts." *Br. Dent. J.* 123(1967): 321-329.
98. Lucas, R.B. *Pathology of Tumors of the Oral Tissues,* 3rd ed. London: Churchill Livingstone, 1976.
99. Shear, M. "Radiological features of mandibular primordial cysts (keratocysts)." *J. Maxillofac. Surg.* 6(1978): 147-154.
100. Pindborg, J.J. and Kramer, I.R.H. *Histological Typing of Odontogenic Tumors, Jaw Cysts and Allied Lesions. International Histological Classification of Tumors.* Geneva: World Health Organization, 1971.
101. Pindborg J.J. and Hansen, J. "Studies on odontogenic cyst epithelium. 2. Clinical and roentgenological aspects of odontogenic keratocysts." *Acta Pathol. Microbiol. Scand.* 58(1963): 283-293.
102. Mosby, E.L. and Sugg, W.E., Jr. "Residual odontogenic keratinizing cyst. Report of a case." *U.S. Navy Medicine* 67(1976): 222-223.

103. Philipsen, H.P. "Om keratocyster (Kolesteatomer) 1 Kaeberne." *Tandlaege-bladet* 60(1956): 963-971.
104. Browne, R.M. "The odontogenic keratocyst: clinical aspects." *Br. Dent. J.* 128(1970): 225-231.
105. Browne. R.M. "The odontogenic keratocyst: histologic features and correlation with clinical behavior." *Br. Dent. J.* 131(1971): 249-259.
106. Wilson, D.F. and Ross, A.S. "Ultrastructure of odontogenic keratocysts." *Oral Surg.* 45(1978): 887-893.
107. Bramley, P.A. "Treatment of cysts of the jaws." *Proc. R. Med. Soc.* 64(1971): 547-555.
108. Greer, R.O. and Carpenter, M. "Surgical oral pathology at the University of Colorado School of Dentistry." *J. Colo. Dent. Assoc.* 54(1976): 13-16.
109. McMillan, M.D. "Ameloblastomas associated with dentigerous cysts. *Oral Surg.* 51(1981): 489-486.
110. Poulson, T.C. "Ameloblastoma: a review of the literature and presentation of five cases associated with odontogenic cysts." *Colorado Oral Cancer Bulletin* 4(1981): 1-13
111. Ritchey, B. and Orban, B. "Cysts of the gingiva." *Oral Surg.* 6(1953): 767-771.
112. Fromm, A. "Epstein's pearls, Bohn's nodules and inclusion-cysts of the oral cavity." *J. Dent. Child.* 34(1967): 275-287.
113. Gorlin et al. "Calcifying odontogenic cyst—a possible analogue of the cutaneous calcifying epithelioma of Malherbe (an analysis of fifteen cases)." *Oral Surg.* 15(1962): 1235-1243.
114. Freedman, P.D.; Lumerman, H. and Gee, J.K. Calcifying odontogenic cyst. A review and analysis of seventy cases." *Oral Surg.* 40(1975): 93-106.
115. Sauk, J.J. "Calcifying and keratinizing odontogenic cyst." *J. Oral Surg.* 30(1972): 893-897.
116. Fejerskov. O. and Krogh, J. "The calcifying ghost cell odontogenic tumor—or the calcifying odontogenic cyst." *J. Oral Pathol.* 1(1972): 273-287.
117. Altini, M. and Farman, A.G. "The calcifying odontogenic cyst. Eight new cases and a review of the literature." *Oral Surg.* 40(1975): 751-759.
118. Farman et al. "Calcifying odontogenic cyst with ameloblastic fibro-odontoma: one lesion or two. *J. Oral Pathol.* 7(1978): 19-27.

Chapter V

Non-Odontogenic Tumors of the Jaws and Facial Skeleton

OSTEOMA

Synonyms

None

INCIDENCE

Traditionally, osteomas have been defined as central, peripheral, or subperiosteal osteogenic tumors containing mature cancellous or compact bone which undergoes slow, but progressive growth. The actual occurrence of osteoma in the jaws, facial bones, and skull is so often misinterpreted that Dahlin did not include this tumor in his statistical review of 6,221 bone tumors;[1] stating that no clear line of distinction between obviously dysplastic lesions of bone and completely benign "true osteomas" can be made.

AGE AND SEX

This point of view notwithstanding, the tumor has been well-characterized in the literature. Most cases have been reported in young adults. Osteomas in children account, in the most extensive reviews, for no more than ten percent of all lesions.[2] Hallberg reported a ratio greater than 2-to-1 of male predominance.

Osteomas are most frequently identified in the mandible. Osteomas of the paranasal sinuses most frequently occur in the frontal and ethmoid sinuses. Lesions of the maxillary sinus are not common; and osteomas only rarely occur in the sphenoid sinus.[3] Salinger[4] quoted Malan[5] who, from a total of 458 cases in the paranasal sinuses, found 41 cases of osteoma in the maxillary sinus.

A rare form of osteoma, termed *osseous choristoma*, has been reported by Cutright[6] in the oral soft tissues, generally beneath ill-fitting dentures. These "tumors" are, in reality, forms of osseous metaplasia and are rarely seen in children.

PATHOGENESIS

The etiology of osteoma is unknown. It has been suggested that they are caused by trauma or infection[1] or that they are, in actuality, hamartomatous lesions and not true neoplasms. Hallberg and Begley[2] suggested that osteomas of the paranasal sinuses arise from the junctional region of membraneous and endochondral bone in that area.

CLINICAL FINDINGS

Osteomas occur as well-circumscribed protuberances of bone or as central, dense, medullary masses (Fig. 5-1). The most common site in the jaws, facial bones, and skull is the mandible. Osteomas generally grow very slowly and produce few symptoms unless they become large enough to produce facial asymmetry.

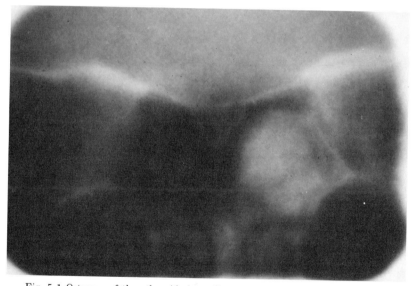

Fig. 5-1 Osteoma of the ethmoid sinus. Courtesy of Dr. Bruce Jafek.

Radiologically, subperiosteal growths appear as dense, radiopaque masses. Endosteal lesions appear as well-circumscribed sclerotic masses.

LIGHT MICROSCOPY

Osteomas have been described as having three relatively distinct histologic patterns. The cancellous type of osteoma is composed of spongy bone trabeculae, arranged in a lamellar fashion and often rimmed by active osteoblasts. Abundant fatty- and fibro-marrow surround the trabecular component. The compact osteoma is composed of dense masses of lamellar bone with little evidence of marrow spaces; osteoblastic activity and connective tissue are sparse. Batsakis[7] described a third variant, osteoma durum. This variant has a histologic pattern that lies between the other two forms in terms of the bone-to-stroma ratio.

DIFFERENTIAL DIAGNOSIS

Multiple osteomas may occur in the jaws and bones of the face, usually as a feature of *Gardner's Syndrome*. This rare, inherited disease is characterized by epidermoid and sebaceous cysts of the skin, multiple skin fibromas, multiple impacted and supernumerary teeth, and intestinal polyposis. The polyps in Gardner's Syndrome, largely confined to the colon, show a tendency toward malignant transformation, often stated to be as great as 40 percent.[8]

On occasion, it may be difficult to distinguish osteoma of the jaw from the so-called *solid odontoma*. Odontoma contains elements of tooth structure, and primitive odontogenic precursors, or so-called osteodentin. Such features are not seen in osteoma.

The relatively common, dense, bony overgrowths of torus palatinus and torus mandibularis are frequently confused with osteoma. These bony protuberances, common to the midline of the palate and lingual surface of the mandible, are probably hereditary in origin and are not neoplastic. They have a limited growth potential and are rarely removed, except for construction of a prosthetic device, or when they are traumatized and become secondarily infected.

Osteoma can mimic osteoblastoma and osteoid osteoma. The marked cellularity of the latter lesions, their frequent association with pain, and their rapid growth potential are significant distinguishing features not seen in osteoma.

TREATMENT AND PROGNOSIS

Symptomatic osteomas are usually treated by complete surgical excision. Lesions rarely recur after complete removal. Brunner[9] has reported secondary intercranial complications following the removal of osteomas from the paranasal sinuses.

OSTEOBLASTOMA

Synonyms

1. Benign osteoblastoma
2. Giant osteoid osteoma

INCIDENCE

Osteoblastoma is a rare, benign, radiographically solitary but progressive, bony neoplasm that was originally described as an "osteoblastic osteoid tissue-forming tumor in the metacarpal bone" by Jaffe and Mayer.[10] Jaffe[11] and Lichtenstein[12] further clarified this entity clinicopathologically in separate reports in 1956. Additional reviews have documented the most frequent sites of occurrence as the vertebral column, long bones, and bones of the hands and feet.[1]

Osteoid osteoma, closely linked to osteoblastoma, is probably no more than a clinical and morphologic variant of the latter.[13] Distinction between the two will be discussed under differential diagnosis.

Osteoblastoma accounted for less than one percent of the 6,221 cases of primary tumors of bone reported by Dahlin.[1] The most common site in the head and neck area is the mandible. In 1967, Borello and Sedano,[14] using the terminology of Dahlin and Johnson,[15] first reported the tumor in the jaws as a "giant osteoid osteoma". Yip and Lee,[16] in 1974, reviewed the literature on osteoblastoma of the jaws and documented only eight cases, including one of their own.[14;17-21]

In an extensive review of the world literature, Greer and Berman[22] were able to document 12 acceptable cases of osteoblastoma of the jaws.[14;16-25] In addition to these 12 reported cases, we were aware that Shafer and Waldron[26] compiled clinicopathological data on nine osteoblastomas that were catalogued as such on the surgical pathology service at the Indiana University School of Dentistry. These data were summarized at the 1975 meeting of the American Academy of Oral Pathology dealing with fibro-osseous lesions of the jaws. Dahlin[1] also referred to seven instances of osteoblastoma in the body of the mandible in his general review of bone tumors, and one case in the calvarium. The paucity of cases in the skull is surprising in view of the fact that Lichtenstein reported it to be a frequent site for osteoblastoma.[27]

AGE AND SEX

According to all published reports, osteoblastoma is a lesion that primarily affects young individuals. Information on age and sex were available in 10 of the 12 published cases reviewed by Greer and Berman.[22] Ages ranged from 6 to 22 years, with a mean age of 14.7 years. Males outnumbered females by a ratio of 7-to-3. Eleven of the 12 case reports included the site of the lesion. Seven were mandibular lesions and four involved the maxilla. The unpublished data gathered by Shafer and Waldron[26] correlates well with the findings in the published cases. They reported that, in nine cases catalogued as osteoblastomas, the ages ranged from 8 to 20 years, with a mean age of 18 years. There was a similar mandibular propensity as only two cases occurred in the maxilla.

PATHOGENESIS

The etiology of osteoblastoma is unknown. Dahlin[1] questioned whether osteoblastoma is correctly classified with true neoplasms as some osteoblastomas seem to regress or become arrested after incomplete surgical removal.

Dahlin also remarked that histologic fields within osteoblastoma are similar to those seen in aneurysmal bone cyst. This histologic feature, in association with rather remarkable clinical similarities between the two lesions, suggested that both are slightly different manifestations of a reaction to some, as yet unknown, agent.[1]

Perhaps osteoblastoma represents an exuberant attempt at repair of a hematoma of bone as proposed by Shafer.[28] Despite these varied etiologic proposals, osteoblastoma is most widely accepted as a true neoplasm of bone.

CLINICAL FINDINGS

Most osteoblastomas begin as painful expansile lesions of bone. The roentgenographic features may be quite varied. In some instances, only a poorly-circumscribed area of bony destruction is evident, while in others, the lesion can be surrounded by a dense sclerotic zone containing central radiolucent and radiopaque mixtures. In two of the cases reviewed by Greer and Berman,[22] the lesions were reported to be so radiodense that they resembled an osteoma (Fig. 5-2). Dahlin[1] reported that occasionally the tumor can be surrounded by a thin layer of bone beneath an expanded periosteum, thereby giving an appearance similar to that of an aneurysmal bone cyst. Greer and Berman,[22] found that all osteoblastomas they reviewed were at least one cm. in diameter at the time of their discovery.

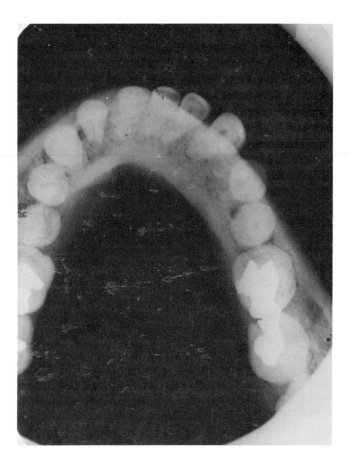

Fig. 5-2 Osteoblastoma of the mandible, characterized by a dome-shaped radiopacity adjacent to the cuspid region.

LIGHT MICROSCOPY

The vast majority of osteoblastomas are characterized histologically by multiple irregular osseous trabeculae set in a highly vascular, connective tissue stroma. Individual trabeculae are usually rimmed by plump, often layered, proliferating osteoblasts (Fig. 5-3). These osteoblasts often have hyperchromatic nuclei but mitotic activity is rare. Multinucleated osteoclasts are frequently seen throughout the supporting stroma.

Variations of this classic appearance include older lesions in which there may be considerable ossification with little stroma and

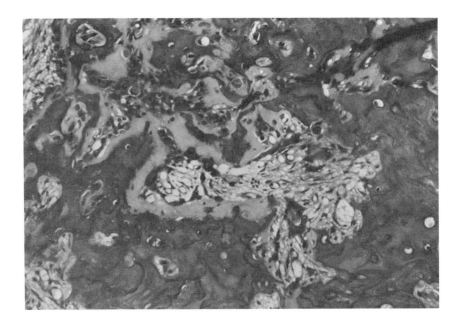

Fig. 5-3 Osteoblastoma showing individual bone trabeculae, surrounded by plump, often layered, osteoblasts. There is considerable remodeling of the bone, and osteoblasts have distinctive hyperchromatic nuclei. (H&E x 300).

much less evidence of osteoblastic activity. Some tumors show considerable remodeling, resulting in incremental zones that resemble cemental resting lines. In fact, Dahlin[1] regarded cementoblastoma and osteoblastoma as so histologically similar, that he included the former lesion among the 43 total osteoblastomas he reviewed.

DIFFERENTIAL DIAGNOSIS

Perhaps the most critical diagnostic challenge one encounters when evaluating a progressively enlarging, central osseous lesion of the jaw, facial bones, or skull, (such as osteoblastoma) is to arrive at an acceptable differential diagnosis from the long list of benign fibro-osseous lesions that occur in those areas. Osteoid osteoma, cementoblastoma, condensing osteitis, fibrous dysplasia, and ossifying fibroma are reasonable considerations.

Cementoblastoma is difficult to distinguish from osteoblastoma. In a 1974 review, Abrams and associates[23] examined seven cases and found an age range of 15 to 22 years. All tumors were seen radiographically as well-demarcated, mottled, opaque areas. The most characteristic feature separating them from osteoblastoma, was their fusion to root surfaces. Histologically, they resembled osteoid osteoma and osteoblastoma. Tooth extraction with enucleation of the tumor is the preferred treatment.

Osteoid osteoma is a slow-growing, generally painful, central osseous lesion that is often confused with osteoblastoma. Osteoid osteoma is rare in the jaws, and most cases occur between the ages of 10 and 25. The criterion of severe pain as a symptom has commonly been used to separate this entity from osteoblastoma. However, from the data we have compiled on all published instances of osteoblastoma of the jaws, in 9 of 13 of these, pain was a prominent finding, quite the opposite of the expected symptom. In our judgement, a more reliable, differential diagnostic parameter is the radiographic appearance. Osteoid osteoma generally appears as a circumscribed sclerotic lesion with a central radiolucent nidus; osteoblastoma has most often been reported as radiolucent with a central sclerotic nidus, or occasionally "ground-glass" appearing. A second, fairly constantly reported feature is that osteoid osteoma rarely attains a size of more than one cm. in diameter before diagnosis, while osteoblastoma may be a much larger lesion and possess unlimited growth potential.

Histologically, osteoid osteoma may be distinguished from osteoblastoma if a central osteoid nidus is identifiable. A highly vascular stroma with trabeculae rimmed by osteoblasts can be seen in both lesions. Conservative surgical excision is the preferred treatment for osteoid osteoma.

Fibrous dysplasia, especially the cranio-facial variety described by Waldron and Giansanti, [24] may be confused with osteoblastoma. The age range of occurrence for both lesions is similar; however, lesions of the jaw occur much more frequently in fibrous dysplasia than in osteoblastoma. Fibrous dysplasia generally has a "ground-glass" or "orange-peel" radiographic appearance. Waldron and Giansanti found this classic radiographic appearance in 16 of 22 cases for which they had complete clinical and radiographic histories. Fibrous dysplasia is poorly-delineated radiographically and tends to become expansile and fan out into adjacent bone. Osteoblastoma, although it certainly may be expansile, only rarely has a "ground glass" radiographic appearance. The most useful means of differentiating between the two is by microscopic examination of the tissue. Woven bone in a fibrous stroma is more characteristic of fibrous dysplasia. This histologic pattern is far from the predominantly blastic, and richly vascular, histologic pattern of osteoblastoma.

Ossifying fibroma is probably a lesion originating from the periodontal ligament. Fairly common in the jaws, ossifying fibroma can occur as a totally radiolucent or totally radiopaque lesion, depending on its stage of development. It is generally circumscribed, similar to osteoblastoma, and occurs in the same age group. Severe pain is seldom a feature. The histopathologic pattern of interlacing osseous trabeculae or globules set in a cellular fibrous stroma is usually the key to diagnosis of this lesion. Complete surgical removal is the preferred treatment.

The distinction between osteosarcoma and osteoblastoma may, at times, be quite difficult. Hajdu and Huvos[25] have suggested several histologic features separating the two entities. These authors maintained that cartilage production is common to osteosarcoma but rare in osteoblastoma, unless a pathologic fracture has occurred.

Fine compact strands of osteoid, poorly-calcified woven bone, and sparse stroma with a paucity of vascular structures are hallmarks of osteosarcoma. Osteoblastoma, in contrast, usually has thick osteoid and woven bone with irregular, serrated margins. Osteoclasts and a richly vascularized stroma are constant features in all but the most sclerotic of osteoblastomas.

TREATMENT AND PROGNOSIS

The treatment of choice for osteoblastoma is a conservative but complete surgical excision, or a nonradical en bloc excision. Recurrence is rare. In 6 of the 12 previously published cases reviewed by Greer and Berman where a follow-up was reported, there had been recurrences of tumors during periods ranging from 1 to 3 years. There has been no recurrence of the tumor added to the series by Greer and Berman[22] during a four-year follow-up period.

OSTEOSARCOMA

Synonyms

1. Osteogenic sarcoma

INCIDENCE

Osteosarcoma is recognized as the most common primary malignancy of bone, accounting for greater than 20 percent of all primary osseous malignancies. However, it is a rather rare neoplasm in the head and neck (jaws, facial bones, and skull). Dahlin[1] found only 83 cases among 962 osteosarcomas of the entire skeletal system, an incidence of less than ten percent for all age groups. Only five of these tumors occurred during the first decade. Garrington,[29] in an analysis of 56 cases of osteosarcoma of the jaws, reported a 6.5 percent incidence in all age groups.

In a review of 60 tumor and tumor-like conditions of the maxilla and mandible in children recorded on the surgical pathology and autopsy services of the Barnes Hospital and Washington University School of Medicine, Dehner[30] documented 14 primary and secondary malignant tumors; and of these, only three osteosarcomas were catalogued as such. To further emphasize the rarity of this tumor in the head and neck area of children, Khanna and Khanna, in an exhaustive review of 122 primary jaw tumors of the maxilla and mandible, found no cases of osteosarcoma during a 17-year-period.[31] Greer and Mierau[32] reported two instances of osteosarcoma, both in the mandible, in their review of 191 childhood tumors of the jaws seen at the University of Colorado.

AGE AND SEX

Osteosarcoma has its greatest incidence in the second decade of life, followed by the third and first decades.[33] In long bones, osteosarcoma has a peak incidence between the ages of 10 and 25. In the jaws, the peak age of onset is approximately a decade later. Osteosarcoma of the skull is rare in children. In the bones of the face, the jaws, and the skull, osteosarcoma can arise in association with pre-existing factors, such as irradiation and fibrous dysplasia, but the transition occurs somewhat later than in the long bones. Most large surveys report a male predisposition for osteosarcoma of the jaws, skull, and bones of the face.[33]

PATHOGENESIS

It is postulated that osteosarcoma can be initiated by irradiation, a pre-existing bone disorder, or trauma. Many authorities believe that the cause of the tumor is related to a disturbance of bone growth and maturation during periods of osteoblastic activity. Experimental support for this concept has been offered by Baserga and co-workers.[34] Recently, a viral etiology has also been suggested.[35] Paget's disease and fibrous dysplasia are the most common pre-existing benign lesions associated with osteosarcoma. Tillman reviewed 24 cases of Paget's disease involving the jaws, and found sarcoma (all types) to be a complication in only three.[36]

Osteosarcoma arises from Paget's disease quite infrequently in the jaws. Rosenmertz and Schare reported a case in a 74-year-old woman, and found only two other adequately documented cases in the literature.[37] A recent case of osteosarcoma arising from pre-existing fibrous dysplasia of the mandible has been reported by Slow.[38]

Osteosarcoma has been produced experimentally in several species of animals, using a variety of physical and chemical agents. A study by Cottier and associates[39] suggested a hormonal factor may be involved in tumor histogenesis.

CLINICAL FINDINGS

The most common symptom of osteosarcoma affecting the jaws and facial skeleton is the presence of a mass, lump, or swelling.[32] Pain is the second most common symptom, which is in sharp contrast to long bone lesions, where pain is almost always the chief complaint. Curtis[40] has recently suggested that mobility of teeth, cortical expansion, and soft tissue swelling are features common to both maxillary and mandibular lesions. However, pain and paresthesia more often accompany mandibular tumors, whereas nasal obstruction, discharge, and epistaxis dominate as symptoms of maxillary tumors.

The localization of osteosarcoma in the jaws is interesting. The tumor is more common in the mandible than in the maxilla, and the body of the mandible is involved more often than the symphysis, angle, or ascending ramus. Maxillary lesions may arise from any portion of that bone, but, they most often occur along the alveolar ridge.

The radiographic appearance of osteosarcoma in the jaws and facial skeleton can be quite variable. The vast majority are perceived as poorly-delineated, unicentric lesions that are either predominantly radiolucent, radiopaque, or an admixture of the two. The classic "sunburst" appearance (Fig. 5-4), so frequently used to describe the radiographic appearance of osteosarcoma, is not always present. When present, it is certainly not uniformly, radiographically diagnostic of the disease as a host of other lesions can induce a similar formation of peripheral laminae of bone deposited around the margins of the tumor in a radiating manner.

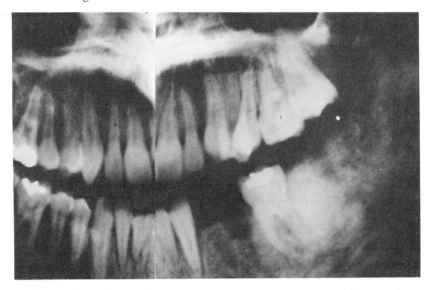

Fig. 5-4 Dense "sunburst" radiopaque osteoblastic osteosarcoma of the posterior mandible in a 15-year-old girl. Courtesy of Dr. Richard Nelson.

Roentgenographic evidence of a symmetrically-widened periodontal membrane space may be a significant early finding in osteosarcoma, according to Garrington,[29] and Gardner.[41] The roentgenographic appearance of *parosteal osteosarcoma* is often remarkably different from that of conventional medullary osteosarcoma. This special variant of osteosarcoma is likely to be present as a large, irregular, and densely radiopaque, ossified tumor mass, adherent to and blending with the regional bony cortex.[1] There is no viable relationship between the radiographic appearance of any form of osteosarcoma and survival statistics.

LIGHT MICROSCOPY

Osteosarcoma shows considerable histologic variability. Nonetheless, both Lichtenstein,[42] and Dahlin[1] noted, rather emphatically, that two essential criteria must be met before a diagnosis of osteosarcoma is rendered. Microscopically, one must find unequivocal sarcomatous stroma and direct production of tumor osteoid and bone from malignant connective tissue (Figs. 5-5, 5-6).

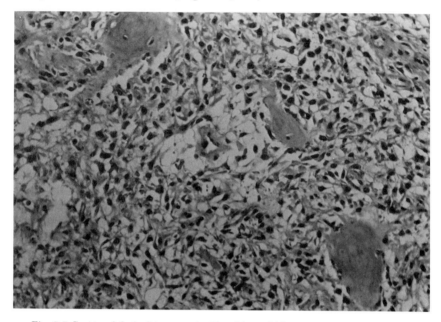

Fig. 5-5 Scattered foci of tumor osteoid, arising within a sarcomatous stroma are seen in this photomicrograph of osteosarcoma. (H&E x 240).

The stroma of the tumor is characteristically composed of anaplastic spindle or oval cells with markedly hyperchromatic nuclei. Tumor foci at the periphery of the specimen tend to contain little calcified product, and central zones are extremely cellular without osseous or chondroid lattices.

Dahlin[1] has described the dominant histologic types of osteosarcoma as osteoblastic, chondroblastic, and fibroblastic. In a review of 962 osteosarcomas in all age groups and anatomic sites, he found the vast majority to be osteoblastic, while among the remaining neoplasms, there was a nearly even division between chondroblastic and fibroblastic tumors.

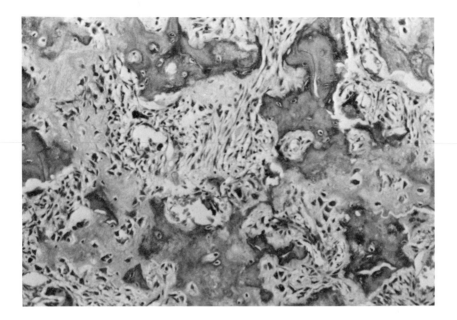

Fig 5-6 Osteosarcoma showing tumor giant cells and a less primitive sarcomatous stroma. (H&E x 270).

There is general agreement among bone pathologists that osteosarcomas of the jaws display an appreciably lesser degree of anaplasia than their long bone counterparts.[1;29] It is also significant to note that there is an apparent greater tendency for osteosarcomas of the jaws in children to show an osteoblastic or chondroblastic histologic dominance with little evidence of fibroblastic types.[30;32]

Multinucleated giant cell forms that are histologically benign may be seen in osteosarcoma; thus, benign giant cell tumors are often difficult to distinguish from the osteosarcoma. The telangiectatic osteosarcoma described by Dahlin is rare in children.[1] In his documentation of 25 instances of this histologic subtype, Dahlin found none in the jaws, facial bones, or skulls of children.

ELECTRON MICROSCOPY

The ultrastructure of osteosarcoma has been well-characterized in several recent reports.[41-45] Malignant osteoblasts, unfortunately, display no specific diagnostic features and, within a given tumor, often exhibit considerable morphologic diversity. Lysosomes, lipid, and glycogen, are variably present. Their most characteristic and consistent feature is that of prominent dilated cisternae of rough endoplasmic reticulum (Fig. 5-7). Although electron microscopy is rarely needed to establish a diagnosis of osteosarcoma, it can be of value, in the occasional problem case, for the purpose of demonstrating early osteoid deposition and mineralization (Fig. 5-8).

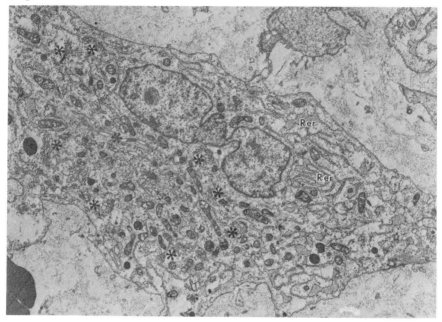

Fig. 5-7 Osteosarcoma cells characteristically display a well-developed Golgi complex (asterisks) and prominent rough endoplasmic reticulum (Rer). (EM x 5,600).

DIFFERENTIAL DIAGNOSIS

Parosteal osteosarcoma is a rare form of osteosarcoma usually separated from classic endosteal osteosarcoma because of its anatomic location and more favorable prognosis. As suggested by the name, this neoplasm grows from the external surface of bone without radiographic evidence of medullary involvement. The tumor is histologically composed of fairly well-formed osseous trabeculae in a malignant fibrocellular stroma that is well-differentiated. The prominent hyperchromatism and mitoses seen in more classical osteosarcoma are conspicuously absent.

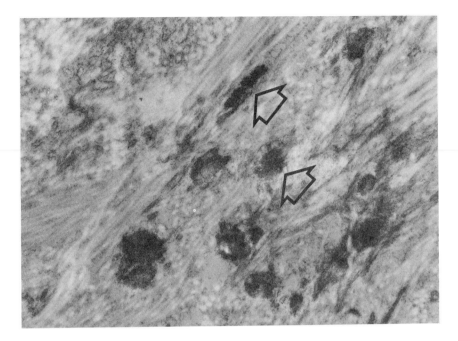

Fig. 5-8 The ultrastructural appearance of osteoid is that of matted collagen fibers, partially obscured by a translucent "glazing"; upon this matrix, hydroxyapaptite crystals (arrows) are deposited. (EM x 28,200).

This special form of osteosarcoma is quite rare in the jaw and facial skeleton. Newland[46] reported only five adequately documented cases of parosteal osteosarcoma of the jaws in a 1977 review, including one of his own. Of all five cases, three findings were in the mandible and two in the maxilla; the youngest patient was 17.

Parosteal osteosarcoma of the jaws and facial skeleton must be distinguished from benign lesions that may occupy a juxtacortical position, such as *osteochondroma* and *myositis ossificans*. Microscopically, these lesions demonstrate a zonal arrangement with active fibroblasts at the center, and maturing bone trabeculae at the periphery. In contrast, parosteal osteosarcoma has bony trabeculae which dominate the base of the lesion.[46]

Parosteal osteosarcoma grows slowly and metastasizes late. Local excision is inadequate and may result in recurrence, regeneration of a more malignant form, or increased potential for metastasis. Surgical therapy in the form of either hemimandibulectomy or wide resection is the most effective treatment for parosteal osteosarcoma.

Many osteosarcomas contain areas that resemble *malignant fibrous histiocytoma* histologically. Dahlin[1] reported areas of "debatable" tumor osteoid found in nearly half of the 35 malignant fibrous histiocytomas he reviewed. However, if one adheres to the postulate that tumor osteoid must be appreciated microscopically to render a diagnosis of osteosarcoma, the distinction should be less difficult.

The distinction between malignant fibrous histiocytoma and osteosarcoma of the jaws and facial skeleton in children is somewhat less perplexing than in adults if one considers that the former tumor nearly always displays: (1) areas of malignant giant cells with nuclei that possess a histiocytic appearance with indentation of nuclei; (2) a fibrogenic storiform pattern; (3) foci of histiocytic mononuclear cells, and (4) marked anaplasia with nuclear anisocytosis and atypical mitoses. These features are rarely prominent in childhood osteosarcomas of the jaws and facial skeleton.

On occasion, osteoid and bone which develop as a reaction to a focus of metastatic carcinoma in the jaws may be quite similar to that produced by osteosarcoma. It may be exceedingly difficult to determine whether the osteoid is indeed produced by malignant cells. A thorough examination of the child to rule out a primary tumor of unsuspected origin is warranted in all such cases.

Telangiectatic osteosarcoma may simulate *aneurysmal bone cyst* at low-power microscopic examination. Although mitotic figures may be numerous in spindle cell areas of an aneurysmal bone cyst, there is a lack of nuclear anaplasia and osteoid material emanating from spindle cell regions and blending into regular osseous trabeculae common to osteosarcoma.

Chondrosarcoma is derived from true cartilage and, in contradistinction to osteosarcoma, does not show neoplastic osteoid or bone developing from a sarcomatous stroma.

Extra-skeletal osteosarcoma can very rarely develop in the oral cavity or adjacent head and neck soft tissues. Parsons[47] has reported a tumor of this type in the lip.

TREATMENT AND PROGNOSIS

Ablative surgery remains the treatment of choice for osteosarcoma of the jaws and facial skeleton. The tumor is exceedingly radioresistant, and although radiation therapy has been employed, it is not the favored primary management modality.

Garrington and associates[29] suggested that while prophylatic neck dissection is unwarranted in osteosarcoma, dissection of nodes involved by the neoplasm may enhance survival.

Hematogenous metastasis is a much less common occurrence from osteosarcoma of the jaws than from long bone sites; correspondingly, survival-rates for osteosarcoma of the jaws are much better than for their long bone counterparts. Garrington and colleagues reported a 35 percent five-year survival-rate in the 34 patient's cases they followed. Curtis and associates reported that approximately 26 percent of their patients with maxillary lesions and 35 percent of their patients with mandibular lesions showed five-year survival-rates.[40] Finklestein reported a 32.3 percent five-year survival-rate in his series of jaw osteosarcomas.[48] These figures are in sharp contrast to the rather routinely reported 20 percent five-year survival-rates for extra-facial and long bone osteosarcomas.[1]

Chemotherapy (principally cyclophosphamide, oncovin, phenylalanine mustard, melphalan, and adriamycin protocols) and immunotherapy have an increasing number of proponents; however, the studies of Uribe-Botero[33] emphasized that chemotherapeutic regimens must be used in conjunction with adequate surgery to be considered as effective therapeutic tools for treating osteosarcoma.

CHONDROSARCOMA

Synonyms

1. Chondrogenic sarcoma

INCIDENCE

Although chondrosarcomas are rare primary tumors of the jaws and facial skeleton, they represent, as in the remainder of the skeleton, the second most common primary malignancy of bone. In a review of 470 chondrosarcomas, Dahlin[1] found 24 in the head and neck area. Pritchard and associates reviewed 358 cases of chondrosarcoma of bone seen at the Mayo Clinic between 1909 and 1975 and found only 24 cases in the head and neck area.[49] The most common sites of origin in this region are the maxilla, mandible, nasal septum, sphenoid sinus, and ethmoid sinuses.

No discussion of chondrosarcoma of the skull, jaws, and facial bones would be complete without a discussion of chondromas in those bones.

Chondromas are well-documented neoplasms of the pelvis, sternum, scapula, long bones, and bones of the head and feet.[50] Acceptance of this tumor as a distinct entity in the jaws and facial bones has been fraught with much controversy, even though numerous reviews of chondromas in these sites have been presented in the literature.[50-52] The source of confusion is the fact that a large percentage of cases initially diagnosed as chondroma eventually assume an aggressive biologic course more consistent with chondrosarcoma. Chaudhry and associates[52] reviewed 52 chondrogenic jaw lesions and found malignant neoplasms outnumbered benign lesions by a ratio of 2-to-1. Blum[53] suggested that chondrogenic neoplasms of the jaws be viewed with a great degree of suspicion, characterized by the assumption that the lesion might be at least potentially malignant. In summarizing his report of lesions, Blum further suggested that radical treatment be employed in all cases.

To further emphasize the rarity of this tumor in the jaws, it is pertinent to note that Dahlin[1] failed to document a single instance of chondroma in the jaws or facial bones in a review of 6,221 tumors. Batsakis[7] suggested that the combination of a paucity of cases in the jaws and in the facial skeleton, linked with both the propensity for recurrence and subsequent aggressive behavior by an apparently benign jaw neoplasm, such as chondroma, lends credence to the supposition that lesions diagnosed as "chondromas" in this location are frequently misdiagnosed chondrosarcomas.

Kilby and Ambegaokar[54] have extensively reviewed a series of benign cartilaginous tumors of the nasal cavity, paranasal sinuses, and nasopharynx. However, there is considerable sentiment suggesting that these lesions, defined as chondromas, were only hypertrophy or hyperplasia of nasal septal cartilage or cartilage-capped exostoses.[7]

Although the debate continues concerning the true nature of chondroma of the jaws, there is no doubt that multiple enchondromatosis (Ollier's disease) of other bones can be accompanied by multiple hemangiomas in the head and neck region, especially the tongue, lips, and cheek.

AGE AND SEX

At the end of 1974, the Armed Forces Institute of Pathology had recorded 60 well-documented cases of chondrosarcoma of the jaws.[55] The age range in their cases was from 12 to 80 years, with an average age of 32. This average age is identical to the age recorded for cases of osteosarcoma of the jaws at that institution. Their youngest patient was a 16-month-old boy. Males and females are affected equally.

Chondrosarcomas of the facial bones and soft tissues, other than the maxilla and mandible, have recently been reviewed by Fu and Perzin.[56] Extra-jaw sites are extremely rare anatomic locations for chondrosarcoma in the child.

PATHOGENESIS

There is considerable doubt about the origin of all cartilaginous tumors, and chondrosarcoma is no exception. The predisposition for chondrosarcoma of the anterior mandible and posterior maxilla has led some authors to postulate that the tumor arises in association with cartilaginous remnants of the nasal capsule and Meckel's cartilage, respectively. However, Shira and Bhaskar[57] have challenged this hypothesis. Jaffe[58] suggested that chondrosarcoma can arise *de novo* from osseous tissues without the presence of cartilaginous rests. Roper, Hall, and Adcock[59] have suggested that chondrosarcomas may arise from portions of nasal septal cartilage that have been entrapped between the palatal shelves as they grow toward the midline. Finally, chondrosarcomas may occasionally arise in previously irradiated benign lesions, such as fibrous dysplasia.[60]

CLINICAL FINDINGS

Swelling is the chief complaint of most children with chondrosarcoma of the jaws or facial skeleton. There is usually an expansion of the cortical plates and a loosening of the teeth when the mandible is affected; nasal stuffiness, pain, nasal discharge, epistaxis, and diplopia are common complaints when the nasal and paranasal sinuses are involved.

Most reports in the literature suggested that when chondrosarcoma occurs in the maxilla, the anterior portion of that bone is the favored location. The posterior (molar-premolar) region is the most common site when the mandible is involved. Until recently, it was uniformly accepted that the mandible was more commonly a site for chondrosarcoma than the maxilla, but, Terezhalmy and Bottomley[61] have suggested that the tumor is found with equal frequency in both arches.

The radiographic picture of chondrosarcoma in the head and neck is variable. Potdar[62] found no specific changes suggestive of a cartilaginous tumor in half of the cases he reviewed. Dahlin found radiographic abnormalities suggesting a chondrosarcomatous change in 8 of 10 cases he reviewed in a 1971 study.[63] The most widely encountered radiographic appearance is that of an osteolytic defect or defects with expansion and resorption of the bone (Fig. 5-9). The defects often have a "ground-glass" appearance, and may show areas of calcification. It is also possible to have a radiographic "sun-burst" appearance. Uniform widening of the periodontal membrane space, similar to osteosarcoma, may also be noted.

LIGHT MICROSCOPY

Chondrosarcomas frequently have a pleomorphic microscopic appearance but the classic histological features remain those suggested by Lichtenstein and Jaffe,[64] which include numerous cartilaginous cells with plump nuclei, cells with more than two such nuclei, and giant cartilage cells with large, single or multiple nuclei and clumps of chromatin.

Evans and co-workers[65] have attempted to associate histological grades of chondrosarcoma with the ultimate biological behavior of the tumor. Lesions regarded as grade 1 by the investigators contain small, dense-staining, chondrocyte nuclei and focal areas with slightly enlarged nuclei and at least a few multinucleated forms. Mineralization, in the form of osseous development at the edge of cartilaginous lobules, is common. Marked cellularity and significant numbers of enlarged nuclei and mitotic figures are rarely observed in grade 1 leions.

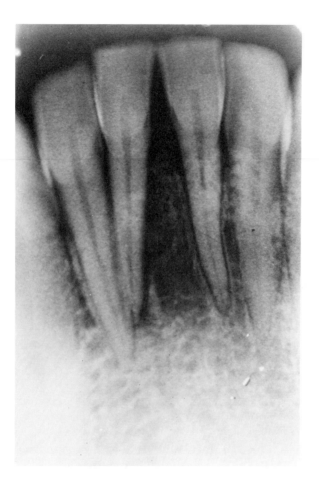

Fig. 5-9 Chondrosarcoma of the anterior mandible showing "moth-eaten" interseptal destruction of bone. Courtesy of Dr. Roy Eversole.

Grade 2 chondrosarcomas contain increased cellularity, sometimes at the periphery of tumor lobules, and nulcei that are much larger than those in grade 1 lesions (Figs. 5-10, 5-11). These alterations, indicative of higher grade lesions, may be focal and therefore not be evident in a small tissue sample.

Grade 3 chondrosarcomas show greater changes than those already described. Nuclear enlargement is more pronounced as is multinucleation. Chondrocytes often have two or more enlarged nuclei. The absence of cartilaginous lobulation and the presence of spindle cell

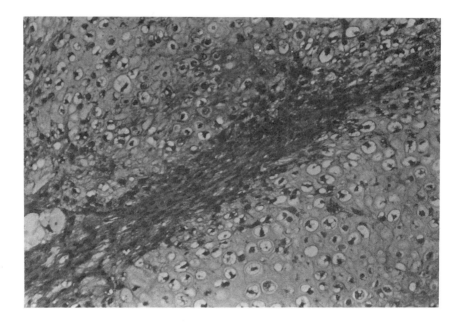

Fig. 5-10 Grade 2 chondrosarcoma of the mandible, showing enlarged nuclei and hypercellularity. (H&E x 250). Courtesy of Dr. Bruce Jafek.

forms is compatible with grade 3 disease in the schema proposed by Evans and associates and suggests a very poor prognosis.[65]

DIFFERENTIAL DIAGNOSIS

Extra-skeletal chondrosarcoma of the head and neck in children is extremely rare. Goldenberg and associates,[66] in a review of the literature on the subject in 1967, presented seven cases of their own, but none were seen in children.

Frequently, the periphery of a chondrosarcoma will appear opaque or fibrous, resembling a fibrosarcoma or osteosarcoma. However, chondrosarcomas produce a matrix substance that ranges in consistency from hyalin-like to mucoid. This mucoid quality is highly suggestive of a malignant cartilaginous neoplasm. Chondrosarcoma, unlike osteosarcoma, never displays tumor osteoid or bone evolving directly out of sarcomatous stroma.

Mesenchymal chondrosarcoma is a decidedly rare malignant neoplasm. Since the tumor was first described in 1959 by Lichtenstein,[67] fewer than 100 cases have been reported in the literature. This

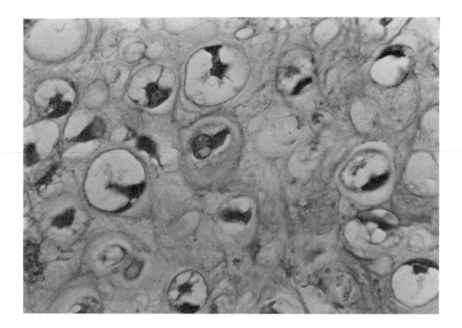

Fig. 5-11 High-power of cellular atypia in chondrosarcoma. (H&E x 400).

neoplasm is characterized by a "bimorphic histologic pattern" consisting primarily of sheets or clusters of highly undifferentiated, small round cells which may have a slight spindling quality, alternating with small zones of chondroid that are well-differentiated and often benign in appearance[68] (Fig. 5-12). Because of its richly vascular component, this lesion is most often confused with hemangiopericytoma, especially in tumors where the cartilaginous component is inconspicuous[69] (Fig. 5-13).

Mesenchymal chondrosarcoma shows a predisposition for the jaws, ribs, and extra-skeletal sites. In a recent review of 81 cases by Joshi and colleagues,[70] 42 percent of the tumors were of an extra-skeletal origin. The tumor is most commonly seen in the second and third decades of life, which is significantly earlier than the common chondrosarcoma. The youngest patient reported by Joshi and associates was a five-year-old girl, and the oldest was a 70-year-old man. Slightly more than half of all reported cases have occurred in females.[71]

Fifteen of the approximately 100 reported cases of mesenchymal chondrosarcoma have occurred in the mandible and maxilla. In a review of reported cases with follow-up, Rollo and associates[69] reported the

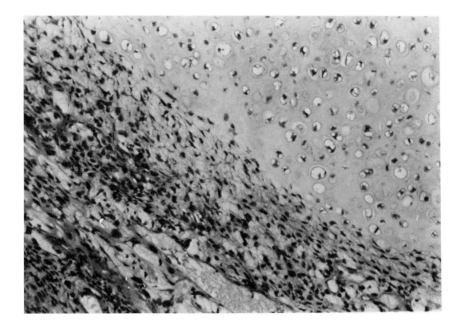

Fig. 5-12 Characteristic appearance of mesenchymal chondrosarcoma with a peripheral chondroid island and highly undifferentiated, round-to-spindle cells immediately adjacent to island. (H&E x 240).

survival rate for mesenchymal chondrosarcoma in all sites to be 68 percent ± 8 percent at five years, and only 32 percent ± 9 percent at 10 years. Since delayed death from the tumor does occur, a five-year survival-rate is of limited significance.[71] In general, cases that show the most favorable course are those in which radical surgical excision is performed. Evidence suggested that mesenchymal chondrosarcoma is a relatively radio-resistant tumor,[68] and there is insufficient evidence to support the primary use of chemotherapy in the treatment of this neoplasm.

Benign chondroblastoma[72] of bone is an infrequently reported neoplasm. The incidence of this tumor is reported to be less than two percent of all primary bone tumors.[73;74] Dahlin and Ivins[73] reviewed 125 cases and estimated that 400 of these tumors have been documented or mentioned in the literature.

Benign chondroblastoma is composed of compact masses of moderate, but variably-sized, round to polyhedral cells. The cells have distinct cytoplasmic and nuclear membranes and slightly eosinophilic

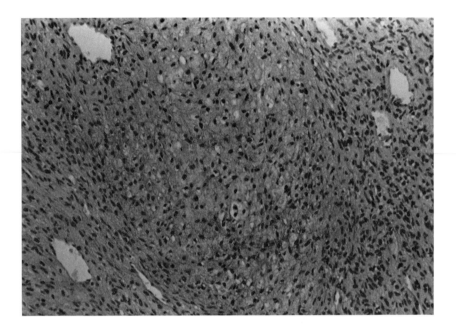

Fig. 5-13 Mesenchymal chondrosarcoma may be confused with hemangiopericytoma because of its rich vascularity and accumulation of clusters of small, undifferentiated round and spindle cells. Careful scrutiny will reveal chondroid matrix, however minimal. (H&E x 200).

cytoplasm. The nuclei are rather large, round or oval, and are often indented. The irregularity of the nuclear membrane is due to invaginations of the cytoplasm.[75] The chondromatous character of the tumor is revealed by transition of tumor cells to areas of mature hyaline cartilage. The outstanding histological feature of the neoplasm is the variable amount of focal calcification within and between the cells. The feature seems to be quite marked in areas of necrosis and chondromatous transformation. Classification of this tumor as a giant-cell tumor by earlier workers was probably due to the presence of osteoclast-like giant cells. Their presence is now believed to be a response to hemorrhage and necrosis. Recent histochemical studies have shown that the tumor cells are capable of producing sulphated acid mucopolysaccharides, a component of cartilage matrix.[75] Presence of glycogen in tumor cells has been reported;[75] however, Levine and Bensch[75] found no diastase digestible PAS positive material in their cases.

The tumor arises mainly in bones developing in cartilage and in the epiphyses of the long bones. An examination of the sites of origin of 182 tumors reviewed by Salver[76] and cited by Dahlin and Ivins[73] revealed only eight chondroblastomas in the jaws, facial, and cranial bones —an incidence of less than two percent.

Chondroblastomas occur mainly in the younger age groups. Over 76 percent of Dahlin's 125 cases,[73] and 88.5 percent of Schajowicz and Gallardo's cases[74] occurred between the ages of 5 and 25 years. However, Dahlin and Ivins[73] have reported that chondroblastoma in unusual sites, such as the skull, facial bones, and jaws, tend to involve older people. A review of eight cases involving cranial bones by Al-Dewachi and co-workers[77] included only one child; a 13-year-old girl. The higher age incidence in head and neck chondroblastomas may be related to slower tumor growth and milder symptoms often ignored by patients.

Chondroblastoma usually behaves as a benign tumor, and cure, in the vast majority of patients, is effected by simple curettage. Recurrences are only occasionally reported, usually following inadequate surgical therapy.

Chondromyxoid fibroma was initially described as a distinct tumor of bone by Jaffe and Lichtenstein in 1948.[27] Since that time only a few cases have been reported in the jaws, facial bones, and skull,[1] with the majority being identified in the mandible. The tumor is primarily a lesion of young adults and not children. Microscopically, it is composed of lobular or spindle-shaped or stellate cells with a myxoid or chondroid intercellular matrix. Multinucleated giant cells are common in this benign tumor, amenable to conservative surgical excision.

TREATMENT AND PROGNOSIS

Chondrosarcoma of the jaws and facial bones is quite refractory to nearly all management modalities except for radical surgery. Radiation therapy in the treatment of chondrosarcoma in this region is generally reserved for those cases in which there is residual disease. Chemotherapy has been employed as an adjuvant, and recently radioactive sulphur (^{35}S) has been introduced as a management modality. The prognosis for chondrosarcoma of the jaws in children is grave, with five-year survival-rates approximating those of osteosarcoma.

FIBROUS DYSPLASIA

Synonyms

1. Osteitis fibrosa cystica
2. Osteodystrophia fibrosa
3. Osteofibroma

INCIDENCE

The term "fibrous dysplasia" was first coined by Lichtenstein in 1938[78] to describe a benign, self-limiting, non-encapsulated lesion of bone that occurs chiefly in young patients. Fibrous dysplasia may be *monostotic* (single or multiple lesions confined to one bone), *polyostotic* (multiple lesions involving more than one bone), or *disseminated* (multiple lesions scattered throughout the skeleton).[79] Monostotic fibrous dysplasia is 20-to- 30 times as common as the polyostotic form.[80] The femur, tibia, fibula, humerus, radius, ulna, and pelvic bones are the most often affected polyostotic sites.[81] Associated skull lesions are found in half the patients with polyostotic fibrous displasia. Zimmerman and associates,[82] and Sherman and Glauser[83] reported that 15 percent of the patients with the polyostotic form of the disease have lesions in the maxilla and mandible. Windholz found that skull lesions accounted for about 10 percent of the cases of monostotic fibrous dysplasia in his review.[84]

In a review of 191 tumors of the oral mucosa and jaws, Greer and Mierau documented a 3.1 percent incidence for fibrous dysplasia.[32] Dehner[85] reviewed all tumors and tumor-like lesions involving the jaws of children in the files of the Division of Surgical Pathology at Barnes Hospital and Washington Unversity School of Medicine over a 23-year-period. A total of 46 histologically benign lesions were diagnosed, and seven (15.2 percent) were fibrous dysplasia.

AGE AND SEX

A definite sex predisposition has been shown in the occurrence of fibrous dysplasia, with females being affected two-to-three times as often as males.[32;86;87] The active form of the disease can be seen throughout adolescence, but it is most prominent in the younger patient. Daramola reviewed 47 cases of fibrous dysplasia of the jaws which were treated over a 15-year-period and found an age range from 5 to 65 years, with an average of 25 years.[87] In a review of a series of jaw lesions, Waldron and Giansanti, coining the now-popular term, *cranio-facial fibrous dysplasia*, documented an age range from 5 to 65 years, with a mean age of 27 years.[88]

Fibrous dysplasia of the cranio-facial region shows a striking tendency to develop early in life. Although the two extensive reviews by Waldron and Giansanti, and Daramola and associates reported a mean age of the mid-twenties, the lesions are most often first diagnosed in childhood or adolescence. Adekeye and associates[89] reviewed 13 lesions involving the cranio-facial complex in Nigerian patients and failed to document a single case in a patient past the second decade of life. Of the four patients older than 20 years of age, the lesions had been present for periods ranging from 5 to 13 years.

PATHOGENESIS

Fibrous dysplasia is best described as a developmental bone defect without a familial or hereditary predisposition. The etiology of the disease process is unknown. The original concept of the disease as first proposed by von Recklinghausen in 1891 has been expanded to include not only monostotic, polyostotic, and disseminated forms of the disease, but also Albright's Syndrome, with its attendant skin pigmentation, precocious puberty, and skeletal abnormalities. Lichtenstein[78] considered the lesions of fibrous dysplasia resulted from "prevented activity of bone forming mesenchyme", whereas Falconer, Cope, and Robb-Smith[90] suggested that the primary change is a marrow fibrosis with subsequent resorption of lamellar bone and aposition of woven bone.

Changus[91] reported that both osteoblasts and stromal fibroblasts in the lesions of fibrous dysplasia are rich in alkaline phosphatase. He concluded that such an elevation of alkaline phosphatase activity suggests that the basic disease defect is one of enhanced osteoblastic activity to stimuli of unknown origin.

CLINICAL FINDINGS

In most cases of fibrous dysplasia where there is jaw involvement, the lesion is a solitary, unilateral one. The maxilla is affected more often than the mandible. Waldron and Giansanti[88] reported an incidence ratio of 13-to-9 for the maxilla in their study. They also noted frequent involvement of the maxillary sinus, orbital floor, and zygoma.

Smith,[92] and Waldron and Giansanti[88] limited the diagnosis of cranio-facial fibrous dysplasia to lesions of undisputed developmental origin, first diagnosed early in life, and tending to stabilize in adulthood.

Pain is an uncommon feature of fibrous dysplasia and symptoms are often very minor. The most typical clinical manifestation is a gradually increasing jaw swelling or mild facial asymmetry. Occasionally, growth may be quite rapid, resulting in considerable cheek swelling, exopthalmos, or nasal obstruction.[86] Lucas reported that such symptoms may account for lesions formerly diagnosed as "leontiases ossea".[86]

Although the cranio-facial lesions of fibrous dysplasia may become quite large, they rarely result in a functional deficit. The most common functional alterations are displaced teeth, malocclusion, and failure of teeth to erupt.

The radiologic features of fibrous dysplasia in the extracranial skeleton are well-established.[93-95] The radiographic features of craniofacial fibrous dysplasia have been more recently delineated by Obisesan and associates.[95] In their review of 25 patients with histologically proven fibrous dysplasia, six roentgenographic types were identified: (1) an "orange-peel" type with alternating areas of granular density and lucency, giving a radiographic appearance resembling the rind of an orange; (2) a whorled, plaque-like type, composed of amorphous material with a radiodensity intermediate between bone and soft tissue arranged in an "onion-peel" pattern; (3) a diffuse, sclerotic type, characterized by a homogenous diffuse radiodensity with indistinct margins; (4) a cystic-like type, featuring a unilocular or multilocular expansile lesion with rather well-defined margins; (5) a pagetoid type, characterized by markedly expanded bone, displaying alternating areas of radiopacity and radiolucency, and (6) an exceedingly rare chalky-type, characterized by amorphous, markedly dense, radiopaque material.

Of the six roentgenographic types described, the "orange-peel" type is by far the most common[95;96] (Fig. 5-14). Obisesan and co-workers suggested that one radiographic type of lesion may change into another during the natural course of the disease. Blood chemistry changes are unusual, except for occasional elevations of serum alkaline phosphatase.

GROSS AND LIGHT MICROSCOPIC FINDINGS

Grossly, the tissue received for pathologic evaluation usually consists of yellow, gray, or brown tissue that has a gritty-cut surface. Normal bone may be replaced by what appears to be yellow-to-white homogeneous areas and occasionally, there may be central areas that appear cystic.

Classically, fibrous dysplasia is composed of a stroma that is fibrous in nature; the stroma may be highly cellular or have the appearance of maturing collagen. Distributed randomly throughout the

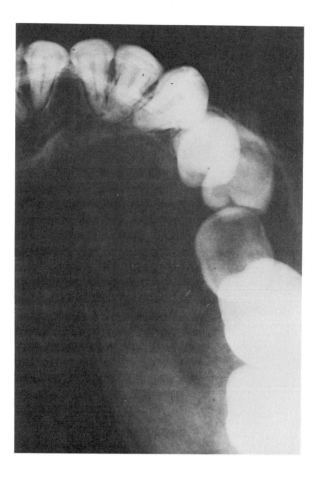

Fig. 5-14 Fibrous Dysplasia. Note "orange-peel" or "ground-glass" quality of bone in this occlusal radiograph.

supporting collagenous stroma are bone trabeculae, usually having large osteocytes within lacunae. The margins of the bone trabeculae often display a streaming of collagen bundles and fibers from the trabeculae into the supporting stroma. The vast majority of the lesions examined will show areas of woven bone. Many authorities consider the presence of woven bone mandatory for a diagnosis of fibrous dysplasia[97] (Fig. 5-15). However, most reports concerning cranio-facial fibrous dysplasia document that it is not necessary to identify woven bone to render a diagnosis.[88;98] In a series of 150 cases of cranio-facial fibrous dysplasia,

Eversole, Sabes, and Rovin[98] were able to identify 19 cases in which there were multiple spheroid calcifications in a connective tissue setting. Of the remaining 131 cases, 85 had woven osteoid, 27 had lamellar bone, and 19 showed osteoblastic rimming. They also reviewed 75 cases of monostotic fibrous dysplasia and found, once again, that there was a variance of the bone pattern in the lesions, ranging from spheroid calcifications to woven osteoid through lamellar bone with areas of osteoblastic rimming (Fig. 5-16).

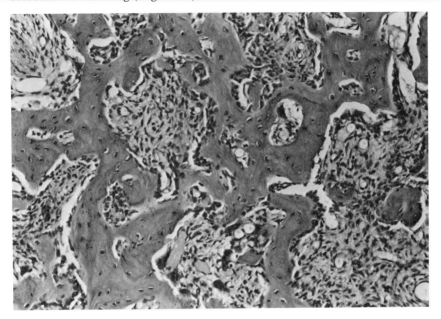

Fig. 5-15 Woven bone trabeculae randomly distributed throughout a loose reticular fibrous stroma, which is characteristic of fibrous dysplasia. Note that bone trabeculae show prominent osteoblastic rimming. (H&E x 260).

Waldron and Giansanti[88] scrutinized relative amounts of woven and lamellar bone from tissue samples in a series of 65 cases of fibrous dysplasia. They also paid considerable attention to evidence of osteoblastic rimming of bone, and while it was discovered that the majority of bone they identified was of the woven character, lamellar bone was constantly seen among the tissue samples.

It is important to realize that fibrous dysplasia represents a dynamic series of events in the maturation of bone as opposed to permanent maturation arrest in the woven bone stage. Spjut and

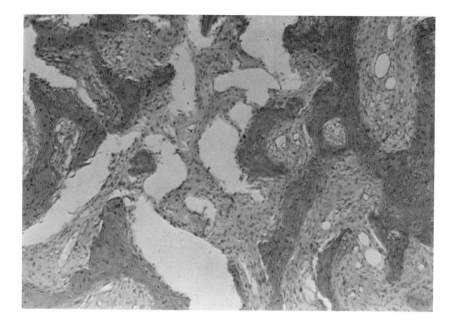

Fig. 5-16 Fibrous dysplasia, showing woven bone but with prominent osteoblastic rimming of trabeculae and more mature fibrous stroma. (H&E x 200).

others[99] have noted that while occasional lamellar transformation can be identified in fibrous dysplasia, this finding should not detract from a diagnosis of fibrous dyplasia if further criteria, especially radiographic and clinical criteria, are fulfilled.

Smith[92] described three histologic types of fibrous dysplasia based upon activity: an active form, a potentially active form, and an inactive form. The active form is most common in the young patient and consists, microscopically, of a highly cellular connective tissue stroma filled with woven bone, arranged in a so-called "Chinese character" arrangement. The potentially active and inactive forms of the disease are seen more frequently in older children, adolescents, and adults. In each state, the bone becomes progressively more prominent and the connective tissue more mature.

Batsakis,[79] and Hamner and Fullmer[100] reported that polarization microscopy may prove useful in separating fibrous dysplasia from other cranio-facial fibro-osseous lesions. Theoretically, under polarization microscopy, a woven bone pattern should remain persistent in fibrous dysplasia and a lamellar component should not be found.

However, in a recent review of six cases of cranio-facial fibrous dysplasia in children by Greer and Mierau,[32] in which all clinical, radiographic, and microscopic features for the diagnosis had been met, only one case failed to demonstrate a total absence of lamellar bone under polarizing microscopy.

DIFFERENTIAL DIAGNOSIS

The histopathologic appearance of cranio-facial fibrous dysplasia is not unique to that disease. Eversole and others[98] have documented a rather broad range of histologic features for fibro-osseous lesions, including the presence of woven bone, lamellar bone, osteoblastic activity around bone trabeculae, globular or spheroid calcifications, immature, highly active, fibrous stroma or mature, avascular, connective tissue. These authors report that all of these histologic features can be seen not only in fibrous dysplasia, but in ossifying fibroma, periapical cemental dysplasia, and chronic sclerosing osteomyelitis. Lucas[86] emphasizes that the distinction between all of these various fibro-osseous lesions is, in fact, clinical rather than histopathological.

To distinguish between fibrous dysplasia and ossifying fibroma is, perhaps the greatest difficulty. In general, lesions diagnosed as ossifying fibroma have a thin, bony shell and a distinct boundary radiographically, whereas the lesions of fibrous dysplasia are more diffuse and tend to extend, in membrane bones, up to suture lines.[86] The histopathologic picture is not pathognomonic for either lesion in our experience.

TREATMENT AND PROGNOSIS

The mere presence of fibrous dysplasia of the cranio-facial bones is not, in itself, an indication for treatment.[79] Ramsey and co-workers,[101] and Waldron[102] maintained that a conservative approach to treatment is of paramount importance for proper management of the disease. Treatment may include cosmetic surgical reduction of bone, curettage, or conservative resection of involved bone. Fibrous dysplasia tends to stabilize following completion of normal skeletal development, although continuous growth has been documented in some cases. The lesions are not radiosensitive. Radiation therapy has, in fact, been shown to render the lesions susceptible to postradiation sarcoma.[103;104]

OSSIFYING FIBROMA

Synonyms

1. Cemento-ossifying fibroma
2. Fibro-osteoma
3. Osteofibroma
4. Cementifying fibroma
5. Juvenile active ossifying fibroma

INCIDENCE

The ossifying fibroma shows varying degrees of occurrence depending upon the population reviewed. In a review of 40 tumors of the mandible and maxilla recorded over a 20-year-period at the Barnes Hospital and the Washington University School of Medicine, Dehner[85] found that 64 percent of the tumors were fibro-osseous lesions and that half of these were ossifying fibromas. However, Greer and Mierau[32] documented only four ossifying fibromas in an extensive review of 191 tumors of the oral mucosa and jaws in infants and children. Waldron and Giansanti[105] reported a total of 43 lesions diagnosed as ossifying fibroma, cementifying fibroma, or cemento-ossifying fibroma of the jaws over a 14.5-year-period at the Emory University School of Dentistry. They did not report the total number of cases accessioned in the School's surgical pathology records.

Regezi and associates[106] reviewed a series of 706 odontogenic tumors submitted to the Department of Oral Pathology at the University of Michigan over a 40-year-period and found cementifying fibroma to account for two percent of their cases.

Khanna and Khanna[107] reviewed a series of primary tumors of the jaws in African children and noted a very high percentage of cemento-ossifying fibromas; with 28.5 percent of 122 primary tumors of the jaws in the children having been diagnosed as cementifying or ossifying fibromas.

AGE AND SEX

Ossifying fibroma can occur in any age group, but the third and fourth decades are, by far, the most common periods of occurrence. Children under 15 years of age certainly can be affected, as documented in the reports of Greer and Mierau,[32] Dehner,[85] and Khanna and Khanna.[107] A so-called *juvenile active ossifying fibroma* has been reported.[26;105;] Juvenile active ossifying fibroma, suggested to be an exceedingly active, aggressive lesion, possesses the potential to kill the patient by local extension into vital structures. There are no well-documented series of cases of this lesion in the literature, and some pathologists regard the tumor to be either a low-grade osteosarcoma or an active cementoblastoma. We have been unable to relate this lesion unequivocally to ossifying fibroma and consider a detailed study of the clinicopathologic features necessary before the lesion is further classified.

PATHOGENESIS

The ossifying fibroma is almost certainly a lesion arising from cells within the periodontal ligament.[105] Most cases are restricted to the tooth-bearing areas of the jaws, and in our opinion, the lesion is probably best-described as a dysplastic condition of membrane bone. There are, however, investigators who consider the lesion to be a true neoplasm, and in rare cases, ossifying fibromas have grown to immense size,[108;109] behaving as pure neoplastic, uncontrolled growths.

Waldron and Giansanti[105] preferred to view ossifying fibroma as one of the preferred lesions within the spectrum of fibro-osseous processes which appear to arise from elements of the periodontal ligament. At one end of the spectrum is a group of reactive, but non-expansile, lesions variously known as periapical cemental dysplasia, periapical cementoma, or periapical osteofibroma. Other growths with an identical histomorphologic appearance possess the property of progressive growth and demonstrate all the features of a benign neoplasm;[105] the ossifying fibroma is probably best placed in the latter category.

CLINICAL FINDINGS

Ossifying fibroma usually occurs as an asymtomatic, monostotic fibrous lesion of the jaws or bones of the face with many features that are similar to fibrous dysplasia. A striking predisposition has been shown for the occurrence of the lesion in the mandible, and occasionally more than one lesion can be present.[105;110;111] Long bone lesions have been reported, but are much less common than jaw lesions.[11] Giansanti and Waldron's extensive review of ossifying fibroma documented that, at the time of diagnostic biopsy or surgical removal, tumor duration ranged from 6 months to 10 years with the duration, in most cases, lasting less than 5 years.

The radiographic appearance of ossifying fibroma can be quite dynamic. The tumor may be predominantly lytic with varying amounts of radiopaque foci, with these opacities varying from slightly to densely sclerotic. A lytic border of variable thickness and well-defined circumscription of the lesion from surrounding bone is nearly always described.[105] Rarely do the lesions have a diffuse, homogenous, radiopaque appearance (Fig. 5-17), although Waldron and Giansanti[105] described only five such lesions in their comprehensive review. Eighty-five percent of these lesions were less than 4 cm. in size. On rare occasions, ossifying fibromas tend to blend into normal bone, causing some difficulty in distinguishing them from fibrous dysplasia. In general, however, fibrous dysplasia lacks the radiographic circumscription of ossifying fibroma.[7]

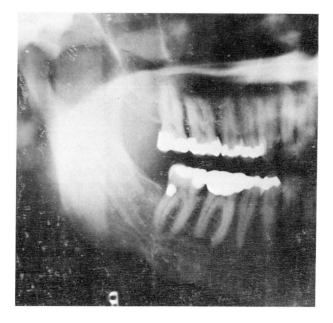

Fig. 5-17 Ossifying fibroma. The lesion is principally radiopaque and surrounded by a peripheral, radiolucent zone at its superior aspect.

LIGHT MICROSCOPY

Ossifying fibroma usually shells out as multiple gritty or partially calcified gray-white pieces of tissue. Histologically, one is usually able to identify a component of fibrous and osseous tissue. The supporting stroma may be composed of interlacing fascicles of collagen or loose, proliferating fibroblasts having a stellate character. The varying amounts of vascularity can be detected not only from areas where there is a total lack of endothelially-lined channels but to areas of extensive capillary proliferation as well.

Lamellar trabeculae may be perceived either as a distinct osseous component, separate from the fibrocellular stroma, or as an anastomosing retiform osseous component which tends to blend into the supporting stroma (Fig. 5-18). Woven bone may also be identified (Fig. 5-19). Globular calcifications, frequently described as cementoid, may be seen in the tissue sample. When such globules are seen, the term *cemento-ossifying fibroma* or *cementifying fibroma* has been employed (Fig. 5-20). In fact, this terminology probably serves to further confuse the spectrum of fibro-osseous lesions. The differentiation between cementoid and osteoid material is, principally, of academic interest, and does not alter the biologic behavior of the tumor.

DIFFERENTIAL DIAGNOSIS

The circumscribed nature of ossifying fibroma helps to distinguish it from fibrous dysplasia. Nonetheless, Lucas[86] pointed out that the histological appearance of lesions described as ossifying fibroma or as fibrous dysplasia by different observers can be identical. Eversole and associates[98] have demonstrated that the histopathology of the fibro-osseous lesion is, indeed, a spectrum and lamellar bone, woven bone, osteoblastic rimming of osseous trabeculae, spheroid calcifications, and "cementicles" can be demonstrated in both ossifying fibroma and fibrous dysplasia.

Waldron and Giansanti[105] maintained that the proper diagnosis of specific fibro-osseous lesions is a clinicopathologic one, but noted that, as a general rule, the stroma of fibrous dysplasia is more collagenous and less cellular than is seen in ossifying fibroma. They also maintained that vascularity tends to be more prominent in the stroma of ossifying fibroma, and the bone trabeculae of fibrous dysplasia are often abortive and haphazard appearing when compared with the more regular retiform pattern of bone noted in ossifying fibroma.

Cementoblastoma may be difficult to distinguish from an actively growing ossifying fibroma. The most characteristic feature

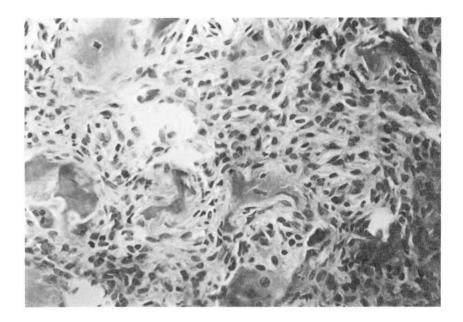

Fig. 5-18 Retiform osseous trabeculae, blending directly into fibrous stroma in ossifying fibroma. (H&E x 220).

separating the two lesions is a fusion of cementoblastoma to root surfaces. While fused globules of cementum or separate areas of layered cementogenesis are seen microscopically in cementoblastoma, these features are absent in ossifying fibroma.

Osteoblastoma and osteoid osteoma are distinct rarities in the jaws.[22] The two lesions are very likely nothing more than variant expressions of a single tumor of osteoblastic origin. The osteoblastoma has a somewhat more limited growth potential than osteoid osteoma or ossifying fibroma, and microscopically, the osteoid trabeculae of osteoblastoma are generally broader, larger, and more widely separated than in osteoid osteoma or ossifying fibroma. Additional salient features of osteoblastoma and osteoid osteoma are discussed under the heading of osteoblastoma.

TREATMENT AND PROGNOSIS

Ossifying fibroma is generally managed by a conservative surgical excision to tumor margins. Since most lesions are rather well-circumscribed, a conservative surgical approach to management usually effects favorable results. The so-called *juvenile active ossifying fibroma* may require more aggressive surgical management, [111] as previously noted. However, these lesions are poorly-delineated clinicopathologically. Single case reports do note that so-called active ossifying fibromas contain an abundance of cementoid material. [111]

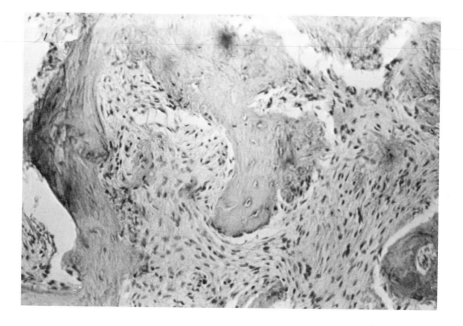

Fig. 5-19 Woven bone fragments set in a loose, reticular stroma are characteristic of ossifying fibroma. (H&E x 200).

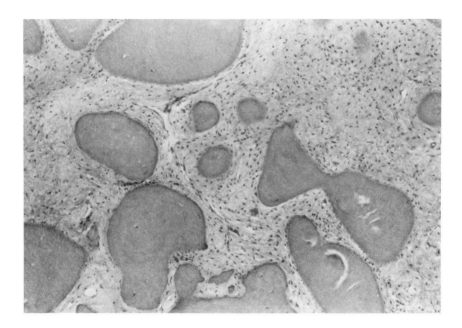

Fig. 5-20 So called "cemento-ossifying" fibroma, showing calcified globules, supported by a fibrocellular stroma. (H&E x 180).

EWING'S SARCOMA

INCIDENCE

Ewing's sarcoma is rare among lesions of the jaws and facial skeleton. Even more rare is its presentation as a soft tissue lesion of the head and neck without osseous involvement (extra-skeletal Ewing's sarcoma). Ewing's sarcoma in all sites may account for up to 40 percent of malignant bone tumors in children.[112]

AGE AND SEX

Although Ewing's sarcoma has been reported in infants, the peak incidence is in the second decade of life. Males are more often affected than females, by a ratio of 1.5-to-1. The tumor is extremely rare in the black population.[112]

PATHOGENESIS

The cell of origin of Ewing's sarcoma remains unknown. Speculations generally center about a primitive bone-marrow-based mesenchymal cell.[113] Early speculations that Ewing's sarcoma was a primitive neural tumor have been dismissed. Whatever the cell of origin, the occurrence of extra-skeletal Ewing's tumors requires that the cell of origin not be confined to bone.

Multiple bone lesions are viewed, by some, as testimony to a multicentric origin of tumor, but this is, very likely, a metastatic disease.

Application of immunological techniques for detection of Factor VIII (endothelium) or other antigens which might assist in determining the histogenesis of this tumor have not been reported, nor have Ewing's sarcoma specific antibodies been developed.

CLINICAL FINDINGS

The disease may have an insidious onset but, among the eventual manifestations, local bone pain is common and is often associated with fever and a sense of ill-health. Leukocytosis, elevated serum LDH levels, and high erythrocyte sedimentation rate may be present. Radiological findings include osteolysis with neo-ossification and periosteal reaction, which may be indistinguishable from osteomyelitis, eosinophilic granuloma, osteosarcoma, lymphoma, and metastatic tumor. Soft tissue extension is usually minimal in lesions of the head and neck skeleton.

In view of the fact that metastatic disease may be found in as many as one-third of all cases at the time of diagnosis, skeletal and pulmonary x-ray survey, bone scan, and bone marrow examination are indicated in pre-operative evaluation.[114] Urine studies for catecholamines and related metabolites are indicated because metastatic neuroblastoma must be included in the differential diagnosis.

GROSS AND LIGHT MICROSCOPIC FINDINGS

Ewing's sarcoma of the head and neck skeleton is rarely amenable to more than an incisional biopsy. Tissue is usually gray and/or red in color, soft, and friable, reflecting hemorrhage and/or necrosis.

Histology is variable, but a uniform population of cells having round nuclei twice the size of those found in small lymphocytes is common. Oval-shaped, larger nuclei are seen in some tumors. Nucleoli are usually indistinct and fine, evenly dispersed chromatin is the rule. Cytoplasmic borders are variably distinct and cytoplasm may be minimal (Fig. 5-21). Some tumors have moderate amounts of clear or vacuolated cytoplasm due to the presence of glycogen, which is best seen with PAS stain or by electron microscopy. This feature is most useful in differentiating Ewing's sarcoma from other small, round cell tumors, although neuroblastomas also contain glycogen, which is best seen by electron microscopy.[115] Mitoses are usually not abundant. Rosette-like aggregates of cells are rarely seen. Cells clinging to connective tissue-stalks give the "grapes on a vine" pattern in some instances.

Extra-skeletal tumors are identical to those in bone, but cells have a tendency to form broad bands or serpentine masses in a loose, fibrous setting.[116;117]

No correlation between histological varieties of Ewing's sarcoma and clinical course and/or response to therapy has been recorded.

ELECTRON MICROSCOPY

The cells of Ewing's sarcoma display no specific features, but their ultrastructure is sufficiently distinctive to usually allow confident identification. Characteristic focal aggregates of glycogen (Fig. 5-22) can be easily demonstrated in most examples, even when light microscopic PAS stains are negative. We were able to convincingly demonstrate cell junctions (Fig. 5-22, inset) in only 14 of 25 specimens examined but, when present, they provide another useful diagnostic feature. Ewing's tumors, arising in extra-osseous sites, are indistinguishable ultrastructurally from those arising in bone.

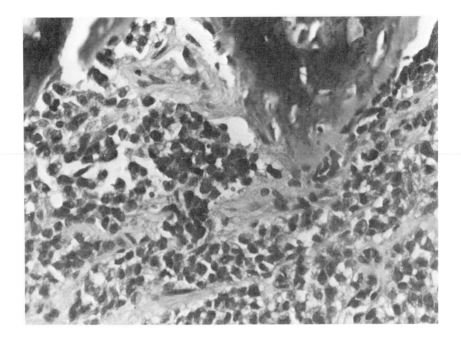

Fig. 5-21 Ewing's sarcoma of bone. (H&E x 250).

The tumor with which Ewing's sarcoma is most likely to be confused, primary lymphoma of bone, virtually never exhibits cell junctions and only rarely displays even small amounts of glycogen. A poorly-differentiated Ewing's tumor, having neither glycogen nor cell junctions, might be difficult to distinguish from lymphoma on ultrastructural grounds alone.

DIFFERENTIAL DIAGNOSIS

Differential diagnosis includes: lymphoma, rhabdomyosarcoma, neuroblastoma, leukemia, small-cell osteosarcoma, and osteomyelitis. The differential diagnosis of these lesions, which constitute the group of so-called small, round cell tumors of bone, is aided by immunologic and electron microscopic evaluations. ·

TREATMENT AND PROGNOSIS

Radiation and chemotherapy are the therapeutic modalities applicable to Ewing's tumors in the head and neck region as surgical resection is usually precluded by location. Prognosis is uncertain as it

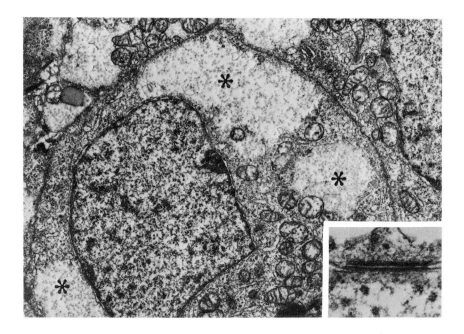

Fig. 5-22 Ewing's sarcoma cells characteristically display large, focally distributed accumulations of cytoplasmic glycogen (asterisks) and cell junctions (inset) of a fairly distinctive appearance. (EM x 14,100), (inset x 43,700).

relates to the site of involvement. The rarity of head and neck tumors precludes comparison with lesions in other sites.[114]

If metastatic disease is present at the onset, a five-year survival-rate might be expected to be less than 20 percent of such cases with modern radiation and chemotherapy.

References

1. Dahlin, D.C. *Bone Tumors. General Aspects and Data on 6,221 Cases,* 3rd ed. Springfield: Charles C. Thomas, 1978.
2. Hallberg, O.E. and Bagley, J.W. "Origin and treatment of osteomas of the paranasal sinuses." *Arch. Otolaryngol.* 51(1950): 750-760.
3. Mikaelian, D.O; Lewis, W.J. and Behringer, W.W. "Primary osteoma of the sphenoid sinus." *Laryngoscope* 86(1976): 728-733.
4. Salinger, S. "The paranasal sinuses. Malignant tumors." *Arch. Otolaryngol.* 30(1939): 633-675.
5. Malan, E. "Chirurgia degli osteomi delle cauita pneumatiche perifacciali" *Arch. Ital. Chir.* 48(1938): 1-124.
6. Cutright, D.E. "Osseous and chondromatous metaplasia caused by dentures." *Oral Surg.* 34(1972): 625-633.

7. Batsakis, J.G. *Tumors of the Head and Neck. Clinical and Pathological Considerations*, 2nd ed. Baltimore: Williams and Wilkins, 1979.
8. Shiffman, M.A. "Familial multiple polyposis associated with soft and hard tissue tumors." *JAMA* 182(1962): 514-518.
9. Brunner, H. and Spiesman, I.G. "Osteoma of the frontal and ethmoid sinuses." *Ann. Otol. Rhinol. Laryngol.* 57(1948): 714-737.
10. Jaffe, H.L. and Mayer, L. "An osteoblastic osteoid tissue-forming tumor of a metacarpal bone." *Arch. Surg.* 24(1932): 550-564.
11. Jaffe, H.L. "Benign osteoblastoma." *Bull. Hosp. Joint Dis.* 17(1956): 141-151.
12. Lichtenstein, L. "Benign osteoblastoma—a category of osteoid and bone-forming tumors other than classical osteoid osteoma, which may be mistaken for giant cell tumor or osteogenic sarcoma." *Cancer* 9(1956): 1044-1052.
13. Steiner, G.C. "Ultrastructure of osteoblastoma." *Cancer* 39(1977): 2127-2136.
14. Borello, E.D. and Sedano, H.O. "Giant osteoid osteoma of the maxilla." *Oral Surg.* 23(1967): 563-566.
15. Dahlin, D.C. and Johnson, S.W., Jr. "Giant osteoid osteoma." *J. Bone Joint Surg.* 36A(1954): 559-572.
16. Yip, W.Y. and Lee, H.T. "Benign osteoblastoma of the maxilla." *Oral Surg.* 38(1974): 259-263.
17. Byers, P.D. "Solitary benign osteoblastic lesions of bone: osteoid osteoma and benign osteoblastoma." *Cancer* 22(1968): 43.
18. Brady, C.L. and Browne, R.M. "Benign osteoblastoma of the mandible." *Cancer* 30(1972): 329-333.
19. Kramer, H.S. "Benign osteoblastoma of the mandible. Report of a case." *Oral Surg.* 24(1967): 842-851.
20. Kent, J.N.; Castro, H.F. and Girotti, W.R. "Benign osteoblastoma of the maxilla." *Oral Surg.* 27(1967): 209-219.
21. Anand, S.V.; Davey, W.W. and Cohen, B. "Tumors of the jaws in West Africa. A review of 256 patients." *Br. J. Surg.* 54(1967): 901-917.
22. Greer, R.O. and Berman, D.N. "Osteoblastoma of the jaws. Current concepts and differential diagnosis." *J. Oral Surg.* 36(1978): 304-307.
23. Abrams, A.M.; Kirby, J.W. and Melrose, R.J. "Cementoblastoma. A clinical-pathologic study of seven new cases." *Oral Surg.* 38(1974): 394-403.
24. Waldron, C.A. and Giansanti, J.S. "Benign fibro-osseous lesions of the jaws. A clinical radiologic and histologic review of sixty-five cases. Part II. Benign fibro-osseous lesions of periodontal ligament origin." *Oral Surg.* 35(1973): 340-350.
25. Hajdu, S.I. and Huvos, A.G. "Surgical Pathology of Tumors of the Extremities." (Paper delivered at the Spring Meeting of the American Society of Clinical Pathology. Committee on Continuing Education, Dallas, April 9, 1978), p. 33.
26. Shafer, W.G. and Waldron, C.A. "Fibro-osseous Lesions of the Jaws." (Paper delivered at the Thirtieth Annual Meeting of the American Academy of Oral Pathology, Atlanta, April 4, 1976).
27. Lichtenstein, L. *Bone Tumors,* 4th ed. St. Louis: C.V. Mosby, 1972.
28. Shafer, W.G.; Hine, M.K. and Levy, B.M. *A Textbook of Oral Pathology*, 3rd ed. Philadelphia: W.B. Saunders, 1974.
29. Garrington et al. "Osteosarcoma of the jaws. Analysis of 56 cases." *Cancer* 20(1967): 337-391.
30. Dehner, L.P. "Tumors of the mandible and maxilla in children. A study of 14 primary and secondary malignant tumors." *Cancer* 32(1973): 112-120.

31. Khanna, S. and Khanna, N.N. "Primary tumors of the jaws in children." *J. Oral Surg.* 38(1979): 800-804.

32. Greer, R.O. and Mierau, G.W. *Tumors of the Oral Mucosa and Jaws in Infants and Children.* Denver: University of Colorado Medical Center Press, 1980.

33. Uribe-Botero et al. "Primary osteosarcoma of bone." *Am. J. Clin. Pathol.* 67(1977): 427-435.

34. Baserga, R.; Lisco, H. and Cater, D. "The delayed effects of external gamma irradiation on the bones of rats. *Am. J. Pathol.* 39(1961): 455-472.

35. Pritchard, D.J. "Evidence for a human osteosarcoma virus." *Nature* 234(1971): 126-137.

36. Tillman, H.H. "Paget's disease of bone." *Oral Surg.* 15(1962): 1225-1234.

37. Rosenmertz, D.K. and Schare, H.J. "Osteogenic sarcoma arising in Paget's disease of the mandible. Review of the literature and report of a case." *Oral Surg.* 28(1969): 304-309.

38. Slow, I.H.; Stern, D. and Friedmana, E.W. "Osteogenic sarcoma arising in a pre-existing fibrous dysplasia: report of a case." *J. Oral Surg.* 29(1971): 126-129.

39. Cottier, R.; Keller, H. and Roos, B. "Generalized hyperostosis interna and osteosarcoma in a total body x-ray; irradiated female swiss albino mice with hormonally active ovarian tumors." *Pathol. Microbiol.* 27(1964): 458-466.

40. Curtis, M.L.; Elmore, J.S. and Sotereanos, G.C. "Osteosarcoma of the jaws. Report of case with review of the literature." *J. Oral Surg.* 32(1974): 125-130.

41. Gardner, D.G. and Mills, D.M. "The widened periodontal ligament of osteosarcoma of the jaws." *Oral Surg.* 41(1976): 652-656.

42. Lichtenstein, L. "Classification of primary tumors of bone." *Cancer* 4(1951): 335-341.

43. Paschall, H.A. and Paschall, M.M. "Electron microscopic observations of 20 human osteosarcomas." *Clin. Orthop.* 111(1975): 42-56.

44. Williams, A.H.; Schwinn, C.P. and Parker, J.W. "The ultrastructure of osteosarcoma. A review of twenty cases." *Cancer* 37(1976): 1293-1301.

45. Riddick et al. "Osteogenic sarcoma. A study of the ultrastructure." *Cancer* 45(1980): 64-71.

46. Newland, J.R. "Parosteal osteosarcoma of the maxilla." *Oral Surg.* 43(1977): 727-733.

47. Parsons, W.H. and Hunthorne, J.C. "Extra-osseous osteogenic sarcoma." *Ann. Surg.* 119(1944): 595-602.

48. Finklestein, J.B. "Osteogenic sarcoma of the jaw bones." *Radiol. Clin. North Am.* 8(1970): 425-447.

49. Pritchard et al. "Chondrosarcoma: a clinicopathologic and statistical analysis." *Cancer* 45(1980): 149-157.

50. Batsakis, J.G. and Dito, W.R. "Chondrosarcoma of the maxilla." *Arch. Otolaryngol.* 75(1962): 55-61.

51. Kragh, L.V.; Dahlin, D.C. and Erich, J.B. "Cartilaginous tumors of the jaws and facial regions." *Am. J. Surg.* 99(1960): 852-856.

52. Chaudhry et al. "Chondrogenic tumors of the jaws." *Am. J. Surg.* 102(1961): 403-411.

53. Blum, T. "Cartilage tumors of the jaws: report of three cases." *Oral Surg.* 7(1954): 1320-1334.

54. Kilby, D. and Ambegaokar, A.G. "The nasal chondroma. Two case reports and a survey of the literature." *J. Laryngol.* 91(1977): 415-426.

55. Krolls, S.O.; Schaffer, R.C. and O'Rear, J.W. "Chondrosarcoma and osteosarcoma of the same patient." *Oral Surg.* 50(1980): 146-150.

56. Fu, Y.S. and Perzin, K.H. "Non-epithelial tumors of the nasal cavity, paranasal sinuses, and nasopharynx: a clinicopathologic study. II. Cartilaginous tumors (chondroma, condrosarcoma). *Cancer* 34(1974): 453-463.

57. Shira, R.B. and Bhaskar, S.N. "Oral Surgery, Oral Pathology Conference No. 6, Walter Reed Army Medical Center." *Oral Surg.* 16(1963): 1255-1260.

58. Jaffe, H.L. *Tumors and Tumorous Conditions of the Bone and Joints.* London: H. Kimpton, 1958.

59. Roper,R.; Hall, H.T. and Adcock, A.H. "Cartilaginous tumors of the palate." *Dental Gazette* 5(1939): 417-421.

60. Feintuch, T.A. "Chondrosarcoma arising in a cartilaginous area of previously irradiated fibrous dysplasia." *Cancer* 31(1973): 877-881.

61. Terezhalmy, G.T. and Bottomley, W.K. "Maxillary chondrogenic sarcoma. Management of a case." *Oral Surg.* 44(1977): 539-546.

62. Potdar, G.G. "Chondrogenic tumors of the jaws." *Oral Surg.* 30(1970): 649-658.

63. Dahlin, D.C. and Bearout, J.W. "Dedifferentiation of low-grade chondrosarcomas." *Cancer* 28(1971): 461-466.

64. Lichtenstein, L. and Jaffe, H.L. "Chondrosarcoma of bone." *Am. J. Pathol.* 19(1943): 553-589.

65. Evans, H.L.; Ayala, A. and Romsdahl, M.M. "Prognostic factors in chondrosarcoma of bone. A clinico-pathologic analysis with emphasis on histologic grading." *Cancer* 40(1977): 818-831.

66. Goldenberg, R.R.; Cohen, P. and Steinlauf, P. "Chondrosarcoma of extraskeletal soft tissues. A report of seven cases and review of the literature." *J. Bone Joint Surg.* 49A(1967): 1487-1507.

67. Lichtenstein, L. "Unusual benign and malignant chondroid tumors of bone." *Cancer* 12(1959): 1142-1157.

68. Dahlin, D.C. *Bone Tumors,* 3rd ed. Springfield: Charles C. Thomas, 1978.

69. Rollo, J.L.; Green, W.R. and Kahn, L.B. "Primary meningeal mesenchymal chondrosarcoma." *Arch. Pathol. Lab. Med.* 103(1979): 239-243.

70. Joshi, K.; Abrol, B.M. and Roy, S. "Extraskeletal mesenchymal chondrosarcoma." *Indian J. Pathol. Microbiol.* 21(1978): 261-264.

71. Salvador, A.H.; Beabout, J.W. and Dahlin, D.C. "Mesenchymal chondrosarcoma—observations on 30 new cases." *Cancer* 28(1971): 605-615.

72. Jaffe, H.L. and Lichtenstein, L. "Benign chondroblastoma of bone: a reinterpretation of the so-called calcifying or chondromatous giant cell tumor." *Am. J. Pathol* 18(1942): 969-991.

73. Dahlin, D.C. and Ivans, J.C. "Benign chondroblastoma: a study of 125 cases." *Cancer* 30(1972): 401-413.

74. Schajowicz, F. and Gallardo, H. "Epiphysial chondroblastoma of bone: a clinicopathological study of sixty-nine cases." *J. Bone Joint Surg.* 52B(1970): 741-759.

75. Levine, G.D. and Bensch, K.G. "Chondroblastoma — the nature of the basic cell." *Cancer* 29(1972): 1546-1562.

76. Salver, M.; Salzer-Kuntschik, M. and Kretschmer, G. "Das benigne chondroblastom." *Archiv. fur Orthopaedische und Unfall-chirurgie* 64(1968): 229-241.

77. Dewachi-Al, H.S.; Haib-Al, N. and Sangal, B.C. "Benign chondroblastoma of the maxilla: a case report and review of chondroblastoma in cranial bones." *Br. J. Oral Surg.* 18(1980): 150-156.

78. Lichtenstein, L. "Polyostotic fibrous dysplasia." *Arch. Surg.* 36(1938): 874-898.

79. Batsakis, J.G. *Tumors of the Head and Neck. Clinical and Pathologic Considerations,* 2nd ed. Baltimore: Williams and Wilkins, 1979.

80. Jaffe, H.L. "Fibrous dysplasia of bone, a disease entity and specifically not an expression of neurofibromatosis." *Journal of Mount Sinai Hospital* 12(1945): 364-381.

81. Reitzik, M. and Lownie, J.F. "Familial polyostotic fibrous dysplasia." *Oral Surg.* 40(1975): 769-774.

82. Zimmerman, D.C.; Dahlin, D.C. and Stafne, E.C. "Fibrous dysplasia of the maxilla and mandible." *Oral Surg.* 1(1958): 55-68.

83. Sherman, R.S. and Glauser, O.J. "Radiological identification of fibrous dysplasia of the jaws." *Pathology* 71(1958): 553-558.

84. Windholz, F. "Cranial manifestations of fibrous dysplasia of bone. Their relation to leontiasis ossea and to simple bone cysts of the vault." *Am. J. Roentgenol. Rad. Therapy and Nuclear Med.* 58(1947): 51-63.

85. Dehner, L.P. "Tumors of the mandibile and maxilla in children. I. Clinico-pathologic study of 46 histologically benign lesions." *Cancer* 31(1973): 364-384.

86. Lucas, R.B. *Pathology of Tumors of the Oral Tissues,* 3rd ed. London: Churchill Livingstone, 1976.

87. Daramola et al. "Fibrous dysplasia of the jaws in Nigerians." *Oral Surg.* 42(1976): 290-300.

88. Waldron, C.A. and Giansanti, J.S. "Benign fibro-osseous lesions of the jaws: A clinical-radiologic-histologic review of sixty-five cases. Part I. Fibrous dysplasia of the jaws." *Oral Surg.* 35(1973): 190-201.

89. Adekeye, E.O.; Edward, M.B. and Goubran, G.F. "Fibro-osseous lesions of the skull, face and jaws in Kaduna, Nigeria." *Br. J. Oral Surg.* 18(1980): 57-72.

90. Falconer, M.A.; Cope, C.C. and Robb-Smith, A.H.T. "Fibrous dysplasia of bone with endocrine disorders and cutaneous pigmentation (Albright's disease)." *Q. J. Med.* 11(1942): 121-154.

91. Changus, G.W. "Osteoblastic hyperplasia of bone. A histochemical appraisal of fibrous dysplasia of bone." *Cancer* 10(1957): 1157.

92. Smith, J.F. "Fibrous dysplasia of the jaws." *Arch. Otolaryngol.* 81(1965): 592-603.

93. Dipson, M.J. and Middlemiss, J.H. "Fibrous dysplasia of bone." *Br. J. Radiol.* 44(1971): 1-13.

94. Jacobs, P. In *A Textbook of Radiology,* edited by David Sutton, pp. 15-16. Edinburgh: E. & S. Livingstone, 1971.

95. Obisesan et al. "The radiologic features of fibrous dysplasia of the craniofacial bones." *Oral Surg.* 4(197): 949-959.

96. Warth, H.N. *Principles and Practice of Oral Radiologic Interpretation.* Chicago: Yearbook Medical, 1963.

97. Reed, R.J. "Fibrous dysplasia of bone." *Arch. Path.* 75(1963): 480-495.

98. Eversole, L.R.; Sabes, W.R. and Rovin, S. "Fibrous dysplasia: a nosologic problem in diagnosis of fibro-osseous lesions of the jaws." *J. Oral Pathol.* 1(1972): 189-220.

99. Spjut et al. *Tumors of Bone and Cartilage. Atlas of Tumor Pathology*, 2nd series, fascicle 5. Washington, DC: Armed Forces Institute of Pathology, 1970.
100. Hamner, J.E. and Fullmer, H.M. "Oxtalon fibers in benign fibro-osseous jaw lesions." *Arch. Pathol.* 82(1966): 35-39.
101. Ramsey, H.E.; Strong, E.W. and Frazell, E.L. "Fibrous dysplasia of the craniofacial bones." *Am. J. Surg.* 116(1968): 542.
102. Waldron, C.A. "Fibro-osseous lesions of the jaws." *J. Oral Surg.* 28(1970): 58-64.
103. Tannere, H.C.; Dahlin, D.C. and Childs, D.S. "Sarcoma conplicating fibrous dysplasia. Probable role of radiation therapy." *Oral Surg.* 14(1961): 837-846.
104. Slow, I.N.; Stern, D. and Friedman, E.W. "Osteogenic sarcoma arising in pre-existing fibrous dysplasia: report of case." *J. Oral Surg.* 29(1971): 126-129.
105. Waldron, C.A. and Giansanti, J.S. "Benign fibro-osseous lesions of the Jaws: a clinical-radiologic-histologic review of sixty-five cases. Part II. Benign fibro-osseous lesions of periodontal ligament origin." *Oral Surg.* 35(1973): 340-350.
106. Regezi, J.A.; Kerr, D. and Courtney, R.M. "Odontogenic tumors: analysis of 706 cases." *J. Oral Surg.* 36(1978): 771-779.
107. Khanna, S. and Khanna, N.N. "Primary tumors of the jaws in children." *J. Oral Surg.* 37(1979): 800-804.
108. Hammer et al. "Cemento-ossifying fibroma of the maxilla." *Oral Surg.* 26(1968): 579-587.
109. Champion, A.H.R.; Moule, A.W. and Wilkenson, F.C. "Case report of an endosteal fibroma of the mandible." *Br. Dent. J.* 86(1949): 3-6.
110. Landon, J.D.; Rapidis, A.D. and Patel, M.F. "Ossifying fibroma — one disease or six? An analysis of 39 fibro-osseous lesions of the jaws." *Br. J. Oral Surg.* 14(1976): 1-11.
111. Kenneth, S. and Curran, J.B. "Giant cemento-ossifying fibroma. Report of a case." *J. Oral Surg.* 30(1972): 513-516.
112. Dahlin, D.C. In *Bone Tumors*, 3rd ed., pp. 274-287. Springfield: Charles C. Thomas, 1978.
113. Kadin, M.D. and Bensch, K.G. "On the origin of Ewing's Tumor." *Cancer* 27(1971): 257-273.
114. Kosloff, C.; Lane, J. and Murphy L. "Ewing's Sarcoma: Ten year experience with adequate chemotherapy." *Cancer* 47(1981): 2204-2213.
115. Yunis et al. "Glycogen in Neuroblastomas: A light and microscopic study of 40 cases." *Am. J. Surg. Pathol.* 3(1979): 313-323.
116. Angervall, L. and Enzinger, F.M. "Extraskeletal neoplasm resembling Ewing's sarcoma." *Cancer* 36(1975): 240-251.
117. Gillespie et al. "Extraskeletal Ewing's Sarcoma." *Am. J. Surg. Pathol.* 3(1979): 99-108.

Chapter VI

Tumors of the Salivary Glands
INTRODUCTION

Salivary gland tumors are relatively uncommon, occurring at a rate of between 1 and 2.5 per 100,000 throughout the world.[1] Only about five percent of all salivary gland tumors occur in children.[2,3]

The major salivary glands include the parotid, submaxillary, and sublingual glands. These structures are actively functional at birth and throughout life; as such, they may undergo neoplastic change and are subject to a myriad of inflammatory conditions much the same as adnexal structures elsewhere throughout the body. Additional minor salivary glands are abundant throughout the oral cavity, nasopharynx, trachea, and bronchi. These collections of minor glands are comparable in development and structure to the major glands and subject to the same untoward changes.

Batsakis[4] reported that the incidence of non-inflammatory tumors of salivary glands in children is quite low, accounting for less than five percent of all salivary gland tumors in childhood. This view is supported by Krolls and associates,[2] who reviewed 9,993 salivary gland lesions and found that 4.3 percent occurred in pediatric patients (patients less than 15 years of age). It is interesting to note that between 25 and 31 percent of all salivary gland neoplasms in the child are malignant.[2,4]

A host of taxonomic classifications have evolved for tumors of salivary gland origin. Table 6-1 reflects a modified version of the classification currently proposed by the World Health Organization.[5] Those tumors highlighted by an asterisk represent the most common epithelial and stromal salivary gland tumors of children, and will be discussed in detail in this chapter. The reader is referred to the differential diagnosis sections for a discussion of those lesions without an asterisk. Stromal tumors are discussed following the discussion of epithelial tumors.

TABLE 6-1

HISTOLOGICAL TYPING OF SALIVARY GLAND TUMORS

I. Epithelial Tumors

    A. ADENOMAS

        *1. Pleomorphic adenoma (mixed tumor)
         2. Monomorphic adenoma
           a. Adenolymphoma (Warthin's tumor)
           b. Oxyphilic adenoma
           c. Other types

    *B. MUCOEPIDERMOID CARCINOMA (TUMOR)

    *C. ACINIC CELL CARCINOMA (TUMOR)

    D. CARCINOMAS

        1. Adenoid cystic carcinoma
        2. Adenocarcinoma
        3. Epidermoid carcinoma
        4. Undifferentiated carcinoma
        5. Carcinoma in pleomorphic adenoma
          (malignant mixed tumor)

II. Non-Epithelial Tumors

    *A. HEMANGIOMA
    *B. NEURAL TUMORS

III. Unclassified Tumors

IV. Allied Conditions

---

*Those tumors with an asterisk are most common to the childhood age group.

Modified from classification of: Pindborg et al. "Histologic Typing of Odonto-genic Tumors, Jaw Cysts and Allied Lesions." In *Histological Classification of Tumors*, No. 5. Geneva: World Health Organization, 1971.

EPITHELIAL TUMORS OF SALIVARY GLAND ORIGIN
PLEOMORPHIC ADENOMA

Synonyms

1. Mixed tumor
2. Complex adenoma
3. Pleomorphic sialadenoma

INCIDENCE

The mixed tumor is unquestionably the most common benign epithelially-derived tumor of salivary glands in children. Howard and associates[6] found that three percent of the pleomorphic adenomas they reviewed in the parotid glands were in children. Krolls and associates[1] reviewed a series of 3,875 mixed tumors accessioned at the Armed Forces Institute of Pathology prior to 1972, and reported that 1.4 percent occurred in children. One percent of 712 mixed tumors reviewed by Kaufman and Stout at the Columbia Presbyterian Medical Center occurred in children.[3] These researchers found the parotid gland to be the most commonly involved, followed by minor salivary glands and the submandibular gland. They reported no examples in the sublingual glands.

AGE AND SEX

The review of the 55 tumors by Krolls and co-workers[2] indicated no statistically significant occurrence towards either sex; 26 were in males and 29 in females. Kaufman and Stout also reported no significant sexual predisposition in their series.[3] Although mixed tumors have been reported at birth,[6] the peak incidence of tumors in children reported in the series of Krolls and co-workers was at the age of ten. Byars and Ackerman[7] reported similar findings in a series of 17 salivary gland tumors in children, noting an age range between 7 and 18 years.

PATHOGENESIS

The origin of the mixed tumor has been a center of controversy since Virchow first discussed the complex histogenesis of salivary gland tumors. Billroth suggested that the tumors arose from connective tissue entrapment within the glands.[8] This original mesenchymal entrapment theory has been replaced by the concept which claims that the genesis of the mixed tumor is truly adult glandular epithelium.[9] Batsakis[4] has further refined the idea of a glandular origin by proposing that the mixed tumor actually develops from undifferentiated excretory and intercalated duct reserve cells.

CLINICAL FINDINGS

The pleomorphic adenoma usually manifests itself as a firm-to-hard, mobile nontender mass (Fig. 6-1). The vast majority of the mixed tumors of major salivary glands occur in the tail of the parotid gland. The most common site for minor salivary gland tumors is the hard palate (Fig. 6-2). The tumor may be round, smooth, lobular, or nodular, and most are recognized when they attain a size of between 2 and 10 cm. in diameter. [10;11]

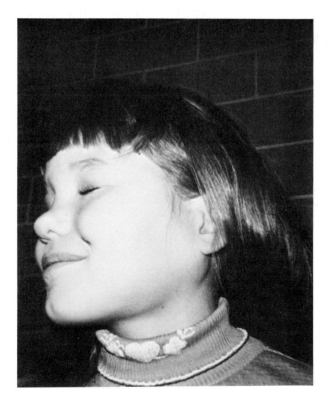

Fig. 6-1 Mixed tumor of the parotid gland. Courtesy of Dr. Bruce Jafek.

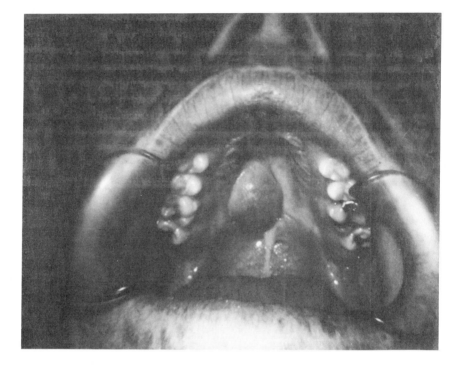

Fig. 6-2 Mid-palatal swelling, representing mixed tumor (pleomorphic adenoma). Courtesy of Dr. Ron Hanawalt.

Pleomorphic adenomas are slow-growing and commonly painless; thus it may be difficult for the clinician to differentiate the lesion from acute or long-standing sialadenitis in the child. The neoplasm has occasionally been reported bilaterally in the palate or parotid glands of adults, but not in children.

GROSS AND MICROSCOPIC FINDINGS

The gross appearance of the pleomorphic adenoma is one of an irregular lobulated tumor mass, surrounded by a connective tissue capsule that may not totally envelop the tumor. Tumor lobules may, in fact, appear quite separate from the central tumor mass, forming small satellite, grape-like clusters. The cut surface can range from gray-white to blue, with random areas of cartilage, bone, or mucoid material.

The connective tissue capsule can vary from a few millimeters in thickness to a leathery, dense peripheral band. Patey and Thackray[12] reported that visualization of the capsule is exceedingly important because the tumor grows by localized infiltration through the capsule, in addition to growth simply by capsular expansion.

Histologically, the tumor displays truly pleomorphic appearances. The most classic of these is a tumor composed of sheets, nests, and cords of epithelial cells distributed throughout a mucoid, chondroid, or mucochondroid matrix (Fig. 6-3). In minor salivary gland tumors, cellular areas dominate the microscopic picture and stromal changes are less prominent. In major salivary gland tumors, stromal changes appear as the most prominent component of the tumor, even to the point where one has to search out the most cellular epithelial component.

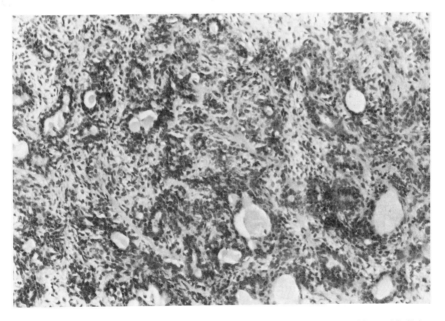

Fig. 6-3 Pleomorphic adenoma composed histologically of ducts lined by epithelial cells with round nuclei and eosinophilic cytoplasm. Occasional darker myoepithelial cells are also visibly distributed throughout the mucoid stroma. (H&E x 280).

Individual epithelial tumor cells are oval, round, or polyhedral with round-to-vesicular nuclei and rich, eosinophilic cytoplasm. Occasionally, the epithelial component of the tumor will take on a spindle-shaped quality. Spindle-shaped cells often interlace into a strand-like meshwork. When this spindle cell pattern dominates the tumor histology, the tumor has been referred to as a myoepithelioma.

Duct-like structures or tubules are commonly seen. They are generally lined by a single layer of cuboidal or columnar cells and filled with eosinophilic coagulum. Fully-developed squamous epithelial islands and keratin pearls may be seen as well. Sebaceous glands can be seen in parotid tumors but are rarely encountered in minor salivary gland neoplasms.

Intercellular stromal material ranges from hyalin-like to fibrillar, with interdispersed areas of mucoid matrix, chondroid material, and occasionally, osteoid material (Fig. 6-4).

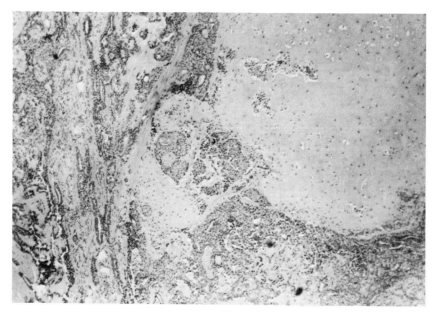

Fig. 6-4 Note the prominent intercellular stromal hyalin and chondroid matrix in pleomorphic adenoma. (H&E x 200).

ELECTRON MICROSCOPY

The ductular epithelial cells (Fig. 6-5) of pleomorphic adenomas rest upon a basal lamina and are interjoined near their luminal surfaces by junctional complexes. Microvilli extend from their apices into the lumina. Both the ductular and myoepithelial components exhibit numerous intermediate, and less commonly, cytokeratin filaments. Well-developed desmosomes are displayed by both cell types.

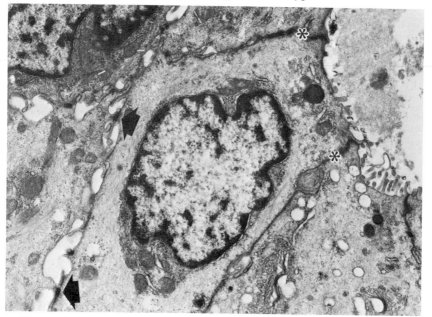

Fig. 6-5 Both epithelial and myoepithelial cells of pleomorphic adenomas typically are packed with cytoplasmic filaments and display numerous desmosomal junctions (arrows). Microvilli and junctional complexes (asterisks) are found at the luminal surface of the ductal epithelium. (EM x 14,100).

Pleomorphic adenomas are indeed mixed tumors in the sense that they may contain a combination of epithelial, myoepithelial, myxoid, and chondroid elements. Electron microscopic [13] [16] and immunohistochemical studies [17;18] have, however, tended to support the contention of Willis, [19] who maintained that the term "mixed tumor" (originally coined to denote a neoplasm consisting of both epithelial and mesenchymal components) is something of a misnomer; recent evidence seems to support his concept that the fibrous, mucinous, and pseudocartilaginous material observed in some examples is produced by metaplastic myoepithelial cells rather than mesenchymal cells.

DIFFERENTIAL DIAGNOSIS

The pleomorphic adenoma is often confused with other salivary gland tumors, the most common tumors being *adenoid cystic carcinoma*, and *monomorphic adenoma*. To render a diagnosis of mixed tumor, one must identify a diverse accumulation of both epithelial and mesenchymal elements. Batsakis[4] remarked that without these biphasic elements, the lesion cannot be regarded as a true mixed tumor. While adenoid cystic carcinomas, with their classic cribiform or cylindromatous pattern, may be confused with the mixed tumor, the presence of myxochondroid or fibroid components occurring in a lesion with a cylindromatous pattern dictates a diagnosis of mixed tumor.[1] A second feature helpful in distinguishing the mixed tumor from adenoid cystic carcinoma is the fact that mixed tumors do not show the high propensity for perineural extension and infiltration displayed by adenoid cystic carcinoma. Pseudocyst development and abundant reduplicated basement membrane substance are common features to adenoid cystic carcinoma; they are much less common in mixed tumors.

Monomorphic adenoma, a term of fairly recent vintage, is now popularly applied to benign salivary gland tumors predominately composed of epithelium.[20] In distinction to the pleomorphic adenoma in which an abundant and prominent stroma constitutes an important part of the growth, monomorphic adenomas possess a scanty, inconspicuous stroma, just sufficient to nourish and hold the tumor together.[20] Alveolar, tubular, trabecular, basaloid, clear cell, and canalicular types of monomorphic adenoma have been described (Fig. 6-6). In contrast to mixed tumors, monomorphic adenomas tend to occur in a somewhat older population, and are rarely, if ever, documented in children. The lesions are slow-growing, seldom attain a size of 2.5 cm., and rarely recur, even following simple enucleation.

Krolls[2] reported one case of monomorphic adenoma that measured approximately 5 cm. in diameter in a seven-day-old boy. A follow-up revealed no recurrence four years after surgical removal of the tumor.

The *malignant mixed tumor* is very rarely reported in children. The only childhood examples of malignant mixed tumors that we were able to identify included one, reported in a series of 38 childhood tumors reviewed by Castro and associates[21] in 1972, and six documented by Schuller and McCabe in 1977.[22] Abrams and Melrose[20] indicated that a diagnosis of malignant mixed tumor should be rendered *only* if one of the following criteria are met:

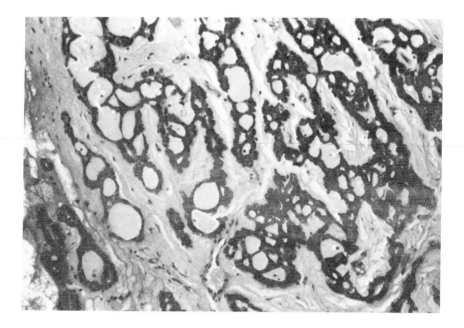

Fig. 6-6 Monomorphic adenoma showing a trabecular pattern of uniform epithelial cells. (H&E x 140).

1. A classical benign mixed tumor which unexpectedly metastasizes.
2. A mixed tumor with cellular abnormalities consistent with an apparent transformation to malignancy, including atypical mitoses, altered nuclear-cytoplasmic cellular ratios, nuclear pleomorphism, and vascular or peripheral invasion.
3. A benign mixed tumor growing in association with a recognized variety of salivary gland malignancy, such as adenoid cystic carcinoma, adenocarcinoma, or squamous cell carcinoma.

Tumor necrosis, excessive hyalinization, stromal ossification, and peripheral infiltration of tumor beyond the capsule should make the surgical pathologist suspect that a benign mixed tumor may have undergone a malignant change. The prognosis for this disease is uniformly poor.

TREATMENT AND PROGNOSIS

To date, no one has been able to correlate the histopathologic appearance of the mixed tumor with its biologic behavior. The ultimate behavior pattern of the tumor depends largely on the therapy rendered. Although surgery is the preferred treatment for this tumor, it is also probably responsible for the rather high recurrence rates due to inadequate excision or spillage of the tumor beyond the often delicate capsule. The recurrence rates for mixed tumors of the major and minor salivary glands in adults ranges from a low of 5 percent[23] to a high of 50 percent. Batsakis[4] attributed this broad recurrence rate range to: (1) inadequate long-term observation of the patient, and (2) inclusion of a large number of cases treated by simple enucleation of tumors in major glands, prior to the acceptance of parotidectomy as a leading mode of treatment. Rankow and Polayes[10] reported that a 10-to-20 percent recurrence rate has been reported in children when tumor cells are known to have spilled beyond the tumor capsule. Long-term judicious observation of the child with a diagnosis of a mixed tumor is mandatory for the proper management of this disease.

RARE BENIGN EPITHELIAL SALIVARY GLAND NEOPLASMS IN CHILDREN

Papillary cystadenoma lymphomatosum (Warthin's tumor) is exceedingly rare in childhood. Krolls and associates[2] have most recently reported the occurrence of such tumors in children. Earlier cases were documented by Lederman.[23] Histopathologically, the tumor is characterized by clusters of cystic spaces, lined by finely granular eosinophilic columnar cells with oval to vesicular nuclei. These cells also line papillary processes that extend into cystic spaces. A supporting lymphoid stroma is prominent (Fig. 6-7).

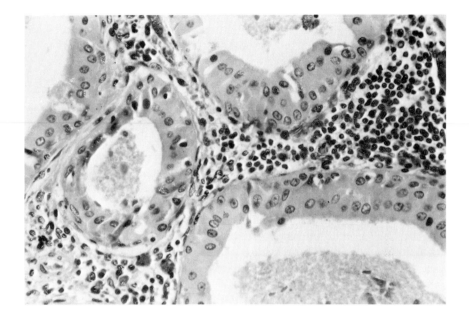

Fig. 6-7 Papillary cystoadenoma lymphomatosum. Ducts lined by a double layer of oxyphilic cells are seen supported by lymphoid tissue. (H&E x 250). Courtesy of Dr. Bruce Jafek.

MUCOEPIDERMOID CARCINOMA

Synonyms

1. Mucoepidermoid tumor
2. Mixed epidermoid and mucus-secreting carcinoma

INCIDENCE

Mucoepidermoid carcinoma is the most common of the malignant epithelially-derived tumors of salivary glands in children. Krolls and associates[2] reported that 20 of 35 malignant salivary gland tumors, seen in a review of AFIP cases occurring in children, were mucoepidermoid carcinomas, and Castro and associates[21] reported that 15 of 18 malignant parotid tumors seen in children were mucoepidermoid carcinomas.

The parotid gland is the most frequently involved site. Fourteen of the 20 tumors reported by Krolls were in the parotid, four in the submandibular gland, and two in minor salivary glands.

AGE AND SEX

There is no sexual predisposition in the tumor's occurrence which peaks at the age of ten.[2;10] The youngest child reported by Krolls and associates was one-year-old.

PATHOGENESIS

Mucoepidermoid tumors are thought to arise from epithelial cells of the duct system in major and minor salivary glands. Foote and Frazell[24] suggested they originate proximal to salivary gland lobules, since the characteristic eosinophilic cells lining the ducts distal to this are rarely seen in mucoepidermoid carcinomas. Bhaskar and Bernier[25] have proposed that minor salivary gland tumors may possibly arise from the epithelium lining the oral mucosa; however, Evans and Cruickshank[1] discounted this theory and suggested it is more probable that mucoepidermoid tumors arise in the subepithelial tissues and ultimately fuse with the overlying epithelium. Interestingly, mucoepidermoid carcinoma is the most common salivary gland tumor to arise centrally within bone. The postulated source of such osseous tumors ranges from the epithelial lining of odontogenic cysts to entrapped embryonic salivary gland tissue within the jaws.[25]

CLINICAL FINDINGS

The great majority of mucoepidermoid tumors occur clinically as slowly growing, painless swellings, similar in growth characteristics to the mixed tumor. Jakobsson and co-workers[26] reported that the period of time between the initial appearance of a mucoepidermoid tumor and the first diagnostic biopsy may be greater than six years. Tumors may be solid, cystic, or an admixture of the two. So-called "high grade" mucoepidermoid tumors grow quite rapidly, are frequently accompanied by pain and ulceration, and tend to be solid rather than cystic. The parotid gland is the most frequent anatomic site for them in children and adults. In our experience, the minor salivary glands of the palate are the next most frequent anatomic location for mucoepidermoid tumors in children and adults, although Krolls reported a greater frequency in the submandibular glands in children.

GROSS AND MICROSCOPIC FINDINGS

Mucoepidermoid tumors appear grossly, as partially encapsulated to non-encapsulated, gray-tan or yellowish nodules. The cut surface of the tumor may appear solid or cystic. When cystic spaces are identified, they are frequently filled with mucus, hemorrhage, or ropy, viscous material. Solid tumors tend to show expansion beyond the peripheral rim of the tumor more frequently than cystic tumors.

Microscopically, the mucoepidermoid tumor is composed of three to six cell types, according to Sikorwa.[27] The most common of these cell types are mucus-secreting, epidermoid, and intermediate cells. The maternal, clear, and columnar cells described by Sikorwa are much less commonly encountered. Foote and Frazell[24] were the first to separate mucoepidermoid carcinoma into three grades of malignancy based on histology: *low grade, intermediate grade, and high grade.*

Low grade tumors are those composed of cystic or glandular spaces which are lined by a single or multiple layer of mucus-producing cells (Fig. 6-8). Portions of cystic walls may also be lined by rather flat epidermoid cells, or occasionally, by intermediate cell types. Because cystic spaces are filled with mucin, cysts often rupture, resulting in extravasation of mucus contents into the hyalinized connective tissue stroma. Tumor cells show no evidence of cellular atypia and there is little extension of tumor cells into adjacent anatomic structures.

Intermediate grade tumors are, more frequently, composed of solid sheets, nests, and cords of intermediate and epidermoid cells (Fig. 6-9). These cells may show focal areas of atypia, including occasional abnormal mitoses and cellular pleomorphism. The large cystic and

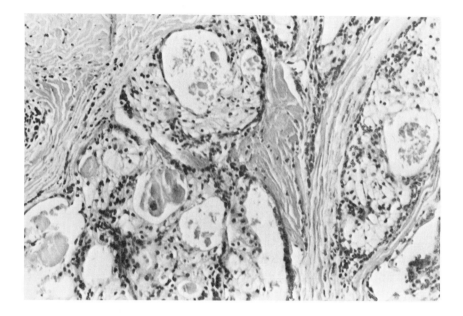

Fig. 6-8 Low-grade mucoepidermoid carcinoma composed predominately of collections of mucous secretory cells with a few intermediate cell types and squamous cells that have undergone hydrophic change. (H&E x 220).

glandular spaces common to the low-grade variant are much less common in the intermediate grade tumor. The stroma is generally composed of interlacing bands of collagen, with an admixture of chronic inflammatory cells. This variant demonstrates a greater tendency toward extension beyond the tumor periphery and into adjacent structures.

High grade mucoepidermoid tumors are composed of mosaic sheets, bands, clusters, and clumps of cells of a prominent squamous character, or a prominent squamous and an equally prominent acellular mucus-like component. Cellular anaplasia, atypical mitoses, and hyperchromatism are prominent. Keratin pearl formation may also be common. Cystic or glandular spaces lined by mucus secreting cells are sparse or totally absent. This histologic variant is locally aggressive and readily extends into peripheral tissues.

There has been considerable debate concerning the question of whether the mucoepidermoid tumor should be considered a carcinoma at all, in light of the fact that the low grade variant most often follows a

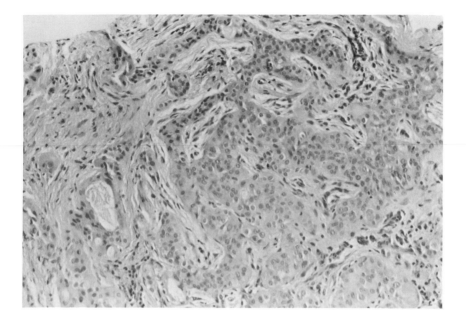

Fig. 6-9 Intermediate-to-high-grade mucoepidermoid carcinoma, showing a mixture of epidermoid and mucous secretory cells. (H&E x 260).

benign biologic course. In fact, the World Health Organization suggested *mucoepidermoid tumor* as the preferred taxonomy. We, nonetheless, favor the view of Batsakis who concluded that "it is not possible by light microscopy to distinguish between a highly differentiated, yet metastasizing tumor and a histologically hypothetically benign mucoepidermoid tumor, thus the patient and the surgeon are best served by regarding all forms of mucoepidermoid tumor as carcinoma."[4]

Our own experience with six mucoepidermoid tumors in children, ranging in age from 10 to 14, showed a predominance of intermediate grade tumors.

DIFFERENTIAL DIAGNOSIS

Distinguishing high grade mucoepidermoid carcinoma from squamous cell carcinoma arising from the oral mucous membranes may prove difficult. Attempts to demonstrate highly PAS-positive cells that are unaltered by hyaluronidase treatment may prove helpful in diagnosing the former.

Mucoepidermoid tumors are sometimes confused with other types of salivary gland tumors, especially adenocystic carcinoma (cylindroma), clear cell carcinoma, and squamous cell carcinoma or adenocarcinoma of ductal origin. Mucinous mixed tumors with squamous metaplasia or keratin pearl formation also have been erroneously called mucoepidermoid tumors.[1] However extensive the epidermoid metaplasia is in a mixed tumor, one always finds the typical spindle or stellate myoepithelial elements extending into diffuse mucinous zones. The mucinous cysts of mucoepidermoid carcinoma are lacking. Hyaline and chondroid areas are also notably lacking in mucoepidermoid carcinomas.

TREATMENT AND PROGNOSIS

The majority of mucoepidermoid carcinomas grow slowly and the five-year survival-rate of all patients with the disease, regardless of age, approaches zero percent.[25;27] Castro and associates[21] reported five-year cures in 96 percent of all their cases of mucoepidermoid carcinoma in the parotid and submandibular glands of children. Intermediate and high grade tumors show lower survival rates. Thorvaldsson[28] reported that in the Mayo Clinic experience, a five-year survival-rate of 41.6 percent has been documented for tumors graded intermediate or high grade. Spiro and associates[29] reported a 44 percent rate of metastasis to regional cervical lymph nodes in their review of intermediate and high grade parotid mucoepidermoid carcionomas.

The primary treatment for mucoepidermoid carcinoma is complete surgical removal of the tumor. Eversole[30] suggested that the extent of surgery should be modulated by the location of the tumor in the gland, the histological appearance of the tumor, and the presence or absence of palpable regional lymph nodes. Some authors suggest that total parotidectomy with regional lymph node dissection is mandatory for high grade tumors.[26.]

Mucoepidermoid tumors are radio-resistant, and although radiotherapy has been employed as an adjunctive form of treatment, it is not considered a primary mode of treatment.

ACINIC CELL CARCINOMA

Synonyms

1. Acinous cell carcinoma
2. Acinic cell tumor
3. Serous acinar adenoma
4. Acinic cell adenocarcinoma

INCIDENCE

Acinic cell carcinoma is the second leading malignant epithelial neoplasm to occur in the salivary glands of children. Krolls and associates,[2] in their extensive review of childhood salivary gland tumors, found that 12 of 35 epithelial malignancies of the salivary glands were acinic cell carcinomas. The most frequent site is the parotid gland. Ten out of twelve tumors reported by Krolls and associates were in this location; two of the tumors arose in minor salivary glands of the oral cavity. Castro and associates,[21] in their review of 38 primary salivary gland tumors in children, also reported that acinic cell carcinoma was the second most frequently encountered epithelial malignancy.

AGE AND SEX

The acinic cell carcinoma of adults occur two to three times more frequently in women than men, but, Krolls found that, in childhood, females with the disease outnumbered males by a ratio of 2-to-1. It is difficult to establish an average age of occurrence for the acinic cell carcinoma in children. Out of the 12 tumors reported by Krolls and associates, an age range from 9 to 14 was recorded. One of the authors (ROG) had the opportunity to diagnose six acinic cell carcinomas in children over the past eight years, where an age range of 10 to 14 has been recorded.

PATHOGENESIS

Acinic cell carcinomas are considered by most authorities to arise from the serous cells of the salivary gland acini.[1] Abrams, however, has postulated that perhaps acinar cells are not the only source for this neoplasm. He supported this concept by noting that transitions between intercalated duct cells and tumor cells can be noted when these lesions are thoroughly scrutinized microscopically, and, as acinar cells themselves originate from terminal portions of salivary ducts, it is probable that acinic cell tumors arise from pluripotential duct cells. Batsakis[4] also supported this theory and has suggested that this pluripotential cell be referred to as a *reserve cell.*

CLINICAL FINDINGS

The clinical presentation of this tumor is rather nonspecific, as the lesion usually has a slow growth pattern which suggests a benign mixed tumor. Pain is not a constant feature in children, although Abrams[31] noted that it has been reported in up to 50 percent of the cases when all age groups are considered. Tumors may grow for a period of 4 to 6 years and attain a diameter of 2 cm. to 5 cm. before patients seek consultation.[1] Facial nerve involvement has been reported in adults, but is rare in children. Tumors range from firm to hard in consistency and although they are most often freely movable and feel well-circumscribed, a true capsule is rarely confirmed microscopically.

GROSS AND LIGHT MICROSCOPIC FINDINGS

Most acinic cell carcinomas are composed of a mixture of round to polygonal cells closely resembling normal acinic cells in terms of their cytoplasmic granularity and basophilia (Figs. 6-10, 6-11). However, intercalated duct, vacuolated, clear, and nonspecific granular cells can grow in microcystic, papillary cystic, and follicular patterns.[20] A prominent lymphocytic infiltrate, especially in parotid tumors, may ramify through the supporting connective tissue stroma, while calcifications may also be quite prominent.

Tumor growth can closely mimic the normal lobular architecture of a salivary gland; atypical mitotic figures are rare and the vast majority of lesions fail to show an infiltrative growth pattern, although perineural invasion may be found on occasion.

Bastsakis[4] divided the tumors into seven growth patterns: (1) acinar lobular; (2) microcystic; (3) follicular; (4) papillary cystic; (5) medullary; (6) ductuloglandular, and (7) primitive tubular. He further attempted to correlate these histologic variants with tumor grade, proposing that high grade, biologically aggressive carcinomas manifest: intravascular extension; local finger-like invasion, and have medullary, ductuloglandular, or primitive tubular foci. Low grade tumors would have a less aggressive biologic potential and display microcystic, follicular, papillary cystic, or acinar lobular patterns of growth.[4] However neat this diagnostic schema may appear, Batsakis[4] and Abrams[20] agreed that acinic cell carcinomas lack histomorphologic features by which local aggressive or metastatic behavior may be routinely predicted. Because of the common, usually benign histological appearance of these tumors and

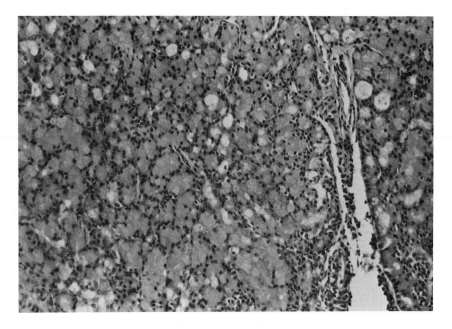

Fig. 6-10 Acinic cell tumor composed of a uniform collection of cells resembling normal acinar tissue. (H&E x 250).

the histomorphologic similarity between local, recurrent, and metastasizing lesions, most investigators believe all tumors to have at least a low grade malignant potential. Thus, the recent trend toward the referral of this lesion simply as an acinic cell tumor is not in the best interest of proper patient management.

DIFFERENTIAL DIAGNOSIS

Acinic cell carcinoma must be distinguished from mucoepidermoid carcinoma, glycogen-rich water-clear cell tumors, and adenocarcinoma of salivary and nonsalivary gland origin. Abrams and Melrose[20] reported that the use of special stains as a method of distinguishing acinic cell carcinoma from other salivary gland neoplasms is of no benefit. However, Evans and Cruickshank reported that the most reliable method of diagnosing acinic cell tumors is to identify typical basophilic cells which react positively with a PAS reagent, after pretreatment with diastase.

Tumors consisting of water-clear cells rich in glycogen may simulate hypernephroma or a parathyroid adenoma, and are possibly of

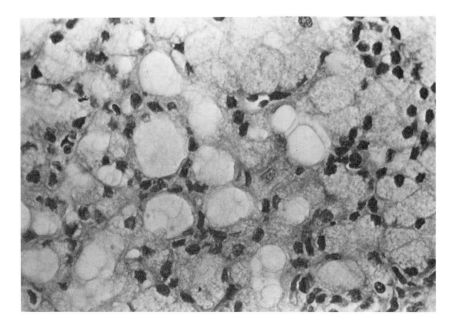

Fig. 6-11 Higher-power photomicrograph of acinic cell tumor. Note the vacuolated as well as granular cytoplasm. (H&E x 350).

myoepithelial origin.[1] They should not be confused with acinic cell tumors that are largely composed of clear cells, containing only very minute traces of glycogen. Interestingly, water-clear cells rich in glycogen occur more often in mucoepidermoid tumors than in acinic cell tumors.

TREATMENT AND PROGNOSIS

Although a great majority of patients with acinic cell carcinoma are cured by initial therapy, the erratic behavior of this tumor may eventually lead to local recurrence, regional lymph node metastasis, and/or in distant metastasis to bone, lung, and liver. Microscopic findings of favorable prognostic significance include tumor encapsulation, multiple large cysts with papillary projections, prominent lymphoid stroma, and tumor origin within lymph nodes. Prognosis is most heavily dependent upon correct initial therapy. Minimally acceptable surgery is parotid lobectomy or submandibulectomy. Measures most often associated with therapeutic failures include: incision in vivo, needle aspiration, excessive palpation, in vivo rupturing of a tumor cyst, and enucleation.

Krolls and associates[2] had excellent follow-up data on the childhood cases they reviewed of all ten acinic cell carcinomas originating in the parotid gland. Only one tumor recurred two years following initial therapy, and there was no recurrence of that tumor after an 11-year follow-up. The other nine cases had been followed for periods ranging from two to nine years. Abrams and Melrose[32] found that 16 of 17 minor salivary gland acinic cell tumors in all age groups (scrutinizd with a follow-up that ranged from 2 to 15 years), showed no recurrence following surgical excision which included removal of a wide margin of apparently normal tissue.

Although the initial post-therapeutic impression concerning acinic cell carcinoma is often very optimistic, Eneroth[33] emphasized that at least a 20- year follow-up is desirable for all cases, if one is to determine the true biologic potential of acinic cell carcinoma.

RARE MALIGNANT EPITHELIAL SALIVARY GLAND NEOPLASMS IN CHILDREN

Adenoid cystic carcinoma is rarely encountered in the salivary glands of children. Schuller and McCabe found six tumors in their 1972 review of the literature.[22] Krolls found nine instances in his review of 430 childhood salivary gland neoplasms.[2] We have seen only two adenoid cystic carcinomas in the head and neck area in children of less than 14 years of age. One occurred in the palate, the other in the trachea. Their histopathology is characterized by classic cylindrical cell clusters set in scanty, connective tissue. Cystic or alveolar-like spaces are prominent throughout the cell clusters (Figs. 6-12, 6-13).

Several cases of *undifferentiated carcinoma* in the parotid glands of children have been reported by Marlowe and Hora,[34] and Schuller and McCabe.[22] These lesions rapidly metastasize and have a lethal potential, equivalent to their counterparts in adults.

Krolls and associates[2] reported three *adenocarcinomas* in children which they were unable to subclassify as acinic cell or adenoid cystic carcinoma. All of these tumors occurred in girls, ranging in age from 6 months to 7 years.

Primary *squamous cell carcinomas* of the salivary glands in children are exceedingly rare. Kauffman and Stout[3] documented only three in a review of the literature that included 712 cases in children.

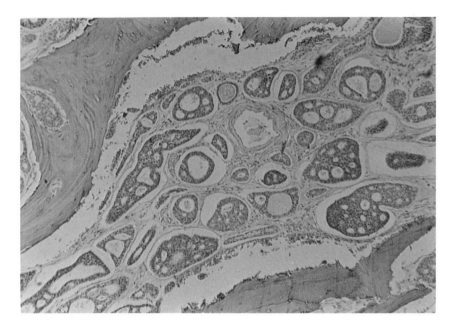

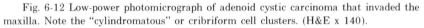

Fig. 6-12 Low-power photomicrograph of adenoid cystic carcinoma that invaded the maxilla. Note the "cylindromatous" or cribriform cell clusters. (H&E x 140).

Salivary gland neoplasms are reported to account for 4 to 8 percent of sinonasal malignancies. Batsakis[4] reported the order of greatest incidence of the sinonasal salivary tumors to be: adenoid cystic carcinoma, adenocarcinoma, pleomorphic adenoma, mucoepidermoid carcinoma, and undifferentiated carcinoma. These tumors occur with distinct rarity in the nose and paranasal sinusues of children.

Aberrant salivary gland tumors, especially mucoepidermoid carcinoma, have been reported to occur centrally within the jaws. These *central mucoepidermoid carcinomas* are rare in children. Browand reported only two cases in a review of 41 previously reported tumors, plus nine cases of his own patients.[35]

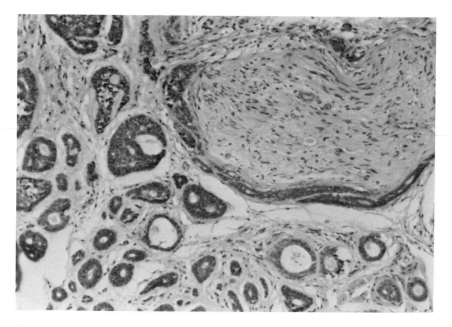

Fig. 6-13 Adenoid cystic carcinoma showing perineural invasion. (H&E x 280).

STROMAL TUMORS OF SALIVARY GLAND ORIGIN

Hemangiomas are the most common neoplasm of the major and minor salivary glands in children. The parotid gland is by far the most common anatomic site for hemangioma in salivary glands. The lesions are most common in the first year of life. Campbell[36] noted that lesions were present during the first year of life in 54 of the 61 reported cases he reviewed.

The parotid gland is also the most common site for the nonvascular mesenchymal neoplasms of salivary glands, although the submandibular, sublingual, and minor salivary glands can also be affected. *Neural tumors* (neurofibroma, and neurilemmoma) are by far the most frequent of these nonvascular neoplasms.[1]

Castro and co-workers,[21] and Krolls[2] reported a total of five *xanthomas* in salivary glands of children, in an exhaustive combined review of 2,565 salivary gland tumors. These benign reticuloendothelial tumors are probably a result of lipid-containing histiocytes which diffusely infiltrate salivary gland tissue, resulting in a tumor mass. They are benign lesions that can be treated by simple surgical excision.

The *ranula*, although more classically a cystic lesion than a neoplasm, is a common expansile growth in children which most frequently affects the sublingual gland as a tumor-like swelling. Galich[37] reported a total of 31 ranulas in a review of 191 benign salivary gland tumors in children. The lesion generally appears as a painless swelling above the mylohyoid muscle in the floor of the mouth. It is thought to arise from obstruction of the sublingual gland, resulting in a localized retention of mucus, an associated inflammatory component, desquamated epithelial cells, and frequently, a mass of granulation tissue. Marsupialization of the cyst or total removal of the gland are the most common modes of treatment. The minor salivary gland *mucocele* is a common variant of the ranula. Mucoceles most commonly involve the lower lip, with the majority of the remainder occurring in the palate, cheek, tongue, and retromolar fossa.[38] Cataldo and Mosadomi[38] reported that more than 25 percent of the 348 mucoceles they reviewed were in patients between the ages of 11 and 20.

The mucocele is characterized, histologically, by extravasation of mucus into surrounding tissues. Retention of mucus is more often associated with the ranula. Minor salivary gland retention cysts with a true epithelial lining are rare; therefore, these lesions are more properly termed pseudocysts.

Mucous retention cysts and mucoceles of the paranasal sinuses are much less common than their oral counterparts. Zizmor and Noyek[39] reported that the frontal and ethmoid sinuses are the most frequently involved sites. Proptosis is the most common clinical finding and radiographically, the vast majority of paranasal sinus mucoceles appear as dome-shaped homogeneous masses, sharply delineated by contrasting air-filled sinuses at the periphery. Sinus mucoceles are usually characterized microscopically by a fibrous soft tissue sac, lined by squamous, columnar, or cuboidal epithelium. Squamous metaplasia appears to be much more common in the wall of paranasal sinus mucoceles than oral mucoceles.

Malignant mesenchymal tumors of the salivary glands are rare in children. Krolls and associates[2] reported that the most commonly encountered tumor in their review was rhabdomyosarcoma, accounting for five out of a total of six malignancies. A sixth tumor was classified as fibrosarcoma. Neurofibrosarcoma has also been reported in the salivary glands of children.[40] In addition, Krolls and colleagues,[2] and Johnson and Samuels[41] have reported a total of seven lymphomas in the parotid, submandibular, and minor salivary glands of children.

References

1. Evans, R.W. and Cruickshank, A.H. *Epithelial Tumors of the Salivary Glands.* Philadelphia: W.B. Saunders, 1970.
2. Krolls, S.O.; Trodahl, J.N. and Boyers, R.C. "Salivary gland lesions in children." *Cancer* 30(1972): 459-469.
3. Kaufman, S.C. and Stout, A.P. "Tumors of the major salivary glands in children." *Cancer* 16(1963): 1317-1331.
4. Batsakis, J.G. *Tumors of the Head and Neck. Clinical and Pathologic Considerations*, 2nd ed. Baltimore: Williams and Wilkins, 1979.
5. Pindborg et al. "Histologic Typing of Odontogenic Tumors, Jaw Cysts and Allied Lesions." In *Histological Classification of Tumors*, No. 5. Geneva: World Health Organization, 1971.
6. Howard et al. "Parotid tumors in children." *Surg. Gynecol. Obstet.* 90(1950): 307-319.
7. Byars, L.T.; Ackerman, L.V. and Peacock, E. "Tumors of salivary gland origin in children. A clinical pathologic appraisal of 24 cases." *Ann. Surg.* 146(1957): 40-52.
8. Billroth, T. "Boebachtugen uber geschwulste der speichiedrusen." *Virchows Archiv.* 17(1859): 357-375.
9. Willis, R.A. *Pathology of Tumors*, 4th ed. London: Butterworth, 1967.
10. Rankow, R.M.N. and Polayes, I. *Diseases of the Salivary Glands.* Philadelphia: W.B. Saunders, 1976.
11. Saunders, B. *Pediatric Oral and Maxillofacial Surgery.* St. Louis: C.V. Mosby, 1979.

12. Patey, D.H. and Thackray, A.C. "The treatment of parotid tumors in the light of a pathological study of parotidectomy material." *Br. J. Surg.* 45(1958): 477-487.

13. Hubner et al. "Role of myoepithelial cells in the development of salivary gland tumors." *Cancer* 27(1971): 1255.

14. Varela-Duran, J.; Diaz-Flores, L. and Varela-Nunez, R. "Ultrastructure of chondroid syringoma. Role of the myoepithelial cell in the development of the mixed tumor of the skin and soft tissues." *Cancer* 44(1979): 148.

15. Erlandson, R.A. *Diagnostic Transmission Electron Microscopy of Human Tumors.* New York: Masson, 1981.

16. Mills, S.E. and Cooper, P.H. "An ultrastructural study of cartilaginous zones and surrounding epithelium in mixed tumors of salivary glands and skin." *Lab. Invest.* 44(1981): 6.

17. Franke et al. "Intermediate-sized filaments of the prekeratin type in myoepithelial cells." *J. Cell Biol.* 84(1980): 633.

18. Caselitz, J. and Loning, T. "Specific demonstration of actin and keratin filaments in pleomorphic adenomas by means of immunoelectron microscopy." *Virchows Archiv. (Pathol. Anat.)* 393(1981): 153.

19. Willis, R.A. *Pathology of Tumors*, 3rd ed. Washington: Butterworth, 1960.

20. Abrams, A. and Melrose, R.J. "Jaw and salivary gland neoplasms." (Paper delivered at the Spring Meeting of the American Society of Clinical Pathology, Dallas, April 9, 1978).

21. Castro et al. "Tumors of major salivary glands in children." *Cancer* 29(1972): 312-317.

22. Schuller, D.E. and McCabe, B.F. "The firm salivary mass in children." *Laryngoscope* 85(1977): 189-191.

23. Lederman, M. "Adenolymphoma of the salivary gland." *Br. J. Radiol.* 16(1943): 383-385.

24. Foote, F.W. and Frazell, E.L. "Tumors of the major salivary glands." *Cancer* 6(1953): 1065-1133.

25. Bhaskar, S.N. and Bernier, J.L. "Mucoepidermoid tumors of major and minor salivary glands. Clinical features, histology, variations, natural history and results of treatment of 144 cases." *Cancer* 15(1962): 801-816.

26. Jakobsson, P.A.; Blanck, C. and Eneroth, C.M. "Mucoepidermoid carcinoma of the parotid gland." *Cancer* 22(1968): 111-124.

27. Sikorwa, L. "Mucoepidermoid tumors of salivary glands." *Pol. Med. J.* 3(1964): 1345-1367.

28. Thorvaldsson et al. "Mucoepidermoid tumors of the major salivary glands." *Am. J. Surg.* 120(1970): 432-438.

29. Spiro, R.H.; Huvos, A.G. and Strong, E.W. "Cancer of the parotid gland. A clinicopathologic study of 288 primary cases." *Am. J. Surg.* 130(1975): 452-459.

30. Eversole, L.R. "Mucoepidermoid tumor: review of 815 reported cases.": *J. Oral Surg.* 28(1970): 490-494.

31. Abrams et al. "Acinic cell adenocarcinoma of the major salivary glands. A clinicopathologic study of 77 cases." *Cancer* 18(1965): 1145-1162.

32. Abrams, A.M. and Melrose, R.J. "Acinic cell tumors of minor salivary gland origin." *Oral Surg.* 46(1978): 220-223.

33. Eneroth, C.M.; Jakobsson, P.A. and Blanck, C. "Acinic cell carcinoma of the parotid gland." *Cancer* 19(1966): 1761-1772.

34. Marlowe, J.F. and Hora, J.F. "Parotid mucoepidermoid carcinoma in children." *Laryngoscope* 78(1968): 68.

35. Browand, B.C. and Waldron, C.A. "Central mucoepidermoid tumors of the jaws." *Oral Surg.* 40(1975): 631-643.

36. Campbell, J.S. "Congenital capillary hemangiomas of the parotid gland. A lesion characteristic of infancy." *N. Eng. J. Med.* 254(1956): 56-60.

37. Galich, R. "Salivary gland neoplasms in childhood." *Arch. Otolaryngol.* 89(1969): 878-882.

38. Cataldo, E. and Mosadomi, A. "Mucoceles of the oral mucous membranes." *Arch. Otolaryngol.* 91(1970): 360-365.

39. Zizmor, J. and Noyek, A. "Cysts and benign tumors of the paraoral sinuses." *Semin. Roentgenol.* 3(1968): 172-201.

40. Karlan, M.S. and Snyder, W.H. "Salivary gland tumors and sialadenitis in children." *Calif. Med.* 108(1968): 423-429.

41. Johnson, D.B. and Samuels, S.K. "Primary lymphosarcoma of the parotid gland in a child." *J. Pediatr. Surg.* 1(1966): 170-177.

Chapter VII

Tumors of Fibrous and Histiocytic Origin

IRRITATION FIBROMA AND LOCALIZED FIBROUS GROWTHS

Synonyms

1. Fibroma
2. Fibrous hyperplasia
3. Fibroid epulis
4. Fibrous polyp

INCIDENCE

The "irritation" fibroma is probably the most common reactive lesion of the oral cavity in children. Stout[1] reported that approximately 15 percent of mesenchymal tumors identified in all anatomic sites, including the oral cavity, are fibromas. Greer and Carpenter[2] reviewed a series of 40 consecutive oral lesions recorded on the surgical pathology data service at the University of Colorado School of Dentistry and found that 16.9 percent represented irritation fibromas or localized fibrous overgrowths.

AGE AND SEX

The irritation fibroma can occur at any age. Greer and Carpenter found that 14 percent of the lesions diagnosed as irritation fibroma in their series were in patients less than 18 years of age.[2] Barker and Lucas[3] reported that only a small percentage of oral fibrous overgrowths occur during childhood and adolescence. They found that only 7 of 171 fibrous overgrowths of the oral cavity occurred in patients less than 20 years of age. Females were affected more often than males in the studies of Greer and Carpenter,[2] and Barker and Lucas.[3]

PATHOGENESIS

There is little consensus as to the exact nature of these lesions, and there is considerable controversy as to whether these localized fibrous overgrowths represent true neoplasms or reactive hyperplasias. Stout[1] wrestled with this problem in evaluating over 1,000 fibrous lesions in anatomic sites other than the oral cavity. He concluded that while the lesions contained a variety of proliferations of fibrocytes, accompanied by collagen and reticular fibers (which more or less resemble neoplasms), the majority were not true neoplasms, and certainly few, if any, had the potential to develop into malignant growths.

Barker and Lucas evaluated the hyperplasia-versus-neoplasia problem by examining 171 fibrous lesions of the oral cavity. They were able to clearly identify only two lesions as fibroma durum, a true localized fibrous neoplasm, and concluded that the remaining 169 lesions were more appropriately labeled fibrous hyperplasias most likely associated with, or directly evolving from, some type of irritation or trauma.

According to Barker and Lucas, true fibromas show a clear separation from surrounding tissue, a distinctive whorling fiber pattern and a definitive capsule; few oral lesions of fibrous origin show such continuity.

CLINICAL FINDINGS

The irritation fibroma can involve any oral anatomic site, but the interdental gingiva and cheeks are the most commonly affected sites in children.[2;3] The lesions usually manifest themselves as asymptomatic, solitary growths that may be pedunculated or sessile, and range in texture from granular to hard. Multiple growths may occur, but only rarely.[2;4;5]

Lesions of the lips, tongue, and palate are usually very well circumscribed. Ill-fitting prosthetic dental appliances or a badly broken-down tooth frequently can be isolated as the initiating factor.

LIGHT MICROSCOPY

Microscopically, the classic appearance of irritation fibroma is one of a soft tissue nodule covered by keratinizing squamous epithelium overlying a lamina propria which is composed of bundles of well-vascularized collagen fibers often arranged in concentric layers. A pseudocapsule may be present at the periphery of the specimen. On occasion, the hyperplastic connective tissue is exceedingly well-vascularized and it may be difficult to separate the fibroma from a *sclerosing pyogenic granuloma*.

Some authors[6] maintain that pyogenic granulomas tend to become more fibrous as they mature and in fact, the irritation fibroma, in many instances, represents only the terminal stage of pyogenic granuloma.

Calcification is frequently seen in gingival lesions. When the stroma is composed of a delicate accumulation of fibroblasts and numerous small spherical amorphous calcified masses, the term *peripheral odontogenic fibroma* or *peripheral fibroma with ossification* is applied (Fig. 7-1). Occasionally, islands of odontogenic epithelium and giant cells are present. This lesion, almost always seen in the interdental papilla area (Fig. 7-2), has a much greater frequency of recurrence than the typical irritation fibroma. Reported recurrence rates range from 16 to 27 percent. [7;8]

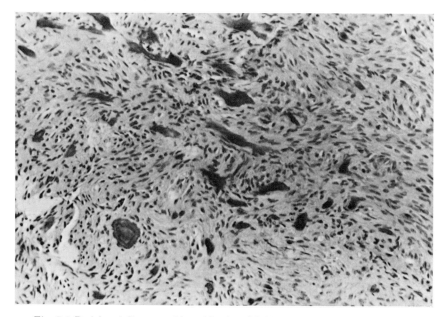

Fig. 7-1 Peripheral fibroma with ossification. Medium-power photomicrograph, illustrating characteristic reactive fibrous proliferation with focal collections of inflammatory cells and scattered calcification. (H&E x 180).

Fibrous lesions that have been continuously traumatized may show surface ulceration, and a variable acute and/or chronic inflammatory component may be present throughout the supporting stroma.

DIFFERENTIAL DIAGNOSIS

A large number of additional benign localized fibrous growths can affect the oral mucous membranes. These lesions must be distinguished from the common "irritation" fibroma. Such lesions may be

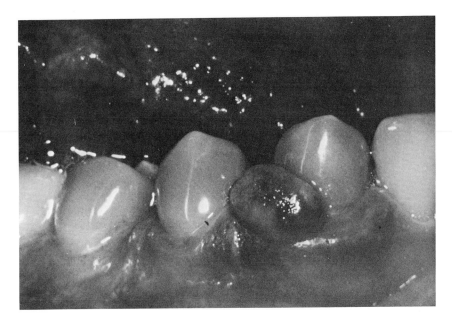

Fig. 7-2 Peripheral fibroma with calcification, showing hyperplastic nodular soft tissue growth, affecting the interproximal gingiva.

drug-induced, idiopathic, hereditary, or traumatic in origin. *Dilantin hyperplasia* is a form of drug-induced or drug-influenced hyperplasia that commonly results in gingival enlargements. The reported incidence of gingival hyperplasia in all users of the drug for epilepsy (diphenylhydantoin) is reported to be about 40 percent. Most cases of diphenylhydantoin gingival hyperplasia are seen in children and adolescents. [9]

Gingival hyperplasia usually begins in the interdental area within three months of the initial administration of the drug. After approximately six months to a year, the lesions will be most severe in appearance, occurring as generalized fibrotic swellings which may overgrow the facial and occlusal surfaces of the teeth. Inflammation is not a constant feature and becomes most obvious only when there is a lack of proper oral hygiene. [10]

Histologically, the classic picture is one of markedly acanthotic penetrating strands of squamous epithelium overlying interlacing, often whorled, hyperplastic collagen bundles. The lesion is typically poorly-vascularized unless there is surface ulceration. Batsakis [11] emphasized that local irritants modify the clinical and microscopic appearance of the process, as they may for all forms of gingival fibromatosis. This concept is most important to remember when reviewing any fibrous overgrowth involving the oral cavity.

The most successful treatment for dilantin hyperplasia is the withdrawal of the drug. Total or partial regression of the gingival fibromatosis usually occurs within six months of withdrawal. In refractory cases, surgical gingivectomy may be required.

Gingival fibromatosis (idiopathic fibromatosis gingivae) is a rare form of hereditary, diffuse hyperplasia of the gingiva. The etiology remains unknown, but there is a well-documented familial tendency, with transmission of the disorder via either an autosomal dominant or recessive gene.[10] Gingival enlargement may be present from birth or it may not be recognized until late in childhood. Most cases are evident at the time of eruption of the permanent dentition. Gingival enlargement may be localized, but it is, in fact, usually so diffuse that it may occasionally cover the crowns of the teeth, causing difficulty in mastication and closing. A host of associated abnormalities, including hypertrichosis and hirsutism, have been reported.[12-14]

Microscopically, the tissue consists of squamous epithelium that overlies coarse bundles of well-formed interlacing collagen fascicles. The epithelium may show mild acanthosis and the supporting connective tissue component may undergo mucoid change. Vascular and inflammatory components are variable. Treatment consists of gingivectomy with gingival recontouring. Recurrence is a possibility, although it decreases with advancing age.

Fibromatosis colli is a disorder of infants, characterized by the formation of a tumor mass of fibrous origin in the sternocleidomastoid muscle. The proliferation, commonly known as wryneck, is not a true neoplasm and lesions gradually undergo remission before the patients reach the age of one. Occasionally, the mass fails to involute and surgical correction is necessary.[15]

Microscopically, the lesion shows a generalized insidious replacement of muscle by fibrous tissue. Fibromatosis colli may be difficult to distinguish from *musculo-aponeurotic fibromatosis (desmoid tumor)*. Batsakis[15] reported that fibromatosis colli is distinguished from the desmoid tumor by its content of relatively large numbers of interspersed residual muscle fibers and the relationship of age of the lesion to the relative amount of collagen.

TREATMENT AND PROGNOSIS

Irritation fibromas and fibrous hyperplasias are generally treated by complete surgical excision with elimination of local irritants. There is little tendency for recurrence except in cases where habitual cheek-biting occurs or where there is a chronic irritant.

Inflammatory fibrous hyperplasia (denture hyperplasia) is a condition associated with ill-fitting or unstable dentures. Single or multiple folds of fibrous tissue overhang denture borders or flanges like a "curtain of excess tissue." This condition has not been reported in children.

THE FIBROMATOSES, INTRODUCTION

The fibromatoses are an interesting group of lesions that arise from human somatic tissues or musculo-aponeuroses. They generally exhibit a localized proliferation of fibroblasts with the formation of their specific products; collagen and reticulin fibers.[16]

There are still numerous unresolved conflicts in the literature regarding the nomenclature, behavior, and clinical management of childhood tumors composed predominately of fibrous tissue,[17] and it remains nearly impossible for the pathologist to routinely predict how these tumors will behave biologically.

McKenzie,[18] Dehner,[17] Enzinger,[19] and Stout[20] have been instrumental in establishing some order to the heretofore chaotic nomenclature established for this group of lesions. Two principle subcategories of fibromatoses have been established: (1) those occurring as congenital lesions or diagnosed principally in childhood, and (2) those that may occur at any time during life, but are found primarily in adults.

Those lesions that may be seen in the head and neck during childhood include: (1) the fibrous hamartoma of infancy; (2) fibromatosis colli; (3) aggressive juvenile fibromatosis; (4) juvenile aponeurotic fibromatosis; (5) congenital generalized fibromatosis; (6) congenital solitary fibromatosis, and (7) desmoid tumor.

Nodular fasciitis and myositis ossificans are frequently included under the heading fibromatosis. We consider nodular fasciitis and focal proliferative myositis to be unique pseudosarcomatous clinicopathological entities which should not be classified under the general heading of fibromatosis.

Those fibromatoses which can be found with some frequency in the head and neck region in children are outlined in Table 7-1 along with their predisposed sites. Only the desmoid tumor (musculo-aponeurotic fibromatosis) and nodular fasciitis will be discussed in detail as they represent a large percentage of those lesions of fibrous origin seen in the head and neck regions of children. Pertinent information concerning additional fibromatoses will be discussed under the differential diagnosis headings.

TABLE 7-1

JUVENILE FIBROMATOSES
THAT MAY AFFECT THE HEAD AND NECK

Lesion	Age	Location
Fibrous hamartoma of infancy	Birth, infancy	Predominately seen in the axillae and shoulder as a lesion of subcutaneous lower dermis and subcutaneous fat.
Fibromatosis colli	Birth, infancy	Sternocleidomastoid muscle, lower third. May be bilateral and associated with congenital anomalies.
Aggressive infantile and juvenile fibromatosis	First year of life through adolescence	Locally aggressive with latent recurrence potential.
Diffuse infantile fibromatosis	First 3 years of life; rarely at birth.	Disorder of arm-shoulder-neck area. Multicentric with inflammatory cell foci.
Congenital generalized and solitary fibromatosis	Multicentric mesenchymal dysplasia with onset in uterine life, infancy, and childhood.	Multiple lesions in subcutaneous tissue, muscle, bone, viscera, and soft tissues.
Desmoid tumor	Children, young adults, and adults.	Shoulder girdle, neck, or extremities.
Hereditary gingival fibromatosis	Children and adolescents.	Attached gingiva.

DESMOPLASTIC FIBROMATOSIS

Synonyms

1. Desmoid tumor
2. Extra-abdominal desmoid tumor
3. Musculo-aponeurotic fibromatosis
4. Juvenile fibromatosis
5. Aggressive infantile fibromatosis
6. Aggressive juvenile fibromatosis

INCIDENCE

The desmoid tumor of the extra-abdominal sites can affect all age groups. Masson and Soule[21] reported that the head and neck region accounted for 12 percent of 284 desmoid tumors in all body locations in their review of these tumors in children and adults.

In an analysis of 250 fibrous tumors occurring in infants and children between birth and 15 years of age, Enzinger[22] reported that the extra-abdominal desmoid tumor accounted for 59 of the tumors. Although Enzinger did not report what percentage of these tumors were in the head and neck, Masson[21] documented that 85 percent of the head and neck desmoid tumors he observed in all age groups, occurred in the supraclavicular region of the neck.

Desmoplastic fibroma is considered a rare disease among primary tumors of bone. Jaffe[23] reported five cases of this tumor in the tibia, femur, and scapula. Later, Whitesides and Ackerman,[24] and Rabhan and Rosai[25] reported a total of 39 cases. In 1972, Kawanishi and co-workers,[26] and Matsumori and associates[27] reviewed the literature and documented a total of 48 cases of desmoid tumor of bone, nine of which occurred in the mandible. Taguchi and Kaneda[28] reviewed these nine cases of mandibular desmoid tumors and added a case of their own. Six of the total of ten cases were in patients less than 15 years of age.

In 1978, Freedman and associates[29] reviewed the world literature concerning desmoplastic fibromas of the jawbones and added a case of their own. They were able to adequately document only 26 cases involving the jaws, since Jaffe first reported the lesion as a separate entity from other central fibrous lesions of bone in 1958.[30]

AGE AND SEX

The extra-abdominal desmoid tumor in the head and neck region is principally a lesion of young adults when soft tissue and bony sites are considered as a group. Masson and Soule[21] reported a fairly uniform distribution of cases during the first five decades of life and noted a 3-to-2 ratio towards females in a survey of 34 cases of desmoid tumor of the head and neck.

When one reviews desmoplastic fibroma as a primary tumor of bone, strikingly different statistics are noted. Freedman and others[29] reported a mean age of 15.7 years, with an age range from birth to 39 years, in a review of 26 cases of desmoid tumor of the jaws. Ninety-two percent of their cases occurred during the patients' first three decades. These findings are similar to those of Sugiura,[31] who found that desmoplastic fibroma was predominately a disease of young persons, with a peak incidence in the second decade. No sexual predisposition was noted in either series. Enzinger[22] noted a peak incidence between the ages of 5 and 15 years for this tumor in a review of 202 fibrous tumors of infancy and childhood.

PATHOGENESIS

Desmoplastic fibromatosis arises as a musculo-aponeurotic fibromatosis with localized proliferative fibroblastic activity. Touraine and Ruel,[32] in 1945, suggested that all the various juvenile fibromatoses, including the head and neck extra-abdominal desmoid tumor, were in some way linked together via an underlying hereditary factor. These authors favored naming all such fibromatoses hereditary polyfibromatosis.

Etiologic factors responsible for desmoplastic fibromatosis in children are difficult to evaluate. The two generally accepted causative factors for desmoids of the anterior abdominal wall (trauma and pregnancy) cannot be invoked in extra-abdominal desmoids.[33] An hormonal factor in the etiology has been postulated but not proven.[33]

CLINICAL FINDINGS

The head and neck extra-abdominal desmoid tumor of the child can occur as a soft tissue mass or as a lesion wholly within bone. The soft tissue lesion usually appears as a progressively enlarging, painless tumor mass that has been present for less than one year.[11] The tumor mass is most often located superficially in the dermis, subcutaneous tissues, or oral mucosa.

When the jaws are involved, the mandible is a much more frequent location than the maxilla. Freedman and co-workers,[29] and Taguchi and Kaneda[28] reported that nearly 70 percent of the lesions they reviewed occurred in the molar-ramus-angle region of the mandible.

By far, the most common clinical manifestation is one of a painless swelling. The most characteristic radiographic appearance of the disease is a loculated, clearly defined radiolucent lesion of bone (Fig. 7-3).[28] Freedman and co-workers reported that 34 percent of the lesions they reviewed showed some degree of root resorption of teeth involved by the lesion.[29] Lesions of the bones of the face are rare; but when present, they generally appear as clearly defined radiolucencies.

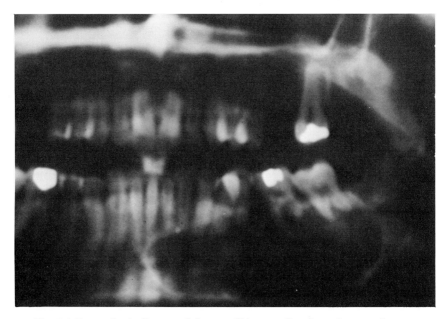

Fig. 7-3 Desmoplastic fibroma of the mandible extending from the ascending ramus to the midline. Courtesy of Dr. Doran Ryan.

LIGHT MICROSCOPY

The desmoid tumor is composed of a rich foundation of abundant collagen fibers that are woven and entangled in layers (Fig. 7-4). Between them, small scattered fibroblasts, following the long axis of collagen bundles, can be identified. The periphery of the tumor may be more heavily collagenized, to the extent that the cells are less prominent and contain narrow, elongated, darkly-staining nuclei. The center of the lesion may contain branching vascular clefts (Fig. 7-5), foci of inflammatory cells, and rarely, scattered, multinucleated giant cells.

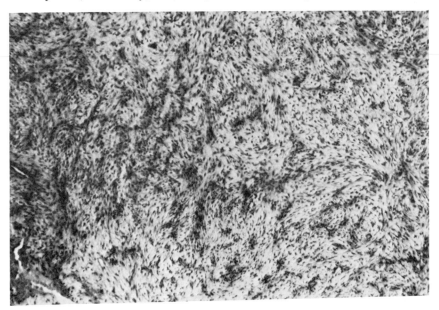

Fig. 7-4 Desmoplastic fibroma of the mandible, showing a rich collagenous stroma, and clusters and interlacing bands of fibroblasts. (H&E x 220).

Individual fibroblasts frequently vary in the appearance of their nuclei and cytoplasmic prominence, and while mitotic activity may be demonstrated, mitotic atypia is not a prominent part of the histopathology of the lesion. Stout[34] coined the term *juvenile fibromatosis*, and Enzinger[22] used the term *aggressive infantile fibromatosis* to describe what we believe to be forms of aggressive desmoplastic fibromatosis. Batsakis[11] has taken a similar view, recognizing that the distinction between the head and neck desmoid tumor and well-differentiated fibrosarcoma, especially in the infant and juvenile patient, is an exceedingly difficult, if not impossible one to make on the basis of histological appearance alone. Mitotic activity is not always a reliable index for malignancy in the infant or child, yet it must be remembered that even

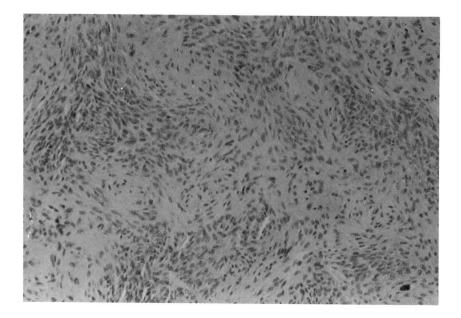

Fig. 7-5 Note branching vascular clefts in this juvenile desmoplastic fibroma of the mandible. (H&E x 280).

if the histological picture is bland, 1 out of 13 cases diagnosed as extra-abdominal desmoid tumor, juvenile fibromatosis, or aggressive infantile fibromatosis will metastasize. [15]

DIFFERENTIAL DIAGNOSIS

When Jaffe[35] first described desmoplastic fibroma of bone, he was quite specific about his histological criteria. He stated that the tumors closely resembled the soft tissue desmoid and were composed of small, inconspicuous fibroblasts set in an abundant collagenous matrix. The fibroblasts showed little, if any, mitotic activity and were uniform in their appearance. More cellular lesions especially those containing plump cells, even if they lacked cellular anaplasia and mitotic activity, were considered to be well-differentiated fibrosarcomas. We tend to agree with the assessment of Jaffe, even though Rabhan and Rosai[36] expanded this original concept to include lesions that are more cellular and contain plumper cells than the tumors Jaffe originally described. Lesions with anaplastic forms or significant numbers of atypical mitoses are more accurately described as *fibrosarcomas*.

Tumors having significant numbers of multinucleated giant cells, along with the xanthomatous areas and hemosiderin deposits characteristic of non-osteogenic fibroma of bone, do not fulfill criteria for desmoplastic fibroma.

Batsakis[11] reported the incidence of fibromatosis in neonates is second only to that of vascular tumors. Among the more common lesions are fibromatosis colli, diffuse infantile fibromatosis, congenital or generalized fibromatosis, and hereditary gingival fibromatosis. Distinctive clinical and histological features which may be helpful in distinguishing these lesions from desmoplastic fibromatosis can be found in Table 7-1.

Accurate diagnosis of desmoplastic fibromatosis in the child should not be a major problem if microscopic features are correlated with history, clinical features, and radiographs. Microscopically, the diagnosis of desmoplastic fibroma should be entertained only when the tumor is composed of heavily collagenized, hypocellular fibrous tissue in which nuclei are small, slender, and spindle-shaped.[37]

Differentiation of desmoplastic fibromatosis from well-differentiated fibrosarcoma may be a more difficult and serious problem. Stout[34] reported that his attempts to find reliable methods of distinguishing between the two diseases and detecting potential metastasizing tumors proved less than successful. He ultimately resorted to arbitrary criteria for diagnosis and noted that even those tumors labeled as well-differentiated fibrosarcomas generally did not behave in a malignant fashion when they occurred in children below the age of 16. If Stout's criteria are followed, the diagnosis of well-differentiated fibrosarcoma should be made only if mitotic activity is prominent, if there is nuclear pleomorphism, or if vascular invasion is observed. It must be remembered that hypercellularity of a fibrous neoplasm in a child does not necessarily imply potential malignant behavior.

We disagree with those who equate differentiated fibrosarcoma with juvenile fibromatosis and use the terms interchangeably. We favor the view of MacKenzie[18] who, in discussing the fibromatoses as a clinicopathological concept stated, "Cumbersome labels such as non-metastasizing fibrosarcoma or fibrosarcoma Grade I are undesirable not only because of the suffix sarcoma but because with the passage of time the qualifying words get lost, leaving the plain fibrosarcoma." The suggestion that the terms fibromatosis and well-differentiated fibrosarcoma are interchangeable would, if accepted, perpetuate a misuse of language and lead to widespread confusion. Conceivably, interchangeable use of the diagnoses could also result in the patient being subjected to excessive therapy.

The principal subclassification problem for some lesions of the fibromatosis group is the distinction between those with a benign nonaggressive natural history (e.g., palmar and plantar fibromatosis) and those with the potential for destruction or aggressive behavior (e.g. desmoids and extra-abdominal desmoids). Many aggressive fibromatoses, especially those located outside the well-recognized abdominal site, present a clinicopathological dilemma because location and clinical presentation do not appreciably aid in the diagnosis. Only through a proper correlation of histological and clinical parameters can these lesions be accurately diagnosed. Juvenile desmoplastic fibromatoses are manifested clinically by local aggressiveness and infiltration beyond palpable margins,[38] thus simulating malignancy. Local recurrence rates as high as 47 percent have been reported, but metastases do not occur.[39] A wide range of cellularity, collagen production, and inflammation can be seen, but it is generally agreed that the mitotic index is low and cellular pleomorphism is not prominent.[37] The latter criteria have, in large part, served to support the concept of benignity in regard to these lesions.

TREATMENT AND PROGNOSIS

The juvenile desmoplastic fibroma of the head and neck must be considered a tumor of aggressive biological potential, with a very high rate of recurrence, and extreme difficulty of eradication. It can prove exceedingly difficult to distinguish this lesion from fibrosarcoma in the child. Stout[16] was of the opinion that in the infant or child whose lesion has metastasized, the lesion was fibrosarcoma at the onset. He maintained that the difficulty in differentiating benign and malignant fibrous tumors in the child often results in the lesion being initially diagnosed conservatively.

The treatment of choice is en bloc surgical resection along with adjacent surrounding normal tissue. Sugiura[31] noted a recurrence of 12 out of 50 cases of desmoid tumors of the jaws. Masson and Soule[21] reported that 70 percent of the patients in their Mayo Clinic series with head and neck desmoid tumors experienced one or more recurrences, while Das Gupta[33] reported a 20 percent recurrence rate of all extra-abdominal desmoid tumors in his study. Although radiation therapy is not the principal procedure of choice, it may be used when anatomical restrictions dictate a non-surgical intervention. It is not recommended when bone involvement is demonstrated.

Masson and Soule[21] suggested that a neck dissection is indicated when a diagnosis of aggressive desmoplastic fibromatosis is obtained for a neck lesion, regardless of tumor size.

NODULAR FASCIITIS

Synonyms

1. Pseudosarcomatous fasciitis
2. Proliferative fasciitis
3. Infiltrative fasciitis
4. Subcutaneous pseudosarcomatous fibromatosis
5. Fasciitis

INCIDENCE

Nodular fasciitis first described by Konwaler[40] in 1955, can occur from early childhood to late adult life. The peak incidence appears to be between the third and fourth decades of life. Approximately 13 percent of all reported cases have occurred in the head and neck.[41;42]

AGE AND SEX

The reports of Allen,[42] Stout,[43] and Price[44] document that males are affected more frequently than females. In Allen's review of 843 consecutive cases of nodular fasciitis, 50 occurred between birth and the age of 9, and 106 occurred between 10 and 19 years of age.

Stout, in a review of 123 cases of pseudosarcomatous fasciitis, documented that 12.2 percent were in children less than 16 years of age. Batsakis reported that approximately half of all reported cases of nodular fasciitis in the head and neck have occurred in children less than 15 years of age.[11]

PATHOGENESIS

Although the specific pathogenesis of nodular fasciitis is unknown, it is most commonly considered to be a reactive inflammatory non-neoplastic fibroproliferative response to injury. At one time, nodular fasciitis was considered to be a form of paniculitis because it often involved adipose tissue. This postulate was largely discounted following the studies by Price and associates[44] who found no evidence of fat necrosis in a clinicopathologic analysis of 65 cases of nodular fasciitis. Konwaler and associates have suggested a possible relationship between fasciitis and nodular subepidermal fibrosis.[40] The microscopic similarities between the two lesions are only superficially similar and we agree with Price and co-workers[44] that subepidermal fibrosis is primarily an entity of the corium and not the fascia. Trauma[45] and viral induction[46] have been suggested as etiologic factors, but remain unsubstantiated.

CLINICAL FINDINGS

The pattern of behavior of nodular fasciitis in children is comparable to that in adults. The vast majority of the lesions appear as small, discrete, subcutaneous or submucosal nodules.

Most nodules measure from 1 to 5 cm. in diameter at the time of removal.[43] Nodular fasciitis is notoriously rapid in growth, and the majority of patients in childhood and adolescence only become aware of the tumor for a short period of time prior to treatment.

Although most patients are aware of a solitary mass, most report only a slight degree of associated pain or tenderness. A definitive history of trauma prior to the appearance of the lesion is rare. Batsakis[11] reported that 60 percent of all lesions are removed within four months of onset, and 40 percent are excised less than three weeks after their onset.

Allen's review of 829 cases of nodular fasciitis documented the following descending frequency of head and neck fasciitis by location: (1) neck; (2) face; (3) forehead; (4) scalp; (5) orbit; (6) conjuntiva; (7) eyelid, and (8) buccal mucosa. The neck, face, and forehead accounted for 70 percent of all lesions.[42]

Batsakis[11] reported that nodular fasciitis shows three distinct patterns of anatomic growth. The tumor can grow from the fascia upward into the subcutaneous tissues, resulting in a well-delineated nodule. A second variant grows primarily along the fascia itself or at the fascia perimeter, and a third anatomic variant grows from the fascia down into underlying muscle.

The first anatomic type with its upward growth is the most common. The characteristic lesion of nodular fasciitis is circumscribed, firm, and when sectioned, shows a variegated cut surface with gelatinous to myxoid areas distributed centrally or irregularly throughout the nodule.

LIGHT MICROSCOPY

The histological features of nodular fasciitis are varied, but four characteristic microscopic features are consistently identified.[42;44] First, there are nodular proliferations of plump to spindle-shaped fibroblasts with variable amounts of cytoplasm, and hyperchromatic nuclei with prominent nucleoli (Fig. 7-6). Second, a stromal meshwork of cell processes, reticulin, and collagen fibers and varying amounts of amorphous ground substances are seen. Third, a vascular component of slit-like spaces and well-formed capillaries in a pattern suggestive of a reparative process is present. Fourth, there is a variable cellular component that includes mononuclear inflammatory cells, extravasated red blood cells, mesenchymal cells not readily distinguishable from fibroblasts, and multinucleated giant cells of various types. Multinucleated giant cells appear in 50 percent of the lesions. Some are definitely of the foreign-body type. Remnants of adipose tissue, fascia, muscle, nerves, and blood vessels may be incorporated by the proliferating cells.

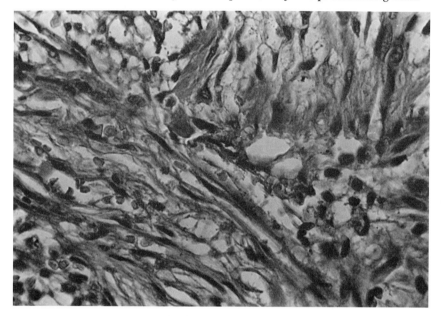

Fig. 7-6 Nodular fasciitis in a 12-year-old boy who had a non-tender swelling at the angle of the mandible for 3 weeks. Plump fibroblasts, collagen fibers, a few vascular spaces, and extravasated red cells are present. (H&E x 340).

The child or adolescent frequently displays a proclivity to harbor lesions that manifest little ground substance and a tendency toward a greater degree of cellularity with a less haphazard arrangement of cells.[44]

DIFFERENTIAL DIAGNOSIS

Nodular fasciitis has been confused with as many as 14 other lesions histologically. Perhaps the best summary of differential diagnostic guidelines has been presented by Allen,[42] in his review of 895 cases of nodular fasciitis. The most common diagnostic challenges will be discussed below.

Clinically, *fibrosarcomas* tend to be larger than the lesion of nodular fasciitis. They have a longer history, and with the exception of myxofibrosarcomas, are usually not subcutaneous in location. Histologically, fibrosarcomas are hypercellular tumors; the nuclear chromatin is coarse and irregularly distributed, and there is often an abundance of bizarre cells with prominent pleomorphic nuclei. Myxofibrosarcomas are a nodular myxoid variant of fibrosarcoma that occur almost exclusively in the subcutaneous tissue of adults more than 40 years of age; such neoplasms closely imitate the pattern of nodular fasciitis, with an S-shaped arrangement of fibroblasts, clefts, extravasated red cells, and myxoid ground substance. Nuclear hyperchromatism and pleomorphism, bizarre multinucleated giant cells, and abnormal mitotic figures are features pointing to myxofibrosarcoma.

Liposarcomas can be readily distinguished from nodular fasciitis on clinical grounds alone, if it is remembered that liposarcomas are usually large, slow-growing tumors and are extremely rare in the subcutaneous tissues. Histologically, myxoid liposarcomas have vacuolated lipoblasts and a prominent pattern of anastomosing and plexiform thin-walled capillaries. Capillaries of nodular fasciitis are never as prominent as in myxoid liposarcomas, and they are arranged in columns and festoons along a linear front. Pleomorphic liposarcomas and sclerosing liposarcomas are both characterized by bizarre pleomorphic hyperchromatic cells, and should cause little confusion with nodular fasciitis. Fat may be demonstrable with special stains in nodular fasciitis, but the presence of adipose tissue is of little value in distinguishing nodular fasciitis from liposarcoma.

Focal proliferative myositis is a benign inflammatory pseudotumor of children that develops rapidly as a painful, localized soft tissue swelling. Those found in the head and neck often involve the masseter muscle and show a microscopic proliferation of large, often atypical, fibroblasts, inflammation, and fibrosis directly into skeletal muscle (Fig. 7-7). The lesion is self-limiting and should be distinguished from polymyositis.

Neurofibromas are characterized by the presence of sharply twisted, spindle-shaped nuclei, thick wave-like bundles of collagen, small round lymphocyte-like cells, and frequently, by mucoid interstitial ground substance. In contrast to neurofibromas, the nuclei of fibroblasts in nodular fasciitis are not sharply twisted, wire-like collagen bundles are absent, and vascular clefts and extravasated red cells are associated with tumor myxoid material and chronic inflammatory infiltrates.

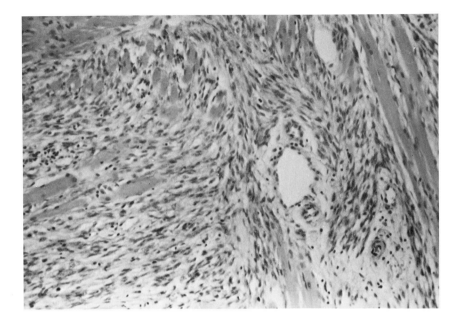

Fig. 7-7 Focal proliferative myositis in a child, showing regenerating muscle fibers, interstitial inflammation, and fibrosis. (H&E x 180).

Nodular fasciitis can be mistaken for a malignant tumor of muscle origin. In sections stained with hematoxylin and eosin, the cytoplasm of rhabdomyoblasts and malignant smooth muscle cells tends to be more eosinophilic and more abundant than that of young fibroblasts, while the cell borders are much more sharply defined. In addition, rhabdomyosarcomas virtually never arise in the subcutaneous tissues.

The distinction between juvenile xanthogranuloma and nodular fasciitis may cause diagnostic difficulty. Slit-like clefts, extravasated red cells, and mucoid interstitial ground substance are findings that suggest a diagnosis of nodular fasciitis. A finding of Touton giant cells favors a diagnosis of xanthogranuloma.

Not infrequently, nodular fasciitis is confused with aggressive fibromatosis (extra-abdominal desmoid). Grossly, aggressive fibromatosis is a large tumor, usually exceeding 5 cm. in diameter, whereas nodular fasciitis is seldom larger than 5 cm. in diameter, and is usually less than 3 cm. Aggressive fibromatoses tend to affect muscles, deep fascia, aponeuroses, and tendons, while sparing the subcutaneous tissues.

Histologically, it may be difficult to differentiate nodular fasciitis from aggressive fibromatosis, particularly in the case of deeply seated intra-muscular lesions. Aggressive fibromatoses rarely have a prominent myxoid ground substance or an S-shaped pattern of fibroblasts, and should not exhibit large cleft-like spaces. On the other hand, extrava-sated red cells or micro-hemorrhages are frequent in aggressive fibro-matoses. Confusion between these two entities is most likely when small and inadequate biopsies are submitted without information concerning the size of the tumor.

The so-called inflammatory pseudotumors of the buccal mucosal tissues of children described by Liston, Dehner, and others[47] are, in our judgement, more properly classified as variants of nodular fasciitis.

TREATMENT AND PROGNOSIS

Superficial lesions of nodular fasciitis are best treated by simple local excision. Deeper lesions, because of their less well-delineated margins, may require a wider or more radical local excision. Nodular fasciitis has been shown to be wholly benign,[43;47] and the prognosis is excellent.

In reviewing the literature on the subject of recurrence, Klein-stiver and Rodriquez[48] reported a 7 percent recurrence rate in 115 cases subjected to a follow-up. Nine of the 895 cases documented in Allen's review[42] (or one percent) recurred; while of the patients followed by Hutter and associates[49] (including 26 cases followed for 5 to 20 years), none recurred.

In patients who do not undergo treatment (no local excision), the nodules do undergo total involution. This behavior pattern clearly suggests that nodular fasciitis is a self-limiting inflammatory reaction of fascia.

FIBROSARCOMA

Synonyms

1. Infantile fibrosarcoma
2. Juvenile fibrosarcoma
3. Congenital fibrosarcoma

INCIDENCE

Fibrosarcoma is a rather uncommon malignancy, accounting for only 0.5 percent of all malignancies and 5.5 percent of malignant soft tissue sarcomas.[50] The head and neck region is an area of relative predisposition for fibrosarcomas occurring in the first 15 years of life. Soule and Pritchard reviewed the clinicopathologic characteristics of fibrosarcoma in 110 infants and children and found that 20 percent of the cases occurred in the head and neck area.[51] Chung and Enzinger[52] reported a 13 percent incidence of fibrosarcoma in the head and neck region in a review of 53 cases of infantile fibrosarcoma.

Fibrosarcoma of the jaws is most common in the mandible. The lesion is extremely rare in soft tissues of the oral cavity. O'Day and co-workers[53] documented only 21 oral soft tissue fibrosarcomas, including six of their own, in a review of the literature.

AGE AND SEX

The vast majority of the fibrosarcomas of infants and children are diagnosed within the first five years of life. Of the 110 patients studied by Soule and Pritchard, 68 patients were in the first five years of life at the time of tumor discovery, 13 were in the second five years of life, and 29 were in the third five years of life. These same authors reported that the number of patients in which tumors were present at birth is probably biased because congenital lesions are likely to be reported as single cases rather than being included in a series encompassing all age groups. Over half of all tumors manifesting in the first five years of life are diagnosed during the first five months of life.[52] The studies of Soule and Pritchard,[51] and Chung and Enzinger[52] document a very slight male predisposition for all childhood fibrosarcomas regardless of anatomic site.

Eversole and associates[54] reviewed four fibrosarcomas affecting the jaws or the soft tissue of the oral cavity in a thorough review of the literature in 1973. Eight out of 34 patients (20 percent) were children, with the youngest being one week old and the oldest, 8 years of age. The mandible was by far the most common site. These authors suggested that the majority of oral fibrosarcomas are not of soft tissue origin, but rather are periosteal fibrosarcomas.

PATHOGENESIS

The cause of fibrosarcoma is unknown although there are occasional reports of fibrosarcoma arising in burn scars or at the site of a chronically draining sinus tract. A hereditary predisposition has been proposed, but remains unproven. The possibility of radiation-induced fibrosarcoma must be considered when, following radiation therapy, a tumor, formerly quiescent for a long time and thus regarded as dormant, suddenly grows. Soule and Pritchard[51] documented one such case in their review of 110 cases. In addition, Hume and associates[55] described the "reactivated fibrosarcoma", following radiation therapy, of a patient originally affected with a lesion in the neck when one-and-a-half-years-old.

CLINICAL FINDINGS

The primary clinical symptom for the vast majority of children with fibrosarcoma is that of a mass or swelling in the soft tissues. Soft tissue fibrosarcomas undergo so rapid an enlargement that the skin overlying the lesion may appear tense, shiny red, or ulcerated. Tumors in the head and neck are usually discovered prior to reaching 4 cm. in diameter.[52] These tumors are usually poorly-circumscribed with a fusiform, polypoid, or disk-like shape. The tumor may extend with multiple processes into surrounding tissue; rarely is there any suggestion of a capsule.

Cut surfaces range from a mixture of pale pink to gray, white, or tan. Myxoid areas may be observed along with areas of tumor necrosis or cystic degeneration.

Children with fibrosarcoma of the jaws will usually experience pain and/or swelling with occasional symptoms of paresthesia, trismus, or pathologic fracture. The tumor's radiographic appearance is usually one of a diffuse destructive radiolucency with root surfaces in the area exhibiting erosion.[56] The site of origin within the jaws remains obscure, although the periodontal ligament has been suggested as the most likely site. We agree with other investigators who consider endosteal mandibular and maxillary fibrosarcoma a distinct, although rare, pathologic entity separate and distinct from all other bone sarcomas.[11;56;57] This concept is not universally shared among pathologists.

Fibrosarcomas of the subcutaneous tissues of the chin and angle of the mandible are more common in children than adults, and they appear to be much more aggressive biologically than fibrosarcomas which arise from the periosteum of the maxilla or mandible.[11]

Fibrosarcomas of the tonsil and hypopharynx are exceedingly rare in adults and children.[11] In contrast to this finding, fibrosarcoma of the larynx is reported to be the most common mesenchymal malignancy of the larynx.[58]

LIGHT MICROSCOPY

Childhood and adult fibrosarcomas show essentially the same histologic features, although Chung and Enzinger reported the cells of the tumors in fibrosarcomas of children tend to be less mature than in adults.[52]

The classic histological features are those of an anaplastic spindle-cell neoplasm with cells primarily arranged in a herringbone pattern. The degree of cellularity and spindling is dependent upon the degree of cellular anaplasia.

Fibrosarcomas may be extremely well-differentiated, undifferentiated, or present a pattern of moderate differentiation somewhere between the two extremes.[59;60] Those tumors that are labeled *well-differentiated* usually show an interwoven texture of well-differentiated cells and fibers. Fibroblasts appear regular in size and shape, and the nuclear and cytoplasmic tinctorial qualities of the cell are usually rather uniform. Well-developed collagen, arranged in bands and fascicles, generally surrounds tumor cells, and mitoses are rare.

Undifferentiated fibrosarcomas are richly cellular and fibroblasts and their product are quite sparse. Typical mitotic figures are frequent and tumor giant cells may be prominent.

Moderately differentiated fibrosarcoma usually shows a so-called herringbone distribution of cells; mitoses are sparse and ground substance and collagen are evident (Fig. 7-8), but not as prominent as in its well-differentiated counterpart (Fig. 7-9).

Some authors reported that a chronic inflammatory infiltrate is nearly always associated with juvenile fibrosarcoma, and that it is so prominent a feature, it enables the most lucid distinction to be made of the juvenile form from the adult form of the disease.[51] Chung and Enzinger reported a striking pericytoma-like vascular pattern in several of their infantile fibrosarcomas, and also commented that, in the majority of their cases, tumor cells appeared much less mature and less well-oriented than in adult type fibrosarcomas.[52]

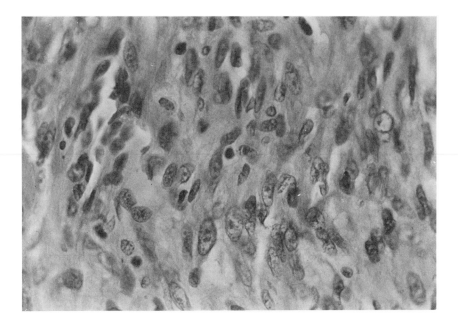

Fig. 7-8 High-power photomicrograph of fibrosarcoma showing abundant ground substance. (H&E x 440).

Dahl and associates[61] have described two forms of fibrosarcoma in children: desmoplastic and medullary. They pointed out that the tumors described as desmoplastic were locally aggressive and histologically similar to fibrosarcoma in adults. They observed no recurrence or metastatic tumor in three of their patients whose tumors were so classified. They classified seven tumors as medullary type and suggested that these tumors were less aggressive biologically than the desmoplastic type. Batsakis[58] emphasized that no histological feature or group of features has been successfully related to the clinical behavior, or the prediction of biologic course, for fibrosarcoma.

ELECTRON MICROSCOPY

Fibroblasts in fibrosarcoma exhibit no specific ultrastructural features. They are, however, characteristically well-endowed with rough endoplasmic reticulum and it is this feature, more than anything else,

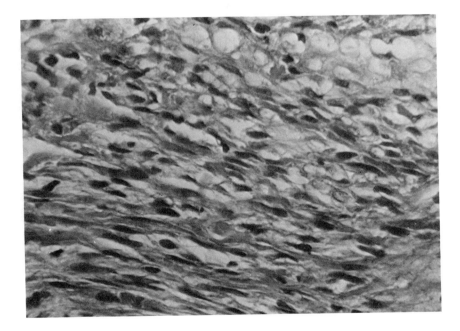

Fig. 7-9 Moderately well-differentiated fibrosarcoma of the neck. (H&E x 260).

that facilitates their identification. Activated fibroblasts (myofibroblasts) often display numerous fine filaments in their peripheral cytoplasm, attachment plaques, foci of basal lamina-like material, pinocytotic vesicles and an occasional poorly-developed cell junction. Fibrocytic neoplasms may display the features of either quiescent or activated cells, or both. Although they tend to be less well-differentiated, the cells of fibrosarcoma (Fig. 7-10) cannot be reliably distinguished from those of the various benign fibrocytic lesions.

Electron microscopy is often helpful in distinguishing fibrosarcoma from other malignant spindle cell tumors.[62] Problems may arise, however, in distinguishing neoplastic myofibroblasts from poorly-differentiated smooth muscle cells, and it is worth mentioning that malignant Schwann cells also tend to lose their characteristic features and more closely come to resemble fibroblasts. Careful integration of the electron microscopic with the light microscopic findings, always advisable, is particularly important when encountering these troublesome lesions.

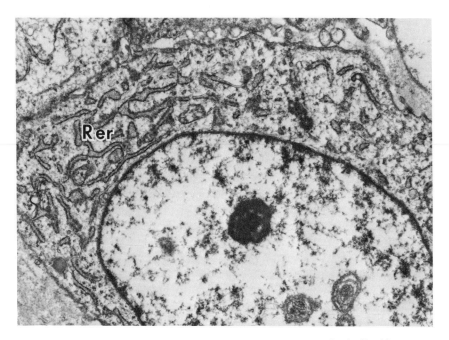

Fig. 7-10 Although somewhat less prominent than in non-neoplastic fibroblasts, abundant rough endoplasmic reticulum (Rer) remains the most distinctive feature of fibrosarcoma cells. (EM x 16,000).

DIFFERENTIAL DIAGNOSIS

The pathologist faced with differential diagnosis of a fibroblastic lesion in the child has a rather broad group of lesions to consider. Rhabdomyosarcoma, liposarcoma, spindle cell lipoma, nodular fasciitis, neurofibrosarcoma, and desmoplastic juvenile fibromatosis (or desmoid tumor of the head and neck) are frequent diagnostic considerations. Differentiation of fibrosarcoma from nodular fasciitis, neurofibrosarcoma, and liposarcoma were discussed under the section Nodular Fasciitis.

Differentiation of juvenile desmoplastic fibromatosis from well-differentiated fibrosarcoma is frequently a very difficult problem. We agree with MacKay[63] who, in discussing the fibromatoses as a clinico-pathological concept, stated that non-metastasizing fibrosarcoma and fibrosarcoma grade I should not be used as synonyms for juvenile fibromatosis. Melrose and Abrams[64] also share this point of view with regard to lesions of the jaws. Very likely, the best rule to follow when faced with a diagnosis of fibrosarcoma versus juvenile desmoplastic fibromatosis is to recall the original histological parameters described by Stout for the latter lesion.[34] He succinctly stated, "...if a fibroblastic tumor has cells that are well differentiated, with no anaplasia and minimal, or no mitoses, and if there is considerable collagen and/or reticulin separating the tumor cells in children less than 16 years of age when the growth first manifests itself, then the lesion represents a juvenile fibromatosis (desmoid fibromatosis)." If Stout's criteria are followed, the diagnosis of well-differentiated fibrosarcoma should be made only if mitotic activity is present, if there is nuclear pleomorphism, or if vascular invasion is observed. It also should be remembered that hypercellularity of a fibrous neoplasm in a child does not necessarily imply potential malignant behavior.

Fibrous histiocytoma probably has been given more synonyms than any other pathologic entity in the medical literature. Common synonyms include: subepidermal nodular fibrosis, dermatofibroma, histiocytoma, and sclerosing hemangioma. The occurrence of this tumor in children indicates a predisposition of the head and neck and is most commonly encountered as a lesion involving the dermis.

The lesion is characterized histologically by a proliferation of foamy histiocytes, multinucleated giant cells, and fibroblast-like cells with little, if any, evidence of a storiform pattern (Fig. 7-11). This lack of a storiform arrangement distinguishes the lesion from the more aggressive, low grade malignancy, *dermatofibrosarcoma protuberans*, which only occasionally occurs in the head and neck of children.

Fibrous histiocytomas of the deep tissues of the head and neck, those involving bone, and the true malignant fibrous histiocytoma described by Batsakis,[11] and Kauffman and Stout,[65] are exceedingly rare in children in the head and neck.

Electron microscopic studies[66-82] have failed to resolve the controversy regarding the histogenesis of fibrous histiocytoma. The spindle cells, in general, closely resemble fibrocytes (Fig. 7-12), but are often somewhat plumper and may contain greater numbers of lysosomes and lipid inclusions than are normally present in this cell type. Myofibrocytic modulation is frequently observed. The amount of collagen present in malignant fibrous histiocytoma is often less than that seen in fibrosarcomas.[68] The larger epithelioid cells and multinucleated giant cells more closely resemble histiocytes (Fig. 7-13). Undifferentiated cells and "transitional forms" (Fig. 7-14) may also be present.

The most common and difficult problem in differential diagnosis is the distinction of malignant fibrous histiocytoma from other neoplasms showing a comparable degree of cellular pleomorphism (e.g.,

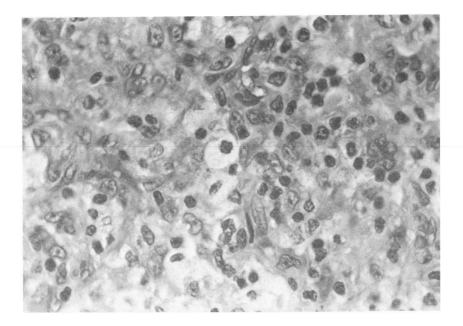

Fig. 7-11 Benign fibrous histiocytoma, showing admixture of foamy histocytes, fibroblastic-appearing cells and hemorrhage. (H&E x 280).

pleomorphic liposarcoma, pleomorphic carcinoma, pleomorphic rhab-domyosarcoma).[83] Pleomorphic rhabdomyosarcoma is the alternative light microscopic diagnosis given most frequent consideration among patients in childhood. Caution must be exercised here, as the deeply eosinophilic giant cells of malignant fibrous histiocytoma (which can exhibit longitudinal striations) may easily be mistaken for rhabdomy-oblasts. The distinction, however, can usually be noted quite easily with electron microscopy. The large cells of pleomorphic rhabdomyosarcoma have been shown to represent the most well-differentiated forms in the spectrum of rhabdomyoblastic differentiations[84] and can be expected to exhibit, even when cross striations cannot be demonstrated by light microscopy, specific myofilaments and Z-band material. The cells of malignant fibrous histiocytoma, on the other hand, display only the nonspecific features commonly associated with histiocytes.

TREATMENT AND PROGNOSIS

Although disagreements over diagnostic terminology persist, fortunately there is general agreement on therapy of fibrosarcoma in

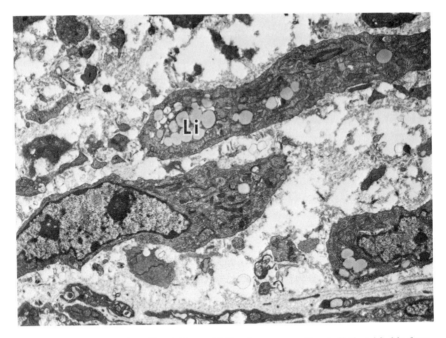

Fig. 7-12 The spindle cells of fibrous histiocytomas are often indistinguishable from those of fibrocytic tumors, but may contain more lipid (Li) and/or lysosomes. Collagen is often relatively sparse. (EM x 6,500).

children. Complete wide local excision with a generous border of clinically or radiographically normal tissue is necessary for primary and recurrent tumors. Soule and Pritchard[51] reported that children with congenital fibrosarcoma and those in whom lesions develop before the first five years of life have a 7.3 percent chance of dying of their tumor or developing metastatic disease even though the local recurrence rate is only 43 percent. Chung and Enzinger[52] reported a five-year survival-rate of 84 percent in their review of 53 cases of infantile fibrosarcoma. These same authors concluded that adjuvant radiotherapy or chemotherapy should be reserved for those rare examples of infantile fibrosarcoma that have recurred or metastasized.

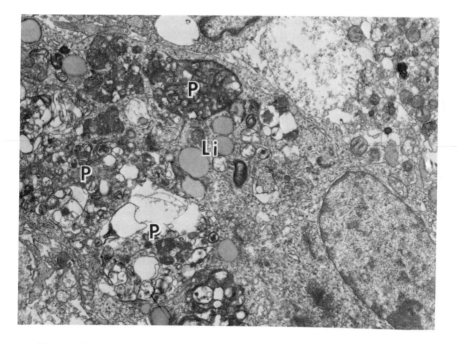

Fig. 7-13 Lysosomes, phagosomes (P) and lipid (Li) are frequently present in large "histiocytes." (EM x 13,100).

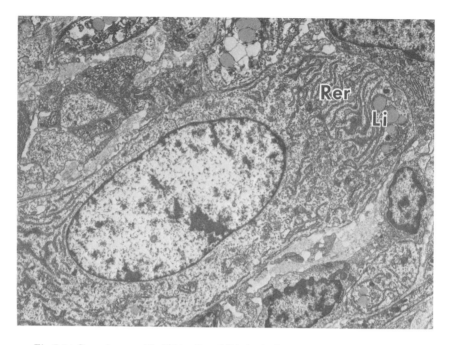

Fig 7-14 Some large epithelioid cells exhibit both the prominent rough endoplasmic reticulum (Rer) characteristic of fibrocytes and the lysosomes and lipid (Li) more commonly associated with histiocytes. (EM x 6,400).

HISTIOCYTOSIS X

Synonyms

1. Eosinophilic granuloma
2. Hand-Schuller-Christian syndrome
3. Letterer-Siwe disease
4. Langerhans cell disease
5. Reticuloendotheliosis (non-lipid)

INCIDENCE

No reliable data exists on the incidence of this disease or group of diseases in the head and neck region. Temporal bone and/or middle ear involvement is said to occur in 15-to-40 percent of cases of multifocal and disseminated disease. In a study of 127 cases between 1941 and 1975, the Boston Children's Hospital group recorded 57 cases (or 45 percent) with lesions of the head and neck region. Gingival lesions occurred in 24 of 63 cases with Stage III disease.[85]

AGE AND SEX

In the same study, generalized or multifocal disease occurred with greatest frequency in children less than three years of age (70 percent) with a male predisposition in a ratio of 1.6-to-1.[85]

PATHOGENESIS

There is great confusion in the nosonomy of these diseases, but, we view a Langerhans cell as a chief element of the pathological process which is not yet classified as neoplasm or reaction. The Langerhans cell is a dendritic histiocyte with an ultrastructurally evident, specific cytoplasmic organelle of undetermined origin and function.[86] The Langerhans cell of Histiocytosis X shares surface antigenic determinants with thymocytes[87] and certain neural cells.[88] Proliferation of Langerhans cells is usually associated with lymphoid cells, including plasma cells and eosinophils in varying numbers. One suspects the Histiocytosis X spectrum of disease of being an aberrant reaction associated with an as yet undefined, abnormal immunological function. The basic cellular disturbance in this syndrome may lie in a lymphoid cell and the Langerhans cell may be recruited secondarily. Thymic abnormalities are probably important in pathogenesis.[89,90]

CLINICAL FINDINGS

Head and neck involvement in Histiocytosis X may take several forms. A draining ear, due to middle ear and/or temporal bone involvement, with or without infection, is common in disseminated disease. Lymph node involvement may be an isolated lesion, part of a more widespread adenopathy, or may be confined to nodes, draining a site of osseous disease (osteo-lymphatic form).[91] Gingival lesions are often associated with adjacent bone involvement and loosening of nearby teeth, with infection, and with radiological changes of suspended teeth (Fig. 7-15).

Evidence of disseminated disease is usually present in patients with Histiocytosis X of the head and neck, who may also manifest rash, diabetes insipidus, hepatosplenomegaly, etc. Eosinophilia and hyper-triglyceridemia may be present. Aberrations of conventional tests of immunologic function are not evident; however, autocytotoxicity may be present without demonstrable quantitative or qualitative aberrations of suppressor T cells.[89] A diagnosis of Histiocytosis X requires careful evaluation of the patient for the extent of disease and detection of organ dysfunction, as disseminated disease (double symptomatic or anatomic site involvement of at least two extraosseous organs) is associated with chronicity and serious sequelae and may be fatal.[85,91]

LIGHT MICROSCOPIC FINDINGS

The lesion is composed of Langerhans cells associated with eosinophils, neutrophils, lymphocytes, plasma cells, and fibroblasts (Figs. 7-16, 7-17). The proportion of cells of each type varies and is influenced by the stage and duration of disease. Multinucleated giant cells (possible fusion products of Langerhans cells) are present and there is often necrosis, variable fibrosis, hemorrhage, and hemosiderosis. Macrophages with vacuoles or nuclear debris in the cytoplasm are present but are rarely prominent in these lesions until late in the course of disease. The Langerhans cell, by light microscopy, is a mononuclear element, approximately 12μ in largest diameter, having a moderate amount of homogeneous pink granular cytoplasm and distinct cell margins. The nucleus is often folded, dented, or polylobulated and has an irregular granular chromatin pattern. One to three basophilic nucleoli of moderate size are the rule.

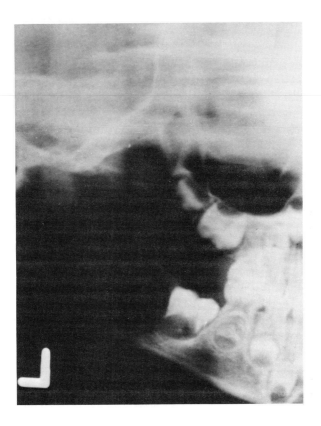

Fig. 7-15 Radiograph showing mandibular lytic lesion and "floating teeth" in case of Histiocytosis X.

ELECTRON MICROSCOPY

Electron microscopy can be of value for the purpose of confirming a diagnosis of Histiocytosis X when it becomes possible for Langerhans-type histiocytes to be identified by the characteristic organelle, the Birbeck granule (Fig. 7-18). These cells are not unique to this disease process and therefore their identification is of relevance only when considered in the proper context. It has been reported that Birbeck granules are not present in all cases of Histiocytosis X, and that their presence might be a favorable prognostic sign. However, our experience

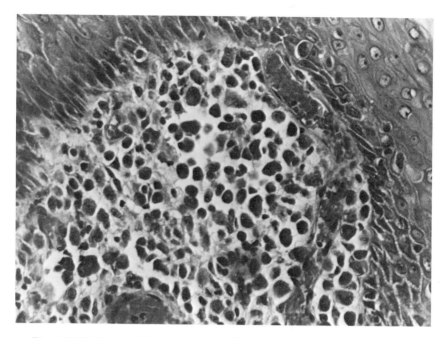

Fig. 7-16 Histiocytosis X: submucosal proliferative and/or infiltrative lesion composed of Langerhans cells and small numbers of leukocytes. Note the junctional involvement. (H&E x 250).

and that of others does not support the preceeding contention, as the Birbeck granule has been found to be a constant feature of this group of diseases.[92]

Ultrastructural findings can play an important role in differentiating other morphologically similar "lymphoreticuloses" from Histiocytosis X. These disorders, which may differ in prognosis, do not feature Langerhans cells.[93]

DIFFERENTIAL DIAGNOSIS

Identification of reactive histiocytic lesions constitutes the most significant of histological differential problems. These lesions lack Langerhans cells and an inciting agent can often be found. Juvenile xanthogranuloma, when disseminated (a rare condition), can be confused with Histiocytosis X.

TREATMENT AND PROGNOSIS

Prognosis is related to age, extent of disease, and evidence of organ dysfunction in the presence of disseminated disease.[85,94] No

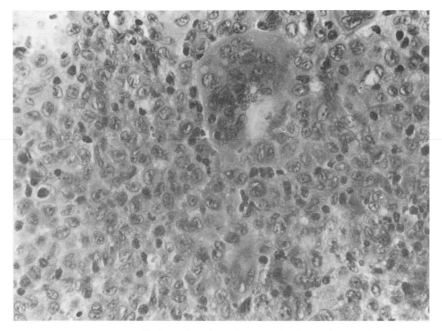

Fig. 7-17 Histiocytosis X: Lymph node replacement by Langerhans cells and leukocytes. Giant cells appear to be of Langerhans cell evolution. (H&E x 250).

histological indicator of prognosis is currently accepted, although attempts have been made to find such indicators.[95] When a diagnosis of Histiocytosis X is made, the patient should be evaluated by skeletal survey for bone lesions (as bone lesions are generally a favorable prognostic indicator) and should have organ function studies performed for Lahey's scoring.[94] In general, disease confined to one organ has a favorable prognosis and the older the patient is at the time of diagnosis, the better the prognosis in disseminated Histiocytosis X. Splenomegaly and thrombocytopenia indicate a bad prognosis.[85,91]

Isolated lesions are radiosensitive and may respond to steroid therapy when non-deforming surgery is not feasible.

There is no proven therapy for disseminated disease and the extremely variable course dictates that prognostic information be given with caution.

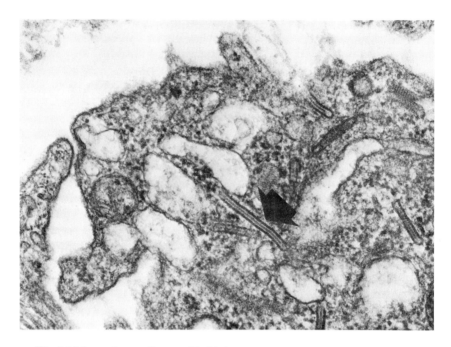

Fig. 7-18 Langerhans cells resemble histiocytes of other varieties, with the exception of their additional feature, a unique cytoplasmic organelle, the Birbeck granule (arrow). (EM x 68,000).

JUVENILE XANTHOGRANULOMA

Synonyms

1. Juvenile xanthoma
2. Nevoxanthoma
3. Nevoxanthoendothelioma

INCIDENCE

Reliable incidence figures are non-existent. In our own pediatric pathology laboratory (The Denver Children's Hospital), we see two to three cases a year out of a total of 2,800 recorded cases. About half of these lesions involve the scalp or other head and neck skin sites.

AGE AND SEX

Most lesions occur in the first year of life. Lesions are not uncommon at birth and some may occur in teenagers. No racial or sexual predisposition is known.

PATHOGENESIS

Pathogenesis is obscure, but there is no relationship to hyperlipidemia or metabolic lipidoses. Endocrine influence is suggested for the incidence of this lesion by virtue of: its occurrence in the newborn; by its commonly occurring spontaneous regression over months or years, and also by a regression usually seen about the time of puberty.

CLINICAL FINDINGS

Lesions may be single or multiple discoid papules of pink-to-red color, ranging from 0.2 to 5.0 cm. in size. The scalp is the most commonly involved site, but extremity lesions are also common. Multiple nodules usually erupt within a short period of time of one another. Lesions of ocular iris,[96] conjunctiva, tongue, vulva, larynx, lung, and pericardium have been reported.[97]

Serum lipid and acute phase reactant levels are normal and patients are usually afebrile. A preoperative diagnosis of hemangioma is commonly made.

The uncommon association between juvenile xanthogranuloma and "cafe au lait" spots in the patient and/or relatives without other stigmata of neurofibromatosis is unexplained.[98]

Gradual involution of lesions over months or years is the rule. However, large lesions may involute incompletely and remain static.

LIGHT MICROSCOPIC FINDINGS

The nodule usually spares epidermis and lies in the mid- to superficial dermis, where cellular elements of the lesions are poorly demarcated from adjacent tissues. An aggregate of spindle fibrocytes, histiocytes, foam cells, and varying numbers of lymphocytes and eosinophils contains the characteristic multinucleated histiocyte, the Touton giant cell (Fig. 7-19).[99] This giant cell has a ring of uniform nuclei and may show varying degrees of cytoplasmic vacuolation between nuclear rings and plasmalemma. Langerhans cells are absent. In early stages of lesion development, histiocytes predominate but, with time, foam cells, fibrocytes, and collagen become more abundant. Well-organized granulomatous morphology is unusual.

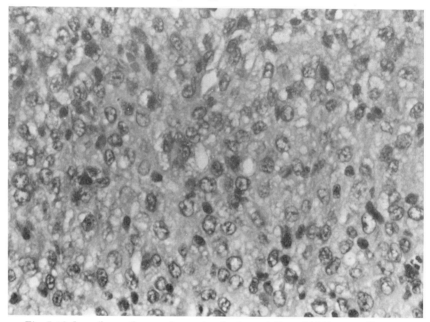

Fig. 7-19 Juvenile xanthogranuloma. A mixed population of histiocytes, fibrocytes, and leukocytes is associated with a poorly-developed giant cell. (H&E x 250).

DIFFERENTIAL DIAGNOSIS

Differential diagnosis includes the various granulomas, sclerosing hemangioma, fibrous histiocytoma, Langerhans cell histiocytoma, and fibromatoses. The presence of foam cells and Touton giant cells forms the basis of distinction, which is rarely difficult. Histiocytes are usually lysozyme positive, in contrast to the lysozyme negative Langerhans cells.

TREATMENT AND PROGNOSIS

The course is benign, with involution of lesions commonly found. Rare visceral involvement may be associated with morbidity, due to mass effect, but is usually self-limited. Surgical excision for diagnostic purposes is curative in solitary lesions, and patience is usually rewarded with regression, when multiple lesions are present.

References

1. Stout, A.P. *Tumors of the Soft Tissues. Atlas of Tumor Pathology*, section 2, fascicle 5. Washington, D.C.: Armed Forces Institute of Pathology, 1953.
2. Greer, R.O. and Carpenter, M. "Surgical oral pathology at the University of Colorado School of Dentistry: a survey of 400 cases." *J. Colo. Dent. Assoc.* 54(1976): 13-16.
3. Barker, D.S. and Lucas, R.B. "Localized fibrous overgrowths of the oral mucosa." *Br. J. Oral Surg.* 5(1967): 86-92.
4. Hayward, J.R. "Multiple recurrent fibro-osseous epulides." *Int. J. Oral Surg.* 2(1973): 115-121.
5. Gusterson, B.A. and Greenspan, J.S. "Multiple polypoid conditions of the oral mucosa." *Br. J. Oral Surg.* 12(1974): 91-95.
6. Shafer, W.G.; Hine, J.K. and Levy, B.M. *A Textbook of Oral Pathology*, 3rd ed. Philadelphia: W.B. Saunders, 1974.
7. Cundiff, E.G. "Peripheral ossifying fibroma. A review of 365 cases." M.S.D. thesis, Indiana University, 1972.
8. Greer, R.O. and Zarlengo, W.D. "Peripheral odontogenic fibroma. A reappraisal of biologic behavior." *J. Colo. Dent. Assoc.* 57(1979): 11-14.
9. Livingston, S. and Livingston, H.C. "Diphenyldydantoin gingival hyperplasia." *Am. J. Dis. Child.* 117(1969): 265-275.
10. Smith, R.M.; Turner, J.E. and Robbins, M.L. *Atlas of Oral Pathology*. St. Louis: C.V. Mosby, 1981.
11. Batsakis, J.G. *Tumors of the Head and Neck. Clinical and Pathologic Considerations*, 2nd ed. Baltimore: Williams and Wilkins, 1979.
12. Winstock, D. "Hereditary gingivo-fibromatosis." *Br. J. Oral Surg.* 2(1965): 59-64.
13. Ramon, Y.; Berman, W. and Bubis, J.J. "Gingival fibromatosis combined with cherubism." *Oral Surg.* 24(1967): 435-448.
14. Giansanti, J.S.; McKenzie, W.R. and Owens, F.C. "Gingival fibromatosis, hypertelorism, antimongoloid obliquity, multiple telangiectases and cafe au lait pigmentation. A unique combination of developmental anomalies." *J. Periodontol.* 44(1973): 299-302.
15. Coventry et al. "Congenital muscular torticollis (wryneck)." *Postgrad. Med.* 28(1960): 383-392.
16. Stout, A.P. "Juvenile fibromatoses." *Cancer* 7(1954): 953-977.

17. Dehner, L.P. and Askin, F.B. "Tumors of fibrous tissue origin in childhood. A clinicopathologic study of cutaneous soft tissue neoplasms in 66 children." *Cancer* 38(1976): 888-899.

18. MacKenzie, D.H. *The Differential Diagnosis of Fibroblastic Disorders.* Oxford: Blackwell Scientific, 1970.

19. Enzinger, F.M. "Fibrous Tumors of Infancy." In *Tumors of Bone and Soft Tissue*, pp. 375-396. Chicago: Year Book Medical, 1965.

20. Stout, A.P. "Pseudosarcomatous fasciitis in children." *Cancer* 14(1961): 1216-1222.

21. Masson, J.K. and Soule, D.H. "Desmoid tumors of the head and neck." *Am. J. Surg.* 112(1966): 615-622.

22. Enzinger, F.M. "Fibrous Tumors of Infancy." In *Tumors of Bone and Soft Tissue*, pp. 375-396. Chicago: Year Book Medical, 1965.

23. Jaffe, H.L. *Tumors and Tumorous Conditions of the Bones and Joints.* Philadelphia: Lea and Febiger, 1958.

24. Whitesides, T.E. and Ackerman, L.V. "Desmoplastic fibroma." *J. Bone Joint Surg.* 42A(1960): 1143-1150.

25. Rabhan, W.N. and Rosai, J. "Desmoplastic fibroma." *J. Bone Joint Surg.* 50(1968): 487-502.

26. Kawanishi et al. "Desmoplastic fibroma of the femur." *Orthop. Surg. Tokyo* 14(1969): 275-280.

27. Matsumori et al. "Primary desmoplastic fibroma of the femur." *Orthop. Surg. Tokyo* 23(1972): 275-281.

28. Taguchi, N. and Kaneda, T. "Desmoplastic fibroma of the mandible. Report of a case." *J. Oral Surg.* 38(1980): 441-444.

29. Freedman et al. "Desmoplastic fibroma (fibromatosis) of the jawbones." *Oral Surg.* 46(1978): 386-395.

30. Jaffe, H.L. *Tumors and Tumorous Conditions of Bones and Joints.* Philadelphia: Lea and Febiger, 1958.

31. Sugiura, I. "Desmoplastic fibroma: case report and review of the literature." *J. Bone Joint Surg.* 58A(1976): 126-130.

32. Touraine, A. and Ruel, H. "La polyfibromatose hereditaire." *Annales de Dermatologie et de Syphiligraphie* 5(1945): 1-5.

33. Das Gupta, T.K.; Grasfield, R.D. and O'Hara, J. "Extra-abdominal desmoids: a clinicopathologic study." *Ann. Surg.* July(1969): 109-121.

34. Stout, A.P. "Fibrosarcoma in infants and children." *Cancer* 15(1962): 1028-1040.

35. Jaffe, H.L. *Tumors and Tumorous Conditions of the Bones and Joints.* Philadelphia: Lea and Febiger, 1958.

36. Rabhan, W.N. and Rosai, J. "Desmoplastic fibroma: report of ten cases and review of the literature." *J. Bone Joint Surg.* 50A(1968): 487-502.

37. MacKenzie, D.H. "The fibromatoses: a clinicopathologic concept." *Br. Med. J.* 4(1972): 277-281.

38. Hunt, R.T.; Morgan, H.C. and Ackerman, L.V. "Principles in the management of extra-abdominal desmoids." *Cancer* 13(1960): 825-836.

39. Conley, J.; Healey, W.V. and Stout, A.P. "Fibromatosis of the head and neck." *Am. J. Surg.* 112(1966): 609-614.

40. Konwaler, B.E.; Keasbey, L.E. and Kaplan, L. "Subcutaneous psuedosarcomatous fibromatosis (fasciitis). Report of 8 cases." *Am. J. Clin. Pathol.* 25(1955): 241-252.

41. Schreiber, M.M.; Shapiro, S.I. and Sampsel, J. "Pseudosarcomatous fibromatosis (fasciitis)." *Arch. Dermatol.* 92(1965):661-665.

42. Allen, P.W. "Nodular fasciitis." *Pathology* 4(1972): 9-26.

43. Stout, A.P. "Pseudosarcomatous fasciitis in children." *Cancer* 14(1961): 1216-1222.

44. Price, E.B.; Silliphant, W.M. and Shuman, R. "Nodular fasciitis. A clinicopathologic analysis of 65 cases." *Am. J. Pathol.* 35(1961): 122-136.

45. Vickers, R.A. "Mesenchymal (Soft Tissue) Tumors of the Oral Region." In *Thomas's Oral Pathology*, 6th ed., edited by R.J. Gorlin and H.M. Goldman, pg. 864. St. Louis: C.V. Mosby, 1970.

46. Shuman, R. *Mesenchymal Tumors of Soft Tissues, Pathology*, 6th ed. St. Louis: C.V. Mosby, 1971.

47. Liston et al. "Inflammatory pseudotumors in the buccal tissues of children." *Oral Surg.* 51(1981): 287-291.

48. Kleinstiver, B.G. and Rodriquez, H.A. "Nodular fasciitis. A study of forty-five cases and review of the literature." *J. Bone Joint Surg.* 50A(1968): 1204-1212.

49. Hutter, R.V.P.; Steward, F.W. and Foote, F.W. "Fasciitis: a report of 70 cases with follow-up proving the benignity of the lesion." *Cancer* 15(1962): 922-1003.

50. Thompson et al. "Soft tissue sarcomas involving the extremities and limb girdles." *South. Med. J.* 64(1971): 33-44.

51. Soule, E.H. and Pritchard, D.J. "Fibrosarcoma in infants and children. A review of 110 cases." *Cancer* 40(1977): 1711-1721.

52. Chung, E.B. and Enzinger, R.M. "Infantile fibrosarcoma." *Cancer* 38(1976): 729-739.

53. O'Day, R.A.; Soule, E.H. and Goresg, R.J. "Soft tissue sarcomas of the oral cavity." *Mayo Clin. Proc.* 39(1964): 169-181.

54. Eversole, L.R.; Schwartz, W.D. and Sabes, W.R. "Central and Peripheral fibrogenic and neurogenic sarcoma of the oral regions." *Oral Surg.* 36(1973): 49-62.

55. Hume, H.A.; Stevens, L.W. and Erb, W.H. "Fibrosarcoma recurrent after forty years. (Letter to the editor)." *JAMA* 202(1967): 71.

56. Van Blarcom, C.W.; Masson, J.M.K. and Dahlin, D.C. "Fibrosarcoma of the mandible." *Oral Surg.* 32(1971): 428-439.

57. Huvcos, A.G. and Higinbotham, N.L. "Primary fibrosarcoma of bone. A clinicopathologic study of 130 patients." *Cancer* 35(1975): 837-847.

58. Batsakis, J.G. and Fox, J.E. "Supporting tissue neoplasms of the larynx." *Surg. Gynecol. Obstet.* 131(1970): 989-997.

59. Stout, A.P. "Fibrous tumors of the soft tissues." *Minn. Med.* 4(1960): 455-460.

60. Stout, A.P. "Fibrosarcoma. The malignant tumor of fibroblasts." *Cancer* 1(1948): 30-63.

61. Dahl, I.; Save-Soderbergh, J. and Angerwall, L. "Fibrosarcoma in early infancy." *Pathol. Eur.* 8(1973): 193-209.

62. Taxy, J.B. and Battifora, H. "The Electron Microscope in the Study and Diagnosis of Soft Tissue Tumors." In *Diagnostic Electron Microscopy*, edited by B.F. Trump and R.T. Jones, pg. 97. New York: John Wiley and Sons, 1980.

63. Chung, E.B. and Enzinger, F.M. "Infantile Fibrosaroma." *Cancer* 38 (1976): 729-739. (McKay, B. therein cited as personal communication to the authors.)

64. Melrose, R.J. and Abrams, A.M. "Juvenile fibromatosis affecting the jaws. Report of three cases." *Oral Surg.* 49(1980): 317-324.

65. Kauffman, S.L. and Stout, A.P. "Histiocytic tumors (fibrous xanthoma and histiocytoma) in children." *Cancer* 14(1961): 469.

66. Merkow et al. "Ultrastructure of a fibroxanthosarcoma (malignant fibroxanthoma)." *Cancer* 28(1971): 372.

67. Fu et al. "Malignant soft tissue tumors of probable histiocytic origin (malignant fibrous histiocytomas): general considerations and electron microscopic and tissue culture studies." *Cancer* 35(1976): 176.

68. Churg, A.M. and Kahn, L.B. "Myofibroblasts and related cells in malignant fibrous and fibrohistiocytic tumors." *Hum. Pathol.* 8(1977): 205.

69. Saito, R. and Caines, M.J. "Atypical fibrous histiocytoma of the humerus. A light and electron microscopic study." *Am. J. Clin. Pathol.* 68(1977): 409.

70. Taxy, J.B. and Battifora, H. "Malignant fibrous histiocytoma. An electron microscopic study." *Cancer* 40(1977): 254.

71. Alguacil-Garcia, A.; Unni, K.K. and Goellner, J.R. "Malignant fibrous histiocytoma. An ultrastructural study of six cases." *Am. J. Clin. Pathol.* 69(1978): 121

72. Kern et al. "Malignant fibrous histiocytoma of the lung." *Cancer* 44(1979): 1793.

73. Lagace, R.; Delage, C. and Seemayer, T.A. "Myxoid variant of malignant fibrous histiocytoma. Ultrastructural observations." *Cancer* 43(1979): 526.

74. Reddick, R.L.; Michelitch, H. and Triche, T.J. "Malignant soft tissue tumors (malignant fibrous histiocytoma, pleomorphic liposarcoma, and pleomorphic rhabdomyosarcoma): an electron microscopic study." *Hum. Pathol.* 10(1979): 327.

75. Tsuneyoshi, M. and Enjoji, M. "Postirradiation sarcoma (malignant fibrous histisocytoma) following breast carcinoma. An ultrastructural study of case." *Cancer* 45(1979): 1419.

76. Chowdhury et al. "Postirradiation malignant fibrous histiocytoma of the lung. Demonstration of alpha ₁-antitrypsin-like material in neoplastic cells." *Am. J. Clin. Pathol.* 74(1980): 820.

77. Harris, M. "The ultrastructure of benign and malignant fibrous histiocytomas. *Histopathology* 4(1980): 29.

78. Mereino, M.J. and LiVolsi, V.A. "Inflammatory malignant fibrous histiocytoma." *Am. J. Clin. Pathol.* 73(1980): 276.

79. Miller, R.; Kreutner, A., Jr. and Kurtz, S.M. "Malignant inflammatory histiocytoma (inflammatory fibrous histiocytoma). Report of a patient with four lesions." *Cancer* 45(1980): 179.

80. Shapiro, F. "Malignant fibrous histiocytoma of bone: an ultrastructural study." *Ultrastructural Pathology* 2(1981): 33.

81. Carstens, P.H.B. and Schrodt, G.R. "Ultrastructure of sclerosing hemangioma." *Am. J. Pathol.* 77(1974): 377.

82. Katenkamp, D. and Stiller, D. "Cellular composition of so-called dermatofibroma (histiocytoma cutis). *Virchows Arch.* [*Pathol. Anat.*] 367(1975): 325.

83. Weiss, S.W. and Enzinger, F.M. "Malignant fibrous histiocytoma. An analysis of 200 cases." *Cancer* 41(1978): 2250.

84. Mierau, G.W. and Favara, B.E. "Rhabdomyosarcoma in children: Ultrastructural study of 31 cases." *Cancer* 46(1980): 2035.

85. Greenberger et al. "Results of Treatment of 127 Patients with Systemic Histiocytosis (Letterer-Siwe Syndrome, Schuller-Christian Syndrome, and Multifocal Eosinophilic Granuloma)." *Medicine* 60(1981): 311-337.

86. Rowden, G. "The Langerhans Cell." *CRC Critical Reviews in Immunology* 3(Issue 2; December, 1981): 95-180.

87. Murphy et al. "Characterization of Langerhans Cell By the Use of Monoclonal Antibodies." *Lab. Invest.* 45(1981): 465-469.

88. Misugi et al. "S-100 protein in neuroblastoma group tumors." *Lab. Invest.* 46(1982): 110.

89. Osband et al. "Histiocytosis X, Demonstration and Successful Treatments with Thymic Extract." *N. Eng. J. Med.* 304(1981): 146-153.

90. Hamoudi et al. "Thymic Changes in Histiocytosis" *Am. J. Clin. Pathol.* 77(1982): 169-173.

91. Nezelof, C.; Frileux-Herbert, F. and Cronier-Sachot, J. "Disseminated Histiocytosis X. Analysis of Prognostic Factors Based on a Retrospective Study of 50 Cases." *Cancer* 44(1979): 1824-1838.

92. Mierau, G.W.; Favara, B.E. and Brenman, J.M. "Electron Microscopy in Histiocytosis X." *Ultrastructural Pathology* (in press).

93. Favara, B.E. "The Pathology of Histiocytosis." *Am. J. Pediatr. Hematol. Oncol.* 3(1981): 45-56.

94. Lahey, E.A. "Histiocytosis X—An Analysis of Prognostic Factors." *J. Pediatr.* 87(1975): 184-189.

95. Newton, W.A., Jr. and Hamoudi, A.B. "Histocytosis: A Histologic Classification with Clinical Correlation." In *Perspectives in Pediatric Pathology*, pp. 251-283. Chicago: Year Book Medical, 1973.

96. Zimmerman, L.E. "Occular lesions of juvenile xanthogranuloma nevoxanthoendothelioma." *Trans. Am. Acad. Ophthalmol. Otolaryngol.* 69(1965): 412-417.

97. Lottsfeldt, F.I. and Good, R.A. "Juvenile xanthogranuloma with pulmonary lesions." *Pediatrics* 33(1964): 233-238.

98. Mihm, M.C., Jr.; Clark, W.H. and Reed, R.J. "The histiocytic infiltrates of the skin." *Hum. Pathol.* 5(1974): 45-54.

99. Helwig, E.B. and Hackney, V.C. "Juvenile xanthogranuloma (nevoxanthoendothelioma)." *Am. J. Pathol.* 30(1954): 525-630.

Chapter VIII

Giant Cell Lesions of the Oral Mucosa, Jaws and Facial Skeleton

PERIPHERAL GIANT CELL GRANULOMA

Synonyms

1. Giant cell epulis
2. Peripheral giant cell tumor
3. Peripheral giant cell reparative granuloma
4. Myeloid epulis

INCIDENCE

The peripheral giant cell granuloma is a reactive soft tissue lesion of childhood and adolescence nearly always occurring on the gingiva or alveolar mucosa. Bhaskar[1] reported that the lesion comprises 7 to 8 percent of oral tumors in childhood. In a review of 191 tumors of the oral mucosa and jaws in infants and children, Greer and Mierau found that peripheral giant cell granuloma represented 8.3 percent of their total.[2]

AGE AND SEX

Although the average age of patients with peripheral giant cell granuloma is approximately 30 years, the lesion occurs not infrequently in children and adolescents. Greer and Mierau documented peak incidence rates in patients between the ages of 6 through 10 and 16 through 20, when they examined 16 peripheral giant cell granulomas occurring in the first two decades of life.[2] The literature documents the fact that females are affected more often than males,[3-6] and Giansanti and Waldron[7] reported that when all age groups are considered, females are affected almost twice as frequently as males. However, Cooke reported incidence by sex is more or less equal between the ages of 6 and 15.[8] Greer and Mierau found an equal distribution of males and females in their review.[2]

PATHOGENESIS

At one time the peripheral giant cell granuloma was considered to be a true neoplasm.[3] Most investigators now consider the lesion to represent an aberrant proliferative response of tissues to injury. Although a history of trauma is a commonly reported etiologic factor, Giansanti and Waldron were able to document associated trauma in only 21 percent of 61 cases they reviewed.[7] Traumatic injury may frequently include recent extractions or injury from severely broken down and decaying teeth, ill-fitting dental restorations, or subgingival calculus, but Waldron and Giansanti have pointed out that the relatively high numbers of extractions and badly decayed teeth in the population in general would seem to indicate the potential for a greater number of these lesions than are reported if trauma alone was the mitigating factor.[7]

Some observers consider the lesion to be part of a reparative process, and as such, it has been popular to designate the lesion a "reparative granuloma". We agree with the conclusions of Sapp,[9] Batsakis,[10] and Waldron and Shafer[11] who reported that the lesions are histologically indistinguishable from central osseous giant cell lesions, and do not contain distinctive microscopic features setting them aside as distinctively reparative in nature. Cooke[8] considered the lesion to arise in the form of excessive osteogenic granulation tissue from alveolar mucoperiosteum, as a result of chronic irritation. Sapp's[9] comprehensive ultrastructural review of four peripheral giant cell granulomas supports the theory of an osseous origin for the lesion, and the author concludes that the lesion represents the periosteal counterpart of the central giant cell granuloma of bone.

CLINICAL FINDINGS

The tooth-bearing areas of the jaws (gingiva and alveolar mucosa) are the most frequent anatomic sites for the peripheral giant cell granuloma. The lesion occurs more frequently as a mucosal lesion of the mandible than of the maxilla,[10;12] while the anterior portions of the jaws, including the region from the central incisor teeth to the cuspids, are more commonly involved than the premolar-molar regions.

The lesion most often appears as a gingival soft tissue overgrowth (Fig. 8-1). The lesion can range in size from a few millimeters in diameter to as great as ten centimeters in diameter.[2] Both Andersen and co-workers,[6] and Shafer and associates[12] reported that the lesion is most often in the range of 1.5 cm. in diameter when first identified. There is no demonstrable correlation between the size of the lesion and its location.

The consistency of the lesion can range from boggy and edematous to spongy or firm. The lesion is usually a rather well-defined

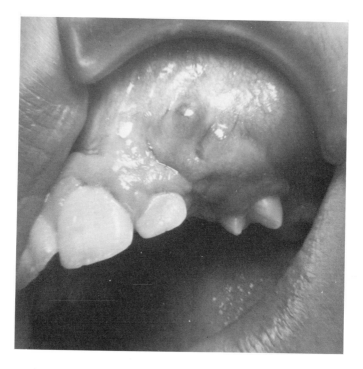

Fig. 8-1 Peripheral giant cell granuloma manifesting as an elevated, hemorrhagic soft tissue nodule. Courtesy of Dr. Sidney Bronstein.

swelling, which is most often sessile, but may rarely be pedunculated. It usually shows a tinctorial mucosal change toward a reddish-blue or deep red color. Surface ulceration is not uncommon, and the lesion frequently bleeds readily upon probing.[6]

Pain is seldom an indicative symptom and only rarely does the presence of a peripheral giant cell granuloma result in local change in the alignment of teeth, delayed tooth eruption, or tooth mobility.

The lesion may cause a radiographically evident "cup- or saucerization" defect in the underlying bone, especially in the edentulous areas;[12] because of this finding, a periapical radiograph may aid in establishing a presumptive clinical diagnosis.

LIGHT MICROSCOPY

Histologically, the peripheral giant cell granuloma consists of a non-encapsulated proliferation of stellate and reticular fibrous connective tissue with a dominance of ovoid or spindle cells and plump endothelial cells. The stroma contains an abundant proliferation of multinucleated giant cells. Supporting stromal cells may show considerable mitotic activity, and capillary proliferation throughout the mass is usually quite prominent. Hemorrhage, chronic inflammatory cells, and hemosiderin are dominant features, and quite frequently, metaplastic bone and calcified structures arranged in globular and trabecular patterns can be identified. The lesion is generally covered totally or partially by stratified squamous epithelium.

Tumor giant cells may show great variation in size, morphology, and the number of nuclei, and the cytoplasm of giant cells can vary from faintly basophilic to deeply eosinophilic. They are commonly intimately associated with small vascular spaces.

ELECTRON MICROSCOPY

Ultrastructurally, the multinucleated giant cells and stromal cells are identical to those found in benign giant cell tumors of other bones.[9] Sapp maintained that the multinucleated cells contain sufficient features in common with osteoclasts to represent a slightly modified form of that cell. Sapp also considered the ultrastructure of stromal cells compatible with the various stages of differentiating osteoprogenitor cells.[9]

DIFFERENTIAL DIAGNOSIS

From a histopathological viewpoint, the peripheral giant cell granuloma holds diagnostic problems, as single giant cells may also be found in other non-neoplastic gingival or alveolar mucosal proliferations. Of the latter, the peripheral fibroma with ossification and the pyogenic granuloma are most notable.[13] The small number of giant cells and lack of erythrocytes and hemosiderin pigment in these two lesions may be helpful in making a distinction between them and the peripheral giant cell granuloma.[6]

TREATMENT AND PROGNOSIS

The peripheral giant cell granuloma is a benign lesion that is usually adequately managed with simple surgical excision to a margin of normal tissue. If only superficial excision is carried out, recurrence is quite possible.[12] Baxter,[3] Cooke,[8] Phillips and Shafer,[14] Standish and Shafer[15] have all reported recurrences in their reviews of large numbers

CENTRAL GIANT CELL GRANULOMA

Synonyms

1. Central giant cell reparative granuloma
2. Giant cell tumor of the jaw

INCIDENCE

Jaffe[16] first suggested the term giant cell reparative granuloma for the intraosseous jaw lesion which had previously been interpreted as benign giant cell tumor. Following his description, the lesion has come to be more commonly called central giant cell granuloma, —the prefix "central" denoting the endosteal origin of the lesion. Its relationship to the so-called true giant cell tumor will be discussed later. The central giant cell granuloma occurs far less commonly than its peripheral soft tissue counterpart. Giansanti and Waldron[7] reported that the soft tissue lesion occurs at least four times as frequently, and Batsakis stated that the central endosteal lesion represents less than one percent of all surgical pathologic accessions.[10] Greer and Mierau documented a 3.6 percent incidence in a review of 191 tumors of the oral mucosa and jaws in children.[2]

AGE AND SEX

The central giant cell granuloma is predominately a disorder of children and young adults, although lesions have been reported in patients in the seventh decade of life.[11] Greer and Mierau recently reviewed the clinicopathologic characteristics of a series of central giant cell granulomas, and found that all of their patients ranged in age from 11 to 20. Waldron and Shafer[11] reported 60 percent of their series of 38 cases occurred in patients less than 30, and Austin and associates[17] reported that 60 percent of the giant cell granulomas they reviewed in a study of 107 giant cell granulomas and related conditions occurred in patients under the age of 20. The lesion is more common in females than males; 68 percent of the 34 cases by Waldron and Shafer were in females, and 59 percent of the 32 cases reviewed by Andersen and co-workers[6] were in females.

PATHOGENESIS

The pathogenesis of central giant cell granuloma has been debated at length since Jaffe proposed that the lesion represented a local reparative reaction, possibly to intramedullary hemorrhage or trauma.[16]

Many individuals consider the benign giant cell tumor of bone and the central giant cell granuloma of the jaws to be similar if not identical lesions.[11;12;18] Batsakis stated that most lesions "diagnosed" as giant cell tumors are in truth giant cell granulomas.[10] Dahlin,[19] however, maintained a clear distinction between the giant cell tumor of bone, which he subdesignated osteoclastoma, and the central giant cell granuloma of the jaws.

Both Dahlin,[19] and Hirschl and Katz[20] have established histological and clinical features that allow for separation of these two entities. These criteria are discussed in detail in the clinical findings and light microscopy sections of this chapter. It is worth noting that in a blind review of microscopic slides from 12 central giant cell granulomas of the jaws and 12 lesions diagnosed as giant cell tumors of long bones accessioned on surgical pathology services at the University of Colorado Schools of Medicine and Dentistry over a 22-year period, one of the authors (ROG) was unable to differentiate between the two lesions using the histologic criteria established by Hirschl and Katz.[20]

However, the aforementioned review did show that age differences between the two lesions were quite distinct. Those lesions diagnosed as central giant cell granulomas were found in patients at least a decade younger than patients in which the lesions were diagnosed as "true giant cell tumors of bone." Follow-up over a six-year-period was available on six of the jaw lesions. None had recurred following excision of the lesion with a margin of normal bone.

Four of the 12 long bone tumor cases were followed for up to 11 years. None had recurred. No consistent surgical procedure was employed to treat the long bone lesions.

In summary, the central giant cell granuloma is thought to result as a response to injury imposed on: the periodontal membrane, osteogenic mesenchyme, dental follicular tissues, or its precursor cells.[10] The giant cell component is considered to be a response to lesional hemorrhage, and as such, the cells are thought to be phagocytic in nature and not neoplastic. On the other hand, true giant cell tumors of long bones are characterized by proliferation of a multinucleated giant cell resulting from fusion of proliferating "neoplastic" mononuclear cells. Thus the lesion is thought by many investigators to be a true neoplasm.[19;21]

CLINICAL FINDINGS

The central giant cell granuloma of the jaws and facial skeleton can appear as innocuously as an asymptomatic lesion discovered on a routine jaw radiographic survey or as boldly as a painful, expansile lesion resulting in considerable jaw deformity. In the vast majority of cases, pain is not a prominent feature.[12] The lesion is common to the tooth-bearing areas of the jaws and occurs far more frequently in the mandible than the maxilla.[6,11] Shafer reported that the anterior segment of the mandible is the most susceptible site, and noted that the lesion not uncommonly crosses the midline.[12]

Lesions of the *facial skeleton* are far less frequent than lesions of the jawbones, although examples have been reported in the ethmoid, sphenoid, and temporal bones.[20] Smith and Ward reviewed a series of 32 "giant cell lesions" of bone treated at the University of California at Los Angeles Medical Center over a 20-year-period and were able to document only three involving the facial skeleton.[22] None occured in infants or children, and after the entire clinicopathologic picture is scrutinized, there is some debate as to whether these lesions were giant cell granulomas or giant cell tumors of bone.

Radiographically, the central giant cell granuloma is a lesion that is quite destructive of bone. Consequently roentgenograms show radiolucencies ranging in size from a few millimeters to several centimeters (Fig. 8-2). Radiolucent zones may be unilocular or multilocular with borders that are generally at least partially well-defined.

Our experience with the radiographic presentation of this tumor in children has been exceedingly consistent. In a review of seven cases in children, six appeared as multilocular or "soap-bubble" type radiolucencies; only one lesion was unilocular. Waldron and Shafer reported similar radiographic findings in a review of 34 giant cell granulomas in all age groups.[11] Long-standing lesions may result in perforation of the cortical plate of bone and displacement of the teeth.[23]

LIGHT MICROSCOPY

The lesion is made up of a very cellular accumulation of spindle-shaped fibroblasts, often arranged into interlacing fascicles of fibrillar connective tissue (Fig. 8-3). Stromal fibroblasts may blend into a densely fibrous or myxomatous stroma, and mitoses in stroma cells are frequent. Distributed throughout this stroma are numerous multinucleated giant cells. The distribution of the giant cell component is quite variable, ranging from diffuse to patchy. Giant cells can range from very small cells with only a few nuclei to exceedingly large cells with 10 to 20 nuclei. Foci of osteoid or new bone as well as extravasated blood and hemosiderin pigment may be seen throughout the stroma.

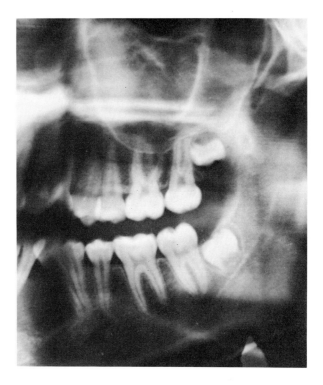

Fig. 8-2 Central giant cell granuloma. Note unilocular radiolucency of the mandible causing expansion of the cortices and separation of teeth. Courtesy of Dr. Don Biggs.

ELECTRON MICROSCOPY

Opinions differ regarding the histogenesis and nature of the various cell types found in giant cell reparative granulomas. It has been variously suggested, for example, that the characteristic giant cells develop from macrophages, bone cells, endothelial cells, or stromal fibroblasts. Understanding of these interesting lesions has been greatly furthered by the work of Scott[24;25] and others who have demonstrated in normal osteogenesis the existence of two distinct types of mononuclear stromal cells, type A and type B. Type A cells resemble differentiating

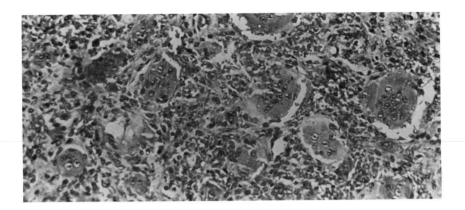

Fig. 8-3 Central giant cell granuloma displaying an admixture of multinucleated giant cells set in a loose cellular fibrous connective tissue stroma. Note extravasated erythrocytes throughout the lesion. (H&E x 200).

osteoblasts. Type B cells exhibit the characteristic cytoplasmic features of osteoclasts; these become multinucleate giant cells through cellular fusion. Ultrastructural studies[9;26;27] point to the conclusion that the same cell types and maturational events occur in giant cell granulomas (Fig. 8-4), providing additional evidence in support of the concept that these are reactive rather than neoplastic lesions.

We find it exceedingly difficult to label the ultrastructural features in any of the three lesions (central giant cell granuloma, peripheral giant cell granuloma and true giant cell tumor of bone) as pathognomonic of any of the lesions specifically.

DIFFERENTIAL DIAGNOSIS

Perhaps the most perplexing differential diagnostic challenge facing the clinician and the pathologist is the distinction of the central giant cell granuloma from "true giant cell tumor of bone." Batsakis[10] summarized the pertinent clinicopathologic differences as follows: (1) true giant cell tumors are rarely identified in bones of the skull, face, and jaws; (2) osteoid formation or other evidence of osteogenic activity is not characteristic of true giant cell tumors, except at the periphery or where there is a fracture or associated injury to adjacent bone; (3) true giant cell tumors are remarkably devoid of hemorrhage, lipid-laden histiocytes, hemosiderin and an inflammatory cellular component, and (4) the incidence of giant cell granulomas demonstrates a distinct predisposition of patients under 20 years of age, whereas giant cell

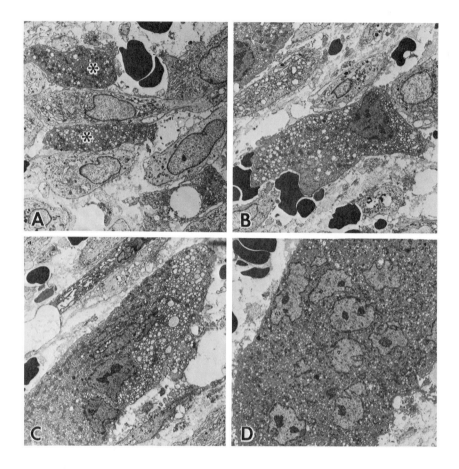

Fig. 8-4 Two distinct types of mononuclear stromal cells are demonstrated in this central giant cell granuloma (A). The osteoblastic elements exhibit prominent Golgi and rough endoplasmic reticulum, while the immature osteoclasts (asterisks) display a characteristic electron-dense cytoplasm with abundant mitochondria. A spectrum of osteoclastic differentiation may be observed; proceeding from the spindle-shaped stromal cell stage (A), they first enlarge (B), then become multinucleate (C), and finally assume their mature giant cell configuration (D). EM x 2,700.

tumors occur most commonly in the 20-to-40-year-old age group. Hamlin and Lund[28] have reported similar findings.

The distinction between the brown tumor of primary and/or secondary hyperparathyroidism and the central giant cell granuloma of the jaws requires consideration of: clinical presentation, anatomic location, roentgenographic features, and the results of metabolic studies. Smith and Ward concluded that the two lesions are indistinguishable on histological appearance alone.[22] Lucas[29] maintained that one striking radiographic feature of note in late-stage hyperparathyroidism which may prove helpful diagnostically, is the absence of a lamina dura around the teeth, a feature not seen with the central giant cell granuloma. The brown tumor of hyperparathyroidism is a distinct rarity in childhood.

Although the *aneurysmal bone cyst* can mimic the central giant cell granuloma clinically and histologically, it is an uncommon lesion in the jaws;[30;31] rather, the dominant sites of involvement are the vertebra and long bones. Daugherty and Eversole[32] reported 80 percent of 17 aneurysmal bone cysts of the jaws were in patients under 20 years of age with a predisposition in females. Microscopically aneurysmal bone cysts may contain zones of giant cells and fibroblastic proliferation similar to the giant cell granuloma, but most authorities consider the lesion primarily a vascular one, dominated by cavernous blood-filled spaces.[10;33-35] Excessive bleeding or welling of blood is usually manifested on surgical exploration of the lesion,[10;12] a feature not seen with central giant cell granuloma.

Cherubism is a rare autosomal dominant developmental disorder, and was first reported in 1933 as a unique type of facial deformity common to children, usually detected between the ages of one-and-one-half and seven years of age.[36;37] The histopathology of cherubism is very similar to that of the central giant cell granuloma, but may be distinguished from the latter by the following clinicopathological features: (1) cherubism usually results in well-defined multilocular jaw radiolucencies involving the retromolar ramus area, whereas the giant cell granuloma favors the anterior mandible; (2) jaw lesions of cherubism are usually bilateral and may affect all four quadrants of the jaws; other bones including the ribs, humerus, femur, and bones of the hands may also be involved; (3) cherubism is familial, affecting parents and siblings; (4) hypertelorism with cherubic facies may be seen, and (5) compared with giant cell granuloma, the lesion of cherubism has a looser, less cellular, delicate fibrous tissue component and does not contain lesional new bone formation.[10]

Chondroblastoma, osteoblastoma, and fibrous dysplasia may all have scant numbers of giant cells when viewed microscopically, but, consideration of the clinical and roentgenographic features along with the histopathology should resolve any uncertainty in differentiating these lesions from the central giant cell granuloma.

This discussion would not be complete without a word about the *malignant giant cell tumor of bone*. Until recently, no such lesion of the jaws had been acceptably described in the literature. In early 1981, Mintz, Abrams, Carlsen and Melrose reported a case in a 55-year-old man.[37] These authors were most adamant in their assertion that any malignant giant cell tumor must show histologic evidence of the benign counterpart in the lesion under study or in material removed previously from the same area, as originally proposed by Dahlin and co-workers.[38] No malignant giant cell tumor of the jaws in children has been reported.

TREATMENT AND PROGNOSIS

The central giant cell tumor of the jaws is essentially a benign condition that can be adequately managed by curettage or complete surgical excision. Following these treatment modalities, the lesion usually fills in with new bone. Andersen and associates[6] reported a 13 percent recurrence rate, while Waldron and Shafer documented six recurrences in an analysis of 38 cases.[11] Recurrences are usually treated by complete surgical excision to margins of normal bone; irradiation is contraindicated.[10]

CHERUBISM

Synonyms

1. Familial fibrous dysplasia
2. Familial cystic multilocular jaw disease
3. Hereditary fibrous dysplasia of the jaws
4. Disseminated juvenile fibrous dysplasia

INCIDENCE

Cherubism is a benign fibro-osseous disease of the jaws, that shows a striking familial incidence. It is, more specifically, a hereditary disorder of an autosomal dominant gene with 100 percent penetrance in males and variable expressivity.[39-41] Penetrance in females ranges between 50 and 70 percent. Incidence figures are difficult to obtain; a comprehensive review by Anderson and McClendon in which the authors investigated the possible mode of inheritance in 65 patients representing 21 families, is probably the largest single documentation of cases since Jones[42] first described the disorder as a familial form of fibrous dysplasia of the jaws in 1933.

AGE AND SEX

The patient with cherubism is usually reported as normal at birth. The disease classically manifests itself between the ages of 1 1/2 and 7,[43] while its characteristic jaw swellings most often appear between the ages of 2 and 4 years. Males are affected about twice as frequently as females.[44]

PATHOGENESIS

The etiology of cherubism remains unknown. A plethora of modes of histogenesis have been reported ranging from the original concept proposed by Jones,[42] —which suggested that the lesions of cherubism represented cystic degeneration of abnormal tooth germs, to the proposal that cherubism is actually a type of fibrous dysplasia.[45;46] Current concepts of pathogenesis support the theory claiming the disease to be a developmental disorder of bone-forming mesenchyme.[47] Associated dental abnormalities are probably secondary to bone changes.

CLINICAL FINDINGS

Cherubism usually manifests clinically as a bilateral, symmetrical, painless enlargement of the jaws with accompanying cheek fullness.

The angle of the mandible is nearly always involved. Unilateral lesions of the maxilla and mandible have been reported but are indeed rare. Hypertelorism and irregularly placed deciduous teeth have been reported as part of the clinical prodrome.[43]

A rim of sclera is commonly visible beneath the iris because of bony orbital floor expansion, skin tightness, and upward displacement of the globe caused by the disease. These findings originally prompted Jones[42] to comment that the patients appeared to be gazing toward heaven in much the same manner as the celebrated cherubs so often depicted in Renaissance art.

Radiographically, cherubism is characterized by multilocular, expansile lesions of the jaws that result in eventual thinning of the labial and lingual cortices (Fig. 8-5). Lesions are most prominent in the posterior regions of the jaws; Batsakis[47] reported that the condyles invariably escape involvement. Delayed eruption of teeth, displacement of teeth, and complete eruption failure of a large percentage of the permanent dentition have all been reported.

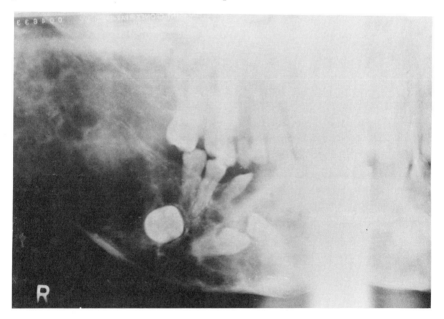

Fig. 8-5 Classic roentgenographic features of cherubism in a 12-year-old boy. Note the prominent multilocular distinctive radiolucency of the posterior mandible. Courtesy of Dr. Roy Eversole.

Multilocular lesions of cherubism have been reported in the ribs, humerus, femur, and carpals.[43] One of the authors (ROG) has had the opportunity to observe lesions in the maxillary sinus, ethmoid sinuses, and frontal bone in a 47-year-old female who had the disease diagnosed at age seven. Such extraoral locations are exceedingly rare.[46;48]

Thorough evaluation of the blood chemistries of these patients are usually normal, although on occasion there may be a slight elevation of alkaline phosphatase. Both the submandibular and cervical lymph nodes may be enlarged, but such findings are not a constant clinical feature of the disease. In rare instances, skin pigmentation may accompany cherubism, suggesting a relationship to disseminated fibrous dysplasia or Albright's syndrome.[47]

The lesions of cherubism increase in size quite rapidly in patients from 7 to 10 years of age,[44;47] whereupon the lesions enter a static phase or progress very slowly until puberty.[44] Following puberty, the occurrence of a gradual improvement, or a limited or total cessation of growth, or a regression becomes possible. Roentgenographic abnormalities tend to remain even after this phase of modulation of the disease.

LIGHT MICROSCOPY

The diagnosis of cherubism is a clinicopathological one and cannot be rendered based upon a group of unique microscopic findings alone. Tissue from bony defects is usually quite friable, granular, and mottled.

The lesions of cherubism classically show a proliferation of plump, spindle-shaped, or stellate fibroblasts with intermittent groups of multinucleated giant cells (Fig. 8-6). Giant cells are frequently clustered around small vascular spaces and often directly abut or appear to actually line vascular spaces. Hemosiderin, inflammatory cells, and perivascular cuffs of eosinophilic material consistent with collagen are common throughout the lesion.[49;50] Reactive bone formation is sometimes seen in the lesion but is not a constant histological feature. As the patient ages, the tissue of the lesion often becomes more fibrous, containing fewer multinucleated giant cells.[51]

DIFFERENTIAL DIAGNOSIS

The histological features of cherubism are not diagnostically distinctive, although Batsakis[47] reported that, compared to giant cell granuloma, the lesion of cherubism has a looser, less cellular, delicate, fibrous tissue component. The aneurysmal bone cyst, brown tumor of

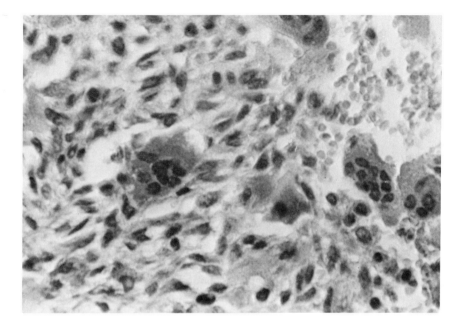

Fig. 8-6 The principal histologic features of cherubism are seen in this photomicrograph: a loose fibrillar stroma, multinucleated giant cells and hemorrhage are prominent. (H&E x 330).

hyperparathyroidism, and occasionally fibrous dysplasia with a giant cell component can be confused with cherubism. Batsakis[47] and Lucas[44] indicated that a combination of the following clinicopathological features should, in most instances, distinguish cherubism from the other giant cell lesions mentioned above: (1) bilateral jaw lesions; (2) affected parents or siblings; (3) almost exclusive occurrence in the jaws; (4) characteristic cherubic facies; (5) involution at puberty, and (6) high incidence of bilateral cervical lymphadenopathy.

TREATMENT AND PROGNOSIS

Patients with cherubism require management based upon the specifics of their disease process, —and not all cases are managed in an identical manner. The lesions tend to show their most active growth period directly following their appearance, with a slower growth period up to puberty.[44] Maxillary lesions show a tendency toward regression earlier than mandibular lesions and may continue to do so until the patient reaches the age of 20.[44] Mandibular lesions may continue to undergo regression until the third or fourth decade of life.

Hammer and Ketcham[50] have analyzed treatment procedures and reported that bony recontouring for cosmetic purposes and thorough curettage are the most common forms of treatment. Radiation therapy is contraindicated under any circumstances.

ANEURYSMAL BONE CYST

Synonyms

1. Aneurysmal giant cell lesion
2. Bone aneurysm
3. Atypical giant cell tumor
4. Hemorrhagic bone cyst

INCIDENCE

Although nearly 75 percent of aneurysmal bone cysts occur in children and young adults, their involvement in the head and neck skeleton is rare with the exception of vertebral lesions.

AGE AND SEX

Although persons in the second and third decades of life are most often affected, cases of patients as young as six-months-old have been reported.[52] Little is reported on racial incidence; however, females seem to be more often affected than males.[53]

PATHOGENESIS

Etiology and pathogenesis of aneurysmal bone cyst remain obscure. Speculations have included a relationship of the lesion to: fibrous dysplasia of bone,[53] nonspecific response to modified osseous lesions of various sorts,[54] and a form of fibrous histiocytoma of bone. The prospects are good for a reactive process.[55]

CLINICAL FINDINGS

Local swelling, pain, and/or tenderness are frequently manifested features of aneurysmal bone cyst. Mass effect on nerves may cause pain and paresthesia. Tumefaction is highly variable as a result of a possible intermittent growth rate with periods of acceleration sometimes exceeding that of a sarcoma; —but in some cases the lesion may remain quite static for months or even years.

Radiographic features are often characteristic. The lesion is lytic, usually polycellular, and expansile with sclerosis of margins. Soft tissue extension is rare but does occur. The general appearance is that of a benign lesion, but on occasion, radiographs are indistinguishable from those of a lytic osteosarcoma.

LIGHT MICROSCOPIC FINDINGS

Lesions are usually hemorrhagic and multicystic but occasionally may be more solid and neoplasm-like.

Histologically, cavernous spaces filled with blood are lined by large endothelial cells. Intercavernous septae are fibrous and may contain multinucleated giant cells, osteoid, and newly-formed bone. Nuclei of giant cells are distinctive in relation to those of the benign-appearing spindle cell stroma. Hemosiderin is commonly seen. (Fig. 8-7).

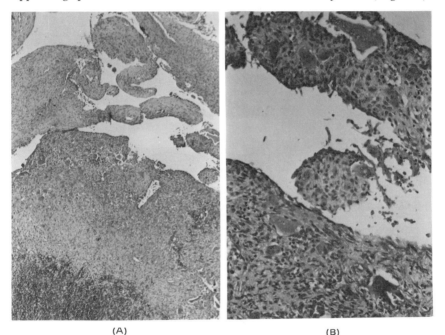

(A)   (B)

Fig. 8-7 Aneurysmal bone cyst. A. Cavernous channels comprise most of the lesion (H&E x 25). B. Intercavernous connective tissues support osteoclast-like giant cells in a benign-appearing stroma. (H&E x 100).

Solid areas of aneurysmal bone cyst lack large vascular spaces and thus interposed septae. Giant cells are more unevenly distributed. Osteoid is sometimes abundant and may have a "lacy" character. Mitoses in stromal cells complete the setting for confusion with osteosarcoma. Useful distinguishing features include: looseness and a prominence of vascularity of the fibrous stroma, absence of cytologic atypia, and association with more typical fields of aneurysmal bone cyst in the same lesion.

In addition, the morphological scope of other bone lesions must be taken into consideration as these may incorporate an associated aneurysmal bone cyst morphology within their own characteristic morphologies. Thus, only in the absence of co-existing lesions may an exclusively aneurysmal bone cyst diagnosis, based upon its characteristic morphology and radiographic features, be made.

DIFFERENTIAL DIAGNOSIS

Aneurysmal bone cyst can be very difficult to distinguish from giant cell tumor, giant cell reparative process (giant cell granuloma), and osteosarcoma, particularly telangiectatic osteosarcoma.

Giant cell tumor is distinctly rare in children, is usually not very vascular, and nuclei of the giant cells resemble those of associated stromal cells. Ossification in giant cell tumors is usually confined to the margins or to areas of degeneration within the tumor.

Telangiectatic osteosarcoma can be misdiagnosed as aneurysmal bone cyst and vice versa. Solid areas of aneurysmal bone cyst may mimic the morphology of osteosarcoma.

Careful evaluation of cytology for atypia is essential to distinguish these lesions. Softer signs are the loose and vascular stroma of aneurysmal bone cyst compared with a more dense stroma of osteosarcoma.

TREATMENT AND PROGNOSIS

Curettage and packing of lesions with bone chips is usually curative, although the recurrence rate may be as high as 30 percent after such procedures. The condition of lesions not amenable to such surgical therapy may require radiation. The risk of post-radiation sarcoma must be kept in mind when radiotherapy is contemplated and that risk weighed against its benefits.[56] No chemotherapeutic procedure has been reported as being successful to date.

References

1. Bhaskar, S.N. "Oral tumors of infancy and childhood. A survey of 293 cases." *J. Pediatr* 63(1963): 195-210.
2. Greer, R.O. and Mierau, G.W. *Tumors of the Oral Mucosa and Jaws in Infants and Children.* Denver: University of Colorado Medical Center Press, 1980.
3. Baxter, G.R. "A study of myeloid epulis and its relationship to myeloid sarcoma of the long bones." *Br. Dent. J.* 51(1930): 49.
4. Bernick, S. "Growths of the gingiva and palate. II. Connective tissue tumors." *Oral Surg.* 1(1948): 1098.

5. Brown, G.N.; Darlington, C.G. and Kupfer, S.R. "A clinicopathologic study of alveolar border epulis with special emphasis on benign giant cell tumors." *Oral Surg.* 9(1956): 765-775.

6. Andersen, L.; Fejerskov, O. and Philipsen, H.P. "Oral giant cell granulomas. A clinical and histologic study of 129 cases." *Acta. Pathol. Microbiol. Scand.* Sect. A 81(1973): 606-616.

7. Giansanti, J.S. and Waldron, C.A. "Peripheral giant cell granuloma: review of 720 cases." *J. Oral Surg.* 27(1969): 787-791.

8. Cooke, B.E.D. "The giant cell epulis: histogenesis and natural history." *Br. Dent. J.* 93(1952): 13-16.

9. Sapp, J.P. "Ultrastructure and histogenesis of peripheral giant cell granuloma of the jaws." *Cancer* 30(1972): 1119-1129.

10. Batsakis, J.G. *Tumors of the Head and Neck. Clinical and Pathological Considerations*, 2nd edition. Baltimore: Williams and Wilkins, 1979.

11. Waldron, C.A. and Shafer, W.G. "The central giant cell reparative cell granuloma of the jaws." *Am. J. Clin. Pathol.* 45(1966): 437-447.

12. Shafer, W.G.; Hine, M.K. and Levy, B.M. *A Textbook of Oral Pathology*, 3rd ed. Philadelphia: W.B. Saunders, 1974.

13. Lee, K.W. "The fibrous epulis and related lesions. Granuloma pyogencium, 'pregnancy tumor,' fibro-epithelial polyp and calcifying fibroblastic granuloma. A clinicopathologic study." *Periodontics* 6(1968): 277-292.

14. Phillips, K.L. and Shafer, W.G. "An evaluation of peripheral giant cell tumor." *J. Periodontol.* 26(1965): 216-222.

15. Standish, S.M. and Shafer, W.G. "Gingival reparative granulomas in children." *J. Oral Surg.* 19(1961): 367-375.

16. Jaffe, H.L. "Giant cell reparative granuloma, traumatic bone cyst and fibrous (fibro-osseous) dysplasia of the jawbones." *Oral Surg.* 6(1953): 159-175.

17. Austin, L.T., Jr.; Dahlin, D.C. and Royer, R.Q. "Giant cell reparative granuloma and related conditions affecting the jawbones." *Oral Surg.* 11(1959): 1285-1295.

18. Mintz et al. "Primary malignant giant cell tumor of the mandible. Report of a case and review of the literature." *Oral Surg.* 51(1981): 164-171.

19. Dahlin, D.C *Bone Tumors. General Aspects and Data on 6,221 Cases.* Springfield: Charles C. Thomas, 1978.

20. Hirschl, S. and Katz, A. "Giant cell reparative granuloma outside the jawbone: diagnostic criteria and review of the literature with the first case described in the temporal bone." *Hum. Pathol.* 5(1974): 171-181.

21. Hanaoka, H.; Friedman, B. and Mack, R.P. "Ultrastructure and histogenesis of giant-cell tumor of bone." *Cancer* 25(1970): 1408-1423.

22. Smith, G.A. and Ward, P.A. "Giant cell lesions of the facial skeleton." *Arch. Otolaryngol.* 104(1978): 186-190.

23. Marble et al. "Central giant cell reparative granuloma with extraosseous manifestations. Report of case." *J. Oral Surg.* 27(1969): 215-220.

24. Scott, B.L. "Thymidine 3H-electron microscope radioautography of osteogenic cells in the fetal rat." *J. Cell Biol.* 35(1967): 115-126.

25. Scott, B.L. "Thymidine-3H study of developing tooth germs and osteogenic tissue." *J. Dent. Res.* 48(1969): 753.

26. Adkins, K.F.; Martinez, M.G. and Hartley, M.W. "Ultrastructure of giant cell lesions. A peripheral giant-cell reparative granuloma." *Oral Surg.* 28(1969): 713-723.

27. Bartel, H. and Piatowska, D. "Electron microscopic study of peripheral giant-cell reparative granuloma." *Oral Surg.* 43(1977): 82-96.

28. Hamlin, W.B. and Lund, P.K. "Giant cell tumors of the mandible and facial bones." *Arch. Otolaryngol.* 86(1967): 658-665.

29. Lucas, R.B. *Pathology of Tumors of the Oral Tissues.* New York: Churchill Livingstone, 1976.

30. Bernier, J.L. and Bhaskar, S.V. "Aneurysmal bone cysts of the mandible." *Oral Surg.* 11(1958): 1018-1028.

31. Gruskin, S.F. and Dahlin, D.C. "Aneurysmal bone cysts of the jaws." *J. Oral Surg.* 26(1968): 523-528.

32. Daugherty, J.W. and Eversole, L.R. "Aneurysmal bone cyst of the mandible: report of case." *J. Oral Surg.* 29(1971): 737-741.

33. Lichtenstein, L. "Aneurysmal bone cyst. Observations of fifty cases." *J. Bone Joint Surg.* 39-A(1957): 873-882.

34. Biesecker et al. "Aneurysmal bone cysts: a clinicopathologic study of 66 cases." *Cancer* 26(1970): 615-625.

35. Buraczewski, J. and Dabska, M. "Pathogenesis of aneurysmal bone cyst: relationship between the aneurysmal bone cysts and fibrous dysplasia of bone." *Cancer* 28(1971): 597-604.

36. Goodman, R.M. and Gorlin, R.J. *Atlas of the Face in Genetic Disorders,* 2nd ed. St. Louis: C.V. Mosby, 1977.

37. Mintz et al."Primary malignant giant cell tumor of the mandible. Report of a case and review of the literature." *Oral Surg.* 51(1981): 164-171.

38. Dahlin, D.C.; Cupps, R.E. and Johnson, E.W., Jr. "Giant cell tumor: a study of 195 cases."*Cancer* 25(1970): 1061-1070.

39. Shafer, W.G.; Hine, M.K. and Levy, B.M. *A Textbook of Oral Pathology,* 3rd ed. Philadelphia: W.B. Saunders, 1974.

40. Anderson, D.E. and McClendon, J.C. "Cherubism — hereditary fibrous dysplasia of the jaws. I. Genetic considerations" *Oral Surg.* 15(1961): 5-16.

41. Kerley, T.R. "Central giant cell granuloma or cherubism. Report of a case." *Oral Surg.* 51(1981): 128-130.

42. Jones, W.A. "Familial Multilocular cystic disease of the jaws." *Am. J. Cancer* 17(1933): 946-950.

43. Goodman, R.M. and Gorlin, R.J. *Atlas of the Face in Genetic Disorders.* St. Louis: C.V. Mosby, 1977.

44. Lucas, R.B. *Pathology of Tumors of the Oral Tissues,* 3rd ed. London: Churchill Livingstoñe, 1976.

45. McDonald, R.E. and Shafer, W.G. "Disseminated juvenile fibrous dysplasia of the jaws." *Am. J. Dis. Child* 89(195): 354-358.

46. McClendon, J.L.; Anderson, D.E. and Cornelius, E.A. "Cherubism — hereditary fibrous dysplasia of the jaws. II-Pathologic considerations" *Oral Surg.* Supp. 215(1962): 17.

47. Batsakis, J.G. *Tumors of the Head and Neck,* 2nd ed. Baltimore: Williams and Wilkins, 1979.

48. Bloom, J.; Chacker, F.M. and Thoma, K. "Multiple cell lesions of bone. Report of a case." *Oral Surg.* 15(1962): 74-83.

49. Hammer, J.E. "The demonstration of perivascular collagen deposition in cherubism." *Oral Surg.* 27(1969): 129-141.

50. Hammer, J.E. and Ketcham, A.S. "Cherubism: an analysis of treatment." *Cancer* 23(1969): 1133.

51. Sanders, B. *Pediatric Oral and Maxillofacial Surgery.* St. Louis: C.V. Mosby, 1979.

52. Spjut et al. *Tumors of Bone and Cartilage. Atlas of Tumor Pathology,* 2nd series, fascicle 5, pp. 357-367. Washington D.C.: Armed Forces Institute of Pathology, 1970.

53. Tillman et al. "Aneurysmal Bone Cyst: an Analysis of Ninety-Five Cases." *Mayo Clin. Proc.* 43(1968): 478-495.

54. Levy et al. "Aneurysmal Bone Cyst Secondary to Other Osseous Lesions." *Am. J. Clin. Pathol.* 63(1975): 1-8.

55. Unni, K.K.; McLeod, R.A. and Dahlin, D.C., "Conditions That Simulate Primary Neoplasms of Bone." *Pathol. Annu.* 15 (1980): 91-131.

56. Weatherby, R.P.; Dahlin, D.C. and Ivins, J.C., "Postradiation Sarcoma of the Bone: Review of 78 Mayo Clinic Cases." *Mayo Clin. Proc.* 56(1981): 294-306.

Chapter IX

Mucocutaneous Pigmented Nevi and Melanoma

INTRODUCTION

A complete discussion of pigmented nevi in the head and neck area, including the proposed pathogenesis, ultrastructure, and myriad of clinical variations is beyond the scope of this text. For a detailed discussion, the reader is referred to a textbook of dermatopathology.

A discussion of the most common types of pigmented nevi encountered in the head and neck region of children follows. To make this information most useful to the reader, information concerning the incidence, age and sex, and clinical features of each entity is compiled under the single heading, clinical findings.

MUCOCUTANEOUS PIGMENTED NEVI

Synonyms

1. Melanocytic Nevus
2. Pigmented Nevus
3. Mole

CLINICAL FINDINGS

Pigmented nevi are exceedingly common lesions of the skin found in all age groups. The average number of pigmented nevi for any one individual is approximately 20. Their greatest frequency is in the head, neck, and trunk. Nevi are usually divided into three principal histological types: (1) *intradermal nevus*; (2) *compound nevus*, and (3) *junctional nevus*. These three subtypes appear clinically as flat or slightly elevated macules, or as papillary or nodular growths (Fig. 9-1). Compound nevi and junctional nevi tend to be somewhat more hyperpigmented than intradermal nevi. Coarse hairs are also somewhat more common to the intradermal nevus.

These histological subtypes account for the greatest number of pigmented nevi in the head and neck area of children, although less frequently encountered nevi, including the spindle cell nevus, blue nevus, cellular blue nevus, halo nevus, and congenital nevus, have been reported in the head and neck area of children.[1-3]

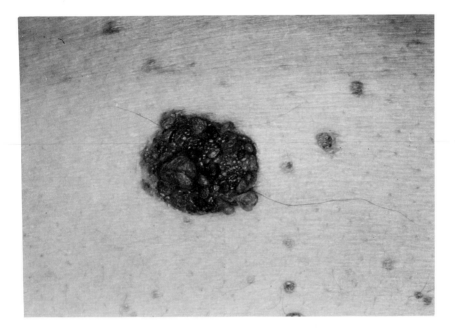

Fig. 9-1 Intradermal nevus of the neck. Courtesy of Dr. Loren Golitz.

Congenital nevi are variants of compound nevi present in 2.5 percent of neonates.[4] Approximately 14 percent of the congenital nevi are located in the head and neck area. They differ from the common variety of nevus because of their great size, (hence the commonly applied name, giant hairy nevus), their tendency to involve the reticular and subcutaneous tissue in an Indian file pattern, and their common involvement of skin appendages, nerves, and vessels. Congenital nevi of the face and scalp may be associated with neurofibromatosis, club foot, and spina bifida.[5] Two to 14 percent of congenital nevi develop foci of melanoma; a much higher percentage than with routine compound nevi.[5]

The *spindle cell nevus*, originally described by Spitz in 1948, is often referred to as juvenile melanoma.[6] Since its original description, this lesion has been shown to be a nevus that can show both epithelioid and spindle cell differentiation. In a review of 2600 nevi, Kernen and Ackerman found only 27 spindle cell and epithelioid cell nevi.[1] The most common location in over half of their cases was the head and neck; and among them, the cheek, forehead, neck, and ears were identified as the most common sites.

The vast majority of spindle cell nevi occur in children. Twenty-one of the 27 cases reviewed by Kernen and Ackerman were in patients less than fourteen. Most lesions appear as small, raised, pink or red nodules on the face that are less than 2 cm. in diameter.[1] There is no apparent sexual predisposition.

The *blue nevus* shows a propensity for development in childhood and adolescence, and the majority are seen in the first two decades of life. The scalp and the face are the most susceptible sites.[2] Rodriguez and Ackerman reported that 34.2 percent of 143 blue nevi they reviewed involved these two areas. Rarely have cases been reported in the palate.[7]

The occurrence of *cellular blue nevus* also indicates a marked predisposition of the first two decades of life. Rodriguez and Ackerman[2] reviewed a series of 45 cellular blue nevi and found that nearly two-thirds of the patients were between the ages of 10 and 39. Their youngest patient was seven-years-old and the oldest was 60. The face and scalp are the second most frequent sites for cellular blue nevi, after the buttocks and sacrococcygeal region. Nearly 18 percent of the cases reviewed by Rodriguez and Ackerman involved the face or scalp.

The true incidence of the blue nevus is unknown; however, Dorsey and Montgomery reported that they had had the opportunity to see more than 500 patients with the lesion.[8] Most patients with blue nevi were aware of a mass or mole, and a large percentage of the patients reported that they had noticed slow long-term growth of the lesion. In a small number of cases, the overlying skin may be ulcerated. The incidence of blue nevus and cellular blue nevus shows a marked female predominance. The female-to-male ratio reported by Rodriguez and Ackerman was 2.2-to-1.

The *halo nevus* is a neurocellular nevus that undergoes a distinctive pattern of regression.[6] This stage-like regression is characterized clinically by initial erythema and edema within subsequent, circumscribed depigmentation, and eventual total regression of the nevus. The halo nevus is most commonly seen in adolescents and young adults. The trunk is the most frequent site, with the head and neck area much less commonly involved. No sexual predisposition has been noted.

PATHOGENESIS

Current dogma supports the concept that nevus cells as well as melanocytes are of neuroectodermal origin. Nevus cells are believed to migrate from the neural crest late in gestation and during the first few months after birth.[9]

The pigmented nevus undergoes a peculiar pattern of development and structural differentiation throughout life. Lund and Stobbe[10] reported that the percentage of nevi with junctional changes decreases as the age of the patient increases. There is also a tendency for nerve clusters and neuroid elements to increase with age. These findings support the concept that melanoblasts tend to migrate away from the epidermis with increasing age, in association with an uninterrupted proliferation of Schwann cells in the dermis.[10]

Although it is generally accepted that melanocytes and nevus cells are of neural crest origin, there is still some debate as to whether all nevus cells develop from epidermal melanocytes, or whether a portion develops from epidermal melanocytes and a portion from the Schwann cells of dermal nerves.[11]

Recent electron microscopic findings tend to complicate the issue further with supportive evidence that an even more primitive cell (the nevoblast), derived from the neurocrest, may be "biopotential" and thus capable of differentiating into an epidermal melanoblastic precursor or a dermal "Schwannian" precursor.[11]

LIGHT MICROSCOPY

The *junctional nevus* is characterized by a proliferation of rather well-circumscribed clusters and nests of nevus cells at the epidermal-dermal interface. The nevus cells range from cuboidal to spindle-shaped to dendritic, and generally show little accumulation of melanin in their cytoplasm. Occasionally, a few clusters of nevus cells are identified below the basement membrane, but the overall nevus cell activity is more or less junctionally linear and often prominent at the arch of rete ridges. Junctional activity of nevus cells may be so great that the appellation, "active junctional nevus", is used.

The *intradermal nevus* is characterized microscopically by an accumulation of nevus cells in the dermis only (Figs. 9-2A, 9-2B). There is little or no evidence of junctional activity at the dermal-epidermal interface, and nevus cells tend to arrange themselves into clusters or strands of epithelioid, giant, or amelanotic nevus cells. When intradermal nevi are composed of spindle-like cells resembling Schwann cells, they are often referred to as *neural nevi*.

The *compound nevus* combines the microscopic characteristics of the junctional and interdermal nevus to the extent that nevus cells are prominent throughout the epidermis and dermis. Papillomatosis is somewhat more common in compound nevi than with the other two types.

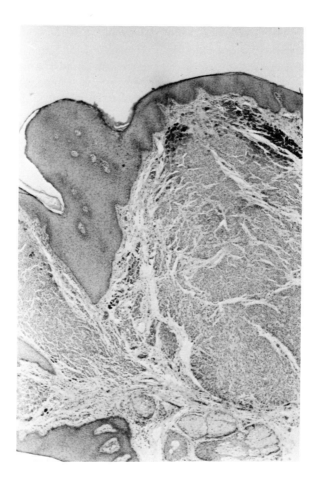

Fig. 9-2A Intradermal nevus showing nevus cells and globular clusters of melanin. (H&E x 120).

Blue nevi are characterized histologically by an accumulation of elongated, spindle-shaped, heavily melanin-laden melanocytes that are confined to the dermis. These cells are generally confined to the deep portions of the dermis and they are frequently most prominent adjacent to blood vessels, nerves, or adnexal structures.

The term *cellular blue nevus* is used to describe the less-common blue nevi which have a striking absence of associated melanin. The cells of the cellular blue nevus are more often round or oval than

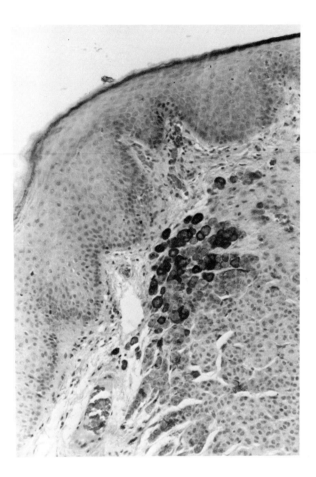

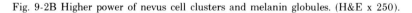

Fig. 9-2B Higher power of nevus cell clusters and melanin globules. (H&E x 250).

dendritic and have very little cytoplasm surrounding their small, centrally-placed nuclei.

The *spindle* or *epithelioid cell nevus* has a growth pattern which mimics that of the compound nevus as both junctional and dermal activity are noted. Either of the two cell types may be dominant. Spindle cell variants are comprised of nests or clusters of tapered, rod-shaped cells with large, elongated nuclei (Fig. 9-3). There is little evidence of melanin within spindle cell clusters, and nuclear pleomorphism and moderate mitotic activity may be present. When epithelioid cells dominate, they also have large nuclei, but individual cells tend to

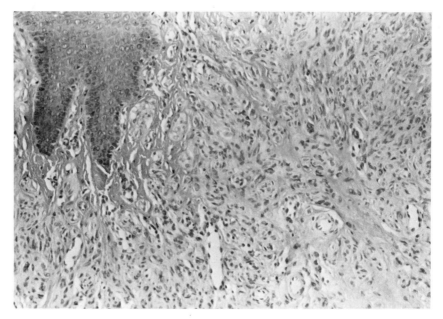

Fig. 9-3 Spindle cell nevus, showing elongated spindle-shaped cells, rich in cytoplasm (H&E X 210).

be polygonal, polyhedral, or cuboidal in shape, with somewhat more abundant cytoplasm. Multinucleated melanocytic giant cells tend to be more common in the epithelioid variant. An admixture of spindle cell and epithelioid types can also occur.

The *halo nevus* is characterized microscopically by two distinct phases. During the early phase, one finds nevus cells dispersed throughout a dermal lymphocytic and histiocytic infiltrate. As the lesion matures, the nevus cells become fewer in number and the inflammatory infiltrate intensifies. Eventually, the lesion may become totally amelanotic and nevus, cells will be totally absent.

DIFFERENTIAL DIAGNOSIS

The most critical distinction that the surgical pathologist must make when reviewing a suspected pigmented nevus is to accurately distinguish the lesion from melanoma. Many lists of criteria have evolved which are helpful in making this distinction, but perhaps none are more useful than the following histologic criteria proposed by Okun and Edelstein[5] for differentiation between the two:

(1) Nuclear atypia is prominent in melanoma, but is uncommon in pigmented nevi. Benign nevi show a progressive diminution of nuclear size with increasing depth; this is not true of melanoma.

(2) Atypical mitoses are common to tumor cells of melanoma.

(3) Transepidermal migration of tumor cells is characteristic of melanoma.

(4) There is a lesser degree of nesting in melanoma; observing melanoma *in situ*, tumor cells are usually diffusely arranged along the epidermal-dermal junction or within the epidermis.

(5) Melanoma shows a greater degree of continuity of epidermal and dermal components.

(6) Primary melanomas show a greater degree of lymphocytic host response in their early phase.

(7) Vascular invasion by tumor cells is prominent in melanoma, but not seen in nevi.

(8) There is a high incidence of spontaneous ulceration associated with melanoma.

TREATMENT AND PROGNOSIS

Most nevi in children become clinically obvious within the second year of life and follow a rather classic benign evolution, rarely differentiating along malignant lines. The recommended treatment for nevus in the head and neck area is complete removal of the nevus, using a cold knife. [12]

A large number of nevi are removed purely for cosmetic reasons; however, nevi subjected to constant trauma in the head and neck, such as those in the collar area and mouth, are often removed as a precautionary measure.

Although electrocautery has been used to remove nevi in the past, it is now considered contraindicated because of the artificial change that occurs in the cells of the tissue sample submitted to the pathologist. It is also disfavored because of the possibility of inducing local metastatic spread from a lesion thought clinically to be a nevus but histologically, is a melanoma. [13]

Recurrence is uncommon for most nevi unless the lesion is incompletely removed. Rodriguez and Ackerman observed no recurrences in their review of 147 blue nevi, all of which were treated by local excision. [2] In this same study, the authors examined 45 cellular blue nevi and performed a follow-up that ranged from 6 months to 17.5 years on 32 of the lesions. One patient developed a recurrence 12 months after the initial treatment.

Spindle cell nevi are adequately managed by local excision. Cautery and irradiation are contraindicated. Kernen and Ackerman[1] reported only one recurrence among 21 spindle cell nevi they reviewed.

MALIGNANT MELANOMA

Synonyms

1. Melanoma
2. Melanocarcinoma
3. Nodular melanoma

INCIDENCE

Malignant melanoma is quite rare in children. McWhorter and Woolner[14] reviewed a total of 172 pigmented lesions seen in children at the Mayo Clinic between 1907 and 1949, and were able to document only five malignant melanomas. Four of the five melanomas they identified occurred in the head and neck area; three in the cheek and one on the ear.

In a review of 1,710 pigmented skin tumors of children seen over a twenty-year-period in Denmark, Skov-Jensen and associates found only 2 melanomas in children under 15.[15] These authors also reviewed the literature on the subject, and were able to glean only 43 cases from the world literature. Twelve of the 43 cases (28 percent) occurred in the head and neck area. Shanon and associates[16] reviewed the world literature concerning melanoma in children in 1976, and reported that nearly half of all cases described in childhood involved various parts of the face. This contrasts with the adult form of the disease, where the scalp is the most susceptible site, followed by the face and neck.[15]

Malignant metastatic melanoma of the head and neck constituted about 21 percent of all childhood melanomas reported in the literature up to 1970.[16] This ratio does not differ substantially from that noted by Conley and Pack in their review of adult melanomas.[17]

AGE AND SEX

Malignant melanoma of the head and neck shows, in its incidence, a slight female predisposition. Nine of fourteen cases reported in children up to 1976 occurred in females.[16] In adults, melanoma of the head and neck is more common in men, except for cases with a facial localization.[17]

Most reported cases of malignant melanoma of the head and neck in children have occurred in patients less than 11 years of age. The oldest patient with a melanoma in this region, as reported by

McWhorter, was 11, as was the oldest patient in the series of Skov-Jensen.[15] The youngest patient in either review was 4 months of age.

Ballantyne[18] reviewed 405 patients with melanoma who were treated at the M. D. Anderson Hospital in Houston covering a 22-year-period and found six of the patients were under the age of 20.

PATHOGENESIS

Most melanomas in childhood develop from the transformation of an apparently benign melanocytic nevus. As such, they are considered to originate from epidermal-dermal junctional melanocytes or their precursors. An exception to this general postulate is observed when, occasionally, in giant pigmented nevi, malignant melanoma may arise in the deep dermis.

Batsakis[19] reported a reinforcing factor to the theory suggesting melanoma transformation from benign nevi by virtue of the fact that a considerable percentage of melanoma patients who were children are known to have had their pigmented lesion for at least 10 years or since birth.

The hereditary aspects of malignant melanoma have been reviewed by Anderson and associates,[20] who suggested melanoma may be inherited through the autosomes, as a dominant characteristic. They also suggested that the hereditary form of melanoma is characterized by a significantly early age of appearance and an increased frequency of multiple primary lesions.

Kahn and Donaldson[21] reported a case of multiple primary melanoma and suggested that an activating factor may be present in the serum of patients with this form of the disease. Melanoma has also been reported to occur in association with generalized melanosis,[22] and Balasanov and colleagues have reported a link between malanoma and lesions resembling vitiligo.[23] There is even recent evidence suggesting that immunological factors are important in the histogenesis of malignant melanoma.[23]

An increased incidence of melanoma in individuals of exceedingly fair complexion who are constantly exposed to actinic radiation over extended periods is a well-known factor in the etiology of the disease.[24]

CLINICAL FINDINGS

Malignant melanoma in children is usually described clinically as a circumscribed, slightly elevated, pink to deeply pigmented lesion with a smooth surface and usually without hair (Fig. 9-4). The tumor is most often found on the face, especially the cheek, and usually develops within a few months. Itching, ulceration, and paresthesia are seldom noted, although bleeding has been reported with considerable frequency.[14] Skov-Jensen and colleagues[15] have suggested that malignant melanoma of children can be divided into 3 categories: (1) congenital malignant melanoma, arising as a transplacental transmission of tumor from a mother with the disease; (2) malignant melanoma, developing before puberty, and (3) malignant melanoma, arising during childhood in nevus pigmentosus giganticus.

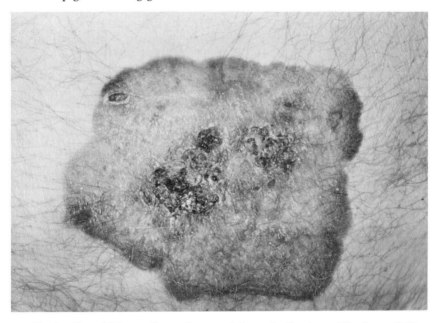

Fig. 9-4 Superficial spreading melanoma of the neck. Courtesy of Dr. Loren Golitz.

Malignant melanoma affects the external ear in approximately 10 percent of head and neck cases in adults;[17] but, it is seen somewhat less frequently in this anatomic location in children. Shanon and associates[16] reported a case in a two-and-one-half-year-old girl, in which the lesion started in the right helix as a brownish nodule that bled easily upon scratching. Malignant melanoma rarely arises in the oral mucosa, nasal mucosa, or nasopharynx.[25;26] Malignant melanoma of the oral cavity has been reported only once in a patient under 20 years of age.[27] One of the authors (ROG) has seen a melanoma of the palate in an 18-year-old male. It is interesting to note that, in this particular instance, the patient had been aware of a "dark spot in the roof of the mouth" since early childhood.

Unilateral nasal obstruction, epistaxis, or a complaint of a foreign body in the throat are the most common initial complaints recorded when the sinuses or pharynx are involved. Pain is seldom an early symptom of the disease in these locations.

LIGHT MICROSCOPY

There are three principal clinicopathologic forms of malignant melanoma. They include: (1) melanoma arising in Hutchinson's freckle; (2) superficial spreading melanoma, and (3) nodular melanoma.[28;29]

Hutchinson's melanotic freckle, also known as lentigo maligna, is not encountered in children and is discussed here only in the interest of comprehensive coverage. Classically, it occurs on the sun-exposed areas of elderly individuals (most often the cheek). It is characterized by a pleomorphic arrangement of atypical anaplastic melanocytes in the basal epithelial layer. The anaplastic melanocytes show little tendency toward nesting or upward epidermal mobility. The supporting dermis usually shows mild to marked solar collagenous degeneration.

Superficial spreading melanoma is considered to be the most common form of melanoma when all anatomic sites are considered; however, McGovern[29] reported the nodular form of this neoplasm to be the most common variant in the tissues of the head and neck.

Microscopically, superficial spreading melanoma is characterized by a pleomorphic arrangement of atypical melanocytes throughout the epidermis, with their greatest concentration in the basal epithelial layer (Fig. 9-5). These tumor cells may have a clear-cell, pagetoid, or cuboidal appearance. Tumor cells show upward mobility in the epidermis and often extend to the superficial keratin layer. The spinous layer may be quite acanthotic and the supporting dermis usually contains some large melanin-laden phagocytic cells.

Nodular melanoma is the most commonly encountered variant in children. The tumor is most often characterized microscopically by an invasion of anaplastic tumor cells into the dermis and upward penetration of tumor cells into the epidermis. Tumor cells are often spindle-shaped or epithelioid and arranged in nests. There is no clear demarcation between junctional and dermal components, and junctional melanocytic activity with atypical mitoses abounds (Fig. 9-6). On occasion, amelanotic spindle cells may be seen, but most often the intensity and quantity of melanin within tumor nests is greater than that seen in spindle cell nevi.

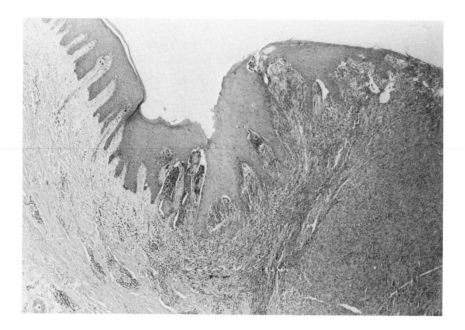

Fig. 9-5 Low-power photomicrograph of superficial spreading melanoma, showing mucosal ulcer and linear spread of atypical melanocytes along the basal layer (left). Nodular vertical invasion of the lamina propria is also seen (right). (H&E x 120).

If the melanoma arises from a pre-exisiting nevus, nests of atypical pleomorphic melanocytes are frequently admixed with clusters of benign nevus cells. Upward extension of anaplastic cells into the epidermis are supportive of melanoma even when benign foci of nevus cells are identified.

Clark and associates[28] have described five levels of invasion of malignant melanoma: Level I. Malignant cells are confined to the epidermis; Level II. There is evidence of invasion of the papillary dermis by malignant cells; Level III. There is microscopic evidence of invasion of malignant cells to the level of subpapillary vessels, but the reticular dermis is spared; Level IV. Invasion of the reticular dermis by malignant cells, and Level V. Invasion of the subcutaneous fat.

ELECTRON MICROSCOPY

Ultrastructural diagnosis of malignant melanoma rests upon the demonstration of a specific organelle, the melanosome. Unmelanized melanosomes exhibit a distinctive substructure (Fig. 9-7), allowing even

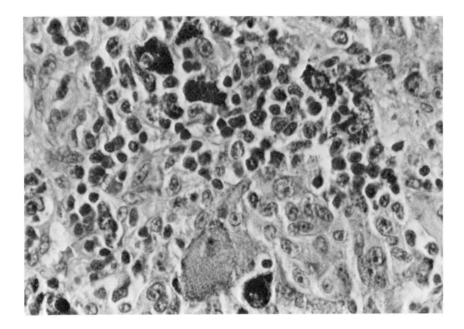

Fig. 9-6 Malignant malanoma, showing a pleomorphic admixture of malignant fusiform cells, small, round neoplastic pigmented cells, and malignant giant cell forms. (H&E x 300).

most amelanotic variants to be identified with reliability. It is important to note, however, that electron microscopy cannot be depended upon to rule out amelanotic melanoma in the problem case. Of the four types of melanoma cells described by Clark and associates,[30] only the first two feature granules exhibiting characteristic melano-filaments. The third type is identified with lesser dependability because its unmelanized melanosomes display only a nonspecific granular or lamellar substructure. The fourth type cannot be identified with any degree of certainty because it does not exhibit melanosomes.

DIFFERENTIAL DIAGNOSIS

Distinction between malignant melanoma and benign pigmented nevi has been discussed under the differential diagnosis section of pigmented nevi earlier in this chapter. There are, however, additional lesions that must be distinguished from malignant melanoma, both clinically and microscopically.

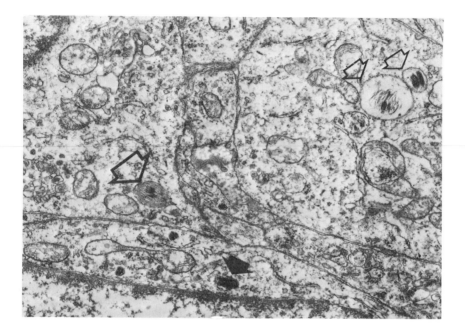

Fig. 9-7 Typical premelanosomes (large open arrow), which appear in sectional profile to contain longitudinally-oriented, cross-striated filaments, can often be found in malignant melanomas, but atypical variants (small open arrows) usually predominate. Some pigmentation may occur even in "amelanotic" examples, obscuring the substructure of the melanosomes affected (solid arrow). (EM x 30,100).

Juvenile xanthogranuloma may be confused with the spindle cell and epithelioid variants of malignant melanoma in the child. The presence of fat-laden histiocytes and Touton giant cells, even with evidence of atypia, supports a diagnosis of xanthogranuloma.

Metastatic melanoma from other anatomic sites to the skin must be a consideration when melanoma is identified without a connection to the overlying epidermis. Lever[31] suggested that the histological appearance of metastic lesions to the skin differs from primary melanoma because metastatic lesions are characterized by an absence of junctional activity and lack of an inflammatory infiltrate. Although most authorities consider that a malignant melanoma located entirely within the dermis is nearly always metastatic,[32] Okun[6] and Bimes[33] have documented cases of malignant melanoma arising from intradermal nevi.

A malignant form of blue nevus has been described[34] but is exceedingly rare. Distinction of malignant blue nevus from metastatic melanoma to the skin may be difficult and no clear-cut rules have been established for differentiating between the two.

Malignant melanoma is often considered, following Levene's report,[35] to be the most pleomorphically variable of all malignant neoplasms, and, as such, can have a pattern of growth that is pseudoglandular, peritheliomatous, trabecular, verrucous, fibroblastic, or neuroid.

In children, a spindle cell pattern of differentiation is often most prominent. Therefore, distinction of spindle cell melanoma from spindle cell carcinoma, sarcoma, and spindle cell nevus is of paramount importance. Microscopic features that favor melanoma include: (1) large numbers of atypical mitotic figures with altered nuclear cytoplasmic ratios; (2) tumor cell melanin; (3) continuity of tumor with the epidermis; (4) a positive Fontana-Masson stain for premelanin or Dopa reaction for melanin, and (5) a lack of desmosomal connections and dyskeratosis.

TREATMENT AND PROGNOSIS

Wide surgical excision or resection is the favored treatment for malignant melanoma. Radiation therapy and adjuvant chemotherapy are used extensively in current experimental management protocols, but they appear to be most effective as therapy for metastatic lesions and are not used as primary management modalities.

Balch and co-workers[36] discussed surgical management of melanoma in a recent paper concerning Stage I melanoma and advocated the following: (1) a surgical margin of 2 cm. is recommended for tumors less than .76 mm. in thickness, and (2) a surgical margin of 3-5 cm. is recommended for thicker lesions.

The removal of fascia adjacent to the tumor, once considered mandatory, is no longer favored by most surgical oncologists.[37] The value of prophylactic lymph node dissection remains a constantly debated issue among surgeons, and although it is a procedure favored by many,[38] there seems to be little evidence that routine lymph node dissection of clinically negative nodes prolongs patient survival.[39]

Childhood malignant melanoma does not differ biologically in any substantial way from its adult counterpart. Shanon suggested that the three-year survival-rate of children with head and neck melanomas is similar to the five-year survival-rate of adults with disease that is similarly staged.[16]

The five-year survival-rate for children with clinical evidence of metastatic melanoma, as reported by Skov-Jensen and colleagues, was

17 percent. A 33 percent five-year survival-rate for children with melanoma has been reported by Lerman and associates.[27]

References

1. Kernen, J.A. and Ackerman, L.V. "Spindle and epithelial cell nevi (so-called juvenile melanomas) in children and adults." *Cancer* 13(1960): 612-625.
2. Rodriguez, H.A. and Ackerman, L.V. "Cellular blue nevus." *Cancer* 21(1968): 393-405.
3. Wayte, D.M. and Helwig, E.G. "Halo Nevi." *Cancer* 22(1968): 69-77.
4. Mark et al. "Congenital melanocytic nevi of the small garment type." *Hum. Pathol.* 4(1973): 395-418.
5. Okun, M.R. and Edelstein, L.M. *Gross and Microscopic Pathology of the Skin. Dermatopathology.* Boston: Foundation Press, 1976.
6. Spitz, S. "Melanoma of childhood." *Am. J. Pathol.* 24(1948): 591-609.
7. Harper, J.C. and Waldron, C.A. "Blue nevus of the palate." *Oral Surg.* 20(1965): 145-149.
8. Dorsey, C.S. and Montgomery, H. "Blue nevus and its distinction from mongolian spot and the nevus of Ota." *J. Invest. Dermatol.* 22(1954): 225-236.
9. Kissane, J.M. In *Pathology of infancy and childhood*, 2nd ed., pg. 1125. St. Louis: C.V. Mosby, 1975.
10. Lund, H.Z. and Stobbe, G.D. "The natural history of the pigmented nevus. Factors of age and anatomic location." *Am. J. Pathol.* 25(1949): 1117-1155.
11. Walton, R.G. "Pigmented nevi." *Pediatr. Clin. North Am.* 18(1971): 897-923.
12. Webster, J.P.; Stevenson, T.W. and Stout, A.P. "Symposium on reparative surgery. Surgical treatment of malignant melanomas of skin." *Surg. Clin. North Am.* 24(1944): 319-339.
13. Amadon, P.D. "Electrocoagulation of melanomas and its dangers." *Surg. Gynecol. Obstet.* 56(1933): 943-946.
14. McWhorter, H.E. and Woolner, L.B. "Pigmented nevi, juvenile melanomas, and malignant melanomas in children." *Cancer* 7(1954): 564-585.
15. Skov-Jensen, T.; Hastrup, J. and Lambrethsen, E. "Malignant melanoma in children." *Cancer* 19(1966): 620-626.
16. Shanon et al. "Malignant melanoma of the head and neck in children. Review of the literature and report of a case." *Arch. Otolaryngol.* 102(1976): 244-247.
17. Conley, J.J. and Pack, G.T. "Melanoma of the head and neck." *Surg. Gynecol. Obstet.* 116(1963): 15-28.
18. Ballantyne, A.J. "Malignant melanoma of the skin of the head and neck. An analysis of 405 cases." *Am. J. Surg.* 120(1970): 425-431.
19. Batsakis, J.G. *Tumors of the head and neck. Clinical and Pathological Considerations,* 2nd ed. Baltimore: Williams and Wilkins, 1979.
20. Anderson, D.E.; Smith, J.L. and McBride, C.M. "Hereditary aspects of malignant melanoma." *JAMA* 200(1967): 81-86.
21. Kahn, L.B. and Donaldson, R.C. "Multiple primary melanoma. Case Report and Study of Tumor Growth *in vitro*." *Cancer* 25(1970): 1162-1169.
22. Sohn et al. "Generalized melanosis secondary to malignant melanoma, report of a case with serum and tissue tyrosinase studies." *Cancer* 24(1969): 893-903.
23. Balasanov, C.V.; Andreev, V.C. and Tchernozenski, I. "Malignant melanoma and vitiligo." *Dermatologica* 139(1969): 211-219.

24. Lewis et al. "Tumour specific antibodies in human malignant melanoma and their relationship to the extent of disease." *Br. Med. J.* 3(1969): 547-552.

25. Trodahl, J.N. and Sprague, W.G. "Benign and malignant melanocytic lesions of the oral mucosa." *Cancer* 25(1970): 812-823.

26. Mesara, B.W. and Burton, W.O. "Primary malignant melanoma of the upper respiratory tract." *Cancer* 21(1968): 217-225.

27. Lerman et al. "Malignant melanoma of childhood, a clinicopathologic study and report of 12 cases." *Cancer* 25 (1970): 436-449.

28. Clark, W.H.; Bernardino, E.A. and Mihn, M.C. "The histogenesis and biologic behavior of primary human malignant melanoma of skin." *Cancer Res.* 29 (1969): 705-726.

29. McGovern, V.J. "The classification of melanoma and its relationship with prognosis." *Pathology* 2(1970): 85-98.

30. Clark, W.H.; ten Heggeler, B. and Bretton, R. "Electron microscope observations of human cutaneous melanomas correlated with their biologic behavior." In *Melanoma and Skin Cancer*, edited by W.H. McCarthy, pp. 121-141. Sydney: Gov. Printer, 1972.

31. Lever, W.F. *Histopathology of skin*, 5th ed. Philadelphia: Lippincott, 1975.

32. Allen, A.C. and Spitz, S. "Malignant melanoma: clinicopathologic analysis of criteria for diagnosis and prognosis." *Cancer* 6(1953): 1-45.

33. Bimes, C. "Histopathologic des maevo-carcinomes." *Bull. Cancer* (Paris) 40(1953): 481-528.

34. Hernandez, F.J. "Malignant blue nevus. A light and electron microscopic study." *Arch. Dermatol.* 107(1973): 741-754.

35. Levene, A. "On the histologic diagnosis and prognosis of malignant melanoma." *J. Clin. Pathol.* 33(1980): 101-124.

36. Balch et al. "Tumor thickness as a guide to surgical management of clinical stage I melanoma patients." *Cancer* 43(1979): 883-888.

37. Stahlin, J.S. "Malignant melanoma: an appraisal." *Surgery* 64(1968): 1149-1157.

38. McNeer, G. "Malignant melanoma." *Surg. Gynecol. Obstet.* 120(1965): 343-344.

39. Sim et al. "A prospective randomized study of the efficacy of routine elective lymphadenectomy in management of malignant melanoma. Preliminary results." *Cancer* 41(1978): 948-956.

Chapter X

Skin Appendage Tumors
INTRODUCTION

Tumors of skin appendages, frequently termed adnexal tumors, arise from the same primitive cells that give rise to the epidermis as a whole. These tumors are classically divided into: (1) tumors with follicular differentiation; (2) tumors with sebaceous differentiation; (3) tumors with apocrine differentiation, and (4) tumors with eccrine differentiation.

Neoplasms in each of the groups may be benign or malignant. The benign variants far outnumber the malignant ones. In terms of histogenesis, the vast majority of these tumors arise in a manner not unlike that of neoplasms of the odontogenic (tooth germ) apparatus. In all likelihood, skin adnexal neoplasms arise from pluripotential cells which have the capacity to differentiate into tumors with hair, sebaceous glands, apocrine, or eccrine components, —a situation very similar to the capacity of odontogenic tumors differentiating to contain enamel, dentin, cementum, pulpal, and periodontal ligament structures.

Although nearly all adnexal tumors of skin have been reported at one time or another in the child, certain of these tumors show a propensity for the head and neck region. The most common of these neoplasms will be discussed in this chapter. Tumors of dermal (mesenchymal) origin are discussed in the chapters dealing with fibrous and fibrohistiocytic lesions.

PILOMATRIXOMA

Synonyms

1. Calcifying epithelioma of Malherbe
2. Calcifying epithelioma

INCIDENCE

The pilomatrixoma is by far the most common of the skin adnexal tumors to occur in the head and neck of children. Moehlenbeck[1] reported that the incidence in dermatohistopathologic material is 1 in 824; this figure was arrived at from a sample of 140,000 skin biopsies subjected to microscopic examination.

Ratios of tumor incidence in histopathologic material found in the literature vary from as low as 1 in 10,500[2] to as high as 1 in 316.[3] These remarkably varied figures are difficult to compare because the number of cases observed by each author is small and because it only partially refers to an entire sample of dermatohistopathological material. Moehlenbeck's[1] review of 1,569 cases indicated that 51.9 percent of the tumors he studied occurred in the head and neck.

AGE AND SEX

Forty percent of the pilomatrixomas arise before the age of 10 and more than 60 percent occur in the first two decades.[1] Moehlenbeck[1] found the highest frequency of occurrence in children to be between 8 and 13 years of age, and the average time between the appearance of the tumors and biopsy to be 4.4 years. The incidence of multiple tumors is reported to be 3.5 percent.[1] Afflicted males outnumber afflicted females by a ratio of 3-to-2.[1;4]

PATHOGENESIS

Numerous authorities have remarked upon the similarity of the tumor cells of the pilomatrixoma to the cells of the hair matrix.[5-7] Recent ultrastructural evidence and histochemical studies have established supporting evidence for derivation of this tumor from the hair matrix.[8-10] The tumor is not hereditary, although a familial occurrence has been reported.[1]

CLINICAL FINDINGS

The pilomatrixoma classically manifests as a solitary, nontender nodule most frequently on the face, neck, or upper extremities (Fig. 10-1). Tumors may reach a size as great as 5 cm.,[11] but the majority vary from 0.5 to 3 cm. in diameter.[12] Occasionally, the lesions are multiple and they are often quite indurated.

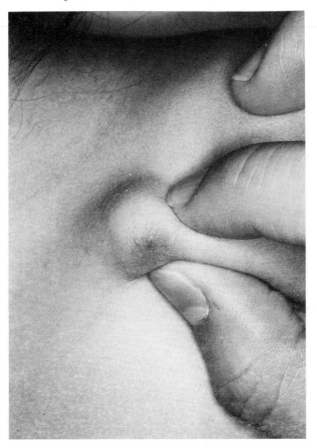

Fig. 10-1 Nodular indurated pilomatrixoma of the neck. Courtesy of Dr. Loren Golitz.

LIGHT MICROSCOPY

The pilomatrixoma is characterized histologically by tumor nests or lobules composed of two cell types: basophilic cells and shadow or ghost cells (Fig. 10-2).

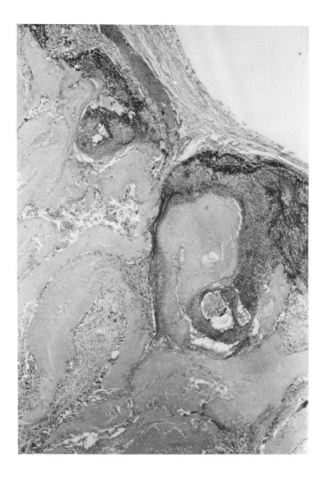

Fig. 10-2 Basophilic epithelial cells surrounding "ghost cells" in pilomatrixoma. (H&E x 200).

Basophilic cells are prominent at the periphery of tumor islands. These cells are similar in character to the cells of the basal epithelial layer of the hair matrix, as they possess round or elongated, deeply-basophilic nuclei and scant cytoplasm, with ill-defined cell borders. In all instances, basophilic cells eventually show foci where they blend into eosinophilic shadow or ghost cells which have clear, vacuolated areas in place of their nuclei. The borders of shadow cells are much more distinct than the borders of basophilic cells. Keratinization, calcification, and giant cells may be found within shadow cell areas.

Turhan and Krainer postulated that the basophilic cells represent hair matrix cells, and the shadow cells, in turn, represent immature hair cortex cells. [13]

DIFFERENTIAL DIAGNOSIS

The *pilar cyst* can resemble the pilomatrixoma as basophilic cells are also commonly seen. However, in pilar cysts, the peripheral layer of basophilic cells shows a characteristic palisading pattern not seen with pilomatrixoma. Interlacing tumor lobules are also absent in pilar cysts. *Basal cell carcinoma* should not be confused with the pilomatrixoma. Ghost or shadow cells are never present in the former.

Only rarely are children or young adults affected by basal cell carcinoma. [14] In most instances, basal cell carcinoma in children is associated with xeroderma pigmentosum, nevus sebaceus, or *nevoid basal cell carcinoma syndrome* with its attenuate palmoplantar pits, odontogenic keratocysts of the jaws, rib and vertebral anomalies, calcification of the falx cerebri, and mental retardation.

Milstone and Helwig [14] reviewed 22 cases of solitary basal cell carcinoma in children, unassociated with the syndrome. They found the patients to vary in age from 7 to 14, and that 82 percent of the tumors involved the head and neck. The most common site was the face. Most tumors were composed of a combination of solid, adenoid, and cystic patterns.

TREATMENT AND PROGNOSIS

The pilomatrixoma is adequately treated by conservative surgical excision with a margin of normal tissue. The incidence of the tumor shows little, if any, predisposition towards recurrence, and malignant degeneration does not occur.

TRICHOEPITHELIOMA

Synonyms

1. Epithelioma adenoides cysticum
2. Multiple benign cystic epithelioma

INCIDENCE

Trichoepithelioma is much less common than pilomatrixoma. Two forms of this disorder have been reported: (1) a solitary type which develops during adult life, and (2) multiple trichoepithelioma first prominent during adolescence. Only the second type will be discussed here.

AGE AND SEX

Gray[15] studied 50 patients with this disease in a review from the Armed Forces Institute of Pathology, and reported an average age of 15 years. The duration of the tumors at the time of biopsy varied from 6 months to 38 years.

The vast majority of patients have lesions of the scalp, face, or back. Gray[15] reported that 37 of the 50 patients he studied had lesions on the scalp or face. A male predisposition has been noted for this disease.[15]

PATHOGENESIS

In 1892, the hair sac was first postulated by Brook[16] as the origin of trichoepithelioma. Since that time, most authors have recognized a differentiation toward hair structures in this tumor and have suggested that pluripotential embryonic adnexal rests give rise to the lesion.[6] Others have suggested that the tumor arises from basal cells of the epidermis.[17] Goldman[18] first found the hereditary pattern of multiple trichoepithelioma to be a regular dominant inheritance without sex linkage.

CLINICAL FINDINGS

This dominantly inherited disorder is characterized clinically by the presence of flesh-colored multiple skin nodules or flesh-colored papules. They generally range in size from 0.2 to 0.5 cm. when identified on the face, neck, or scalp. Occasionally, lesions on the back attain a size of 2 or 3 cm. in diameter. The smaller lesions on the face dominate the nasolabial folds and often coalesce, forming larger telangiectatic nodules. The lesions are generally asymptomatic and only rarely ulcerate. [15]

LIGHT MICROSCOPY

The classic microscopic features are numerous horn cysts, surrounded by a lamellar arrangement of flattened squamous epithelial cells. The walls of horn cysts may contain melanin. When the tumors are less well-differentiated, clusters of basal cells, rudimentary hairs, and granulation tissue filling the adjacent dermis may be noted. A foreign body giant-cell reaction may be prominent in instances where horn cysts have ruptured.

DIFFERENTIAL DIAGNOSIS

Multiple trichoepithelioma must be distinguished from the *nevoid basal cell carcinoma syndrome.* Lever[6] suggested the accomplishment of this distinction to be possible upon the basis that, while both diseases are dominantly inherited, and have multiple lesions, the incidence of trichoepithelioma lesions indicates an anatomic predisposition of the nasolabial folds, with the lesions themselves remaining small and rarely ulcerating; —in contrast to lesions of the nevoid basal cell carcinoma, which are randomly or haphazardly distributed, and, in the late phase of the disease, often attain considerable size, ulcerate, and become locally destructive.

Squamous cell carcinoma may mimic trichoepithelioma, with the exception of keratinization in the latter being abrupt and complete, not gradual and incomplete as in the keratin pearls of squamous cell carinoma.[6] In addition, squamous cell carcinoma of the skin in children occurs almost exlusively in association with xeroderma pigmentosa.

TREATMENT AND PROGNOSIS

Patients with multiple trichoepithelioma have been treated with one or more of several modalities, including surgical excision, electrodessication, currettage, and radiation therapy.[15] None of these management modalities is entirely effective because recurrence or the formation of new lesions in the same area is common.

SYRINGOCYSTADENOMA PAPILLIFERUM

Synonyms

1. Naevus syringocystadenoma papilliferus
2. Papillary syringadenoma

INCIDENCE

The syringocystadenoma papilliferum was originally decribed by Werther in 1913.[19] Since then, over 200 cases have been reported in the literature.[20-25]

AGE AND SEX

This lesion most commonly occurs on the scalp or the face of recently pubescent children where it arises in a nevus sebaceus which has been present since birth. There is a preponderant incidence in females. Of the 100 tumors reviewed by Helwig and Hackney,[23] 58 lesions were reported to be present at birth or were recognized in childhood before the tenth year of life.

PATHOGENESIS

Most scientific evidence suggests that syringocystadenoma papilliferum arises as a result of activation of apocrine cell rests, or from anlage, or primordial epithelial germ cells.

Histochemical and electron microscopic studies of this lesion by Landry and Winkelmann[25] revealed features consistent with an apocrine origin; however, similar studies by Hashimoto[26] support an eccrine derivation.

CLINICAL FINDINGS

The vast majority of these neoplasms in children occur on the scalp, forehead and temple, face, upper lip, and neck as irregular, often corrugated, hyperkeratotic plaques. The lesion may be associated with nevus sebaceous with its attenuate hamartomatous accumulation of sebaceous glands, apocrine glands, and hair follicles.

Less frequently, the syringocystadenoma papilliferum is pedunculated, smooth, pink, or bulbous. Lesions of the scalp are commonly irritated while combing the hair and they may occasionally ulcerate or bleed. Most lesions range in size from 1 to 4 cm. in diameter, develop gradually, and grow slowly. Lesions may have a cystic quality, but only rarely.

LIGHT MICROSCOPY

Syringocystadenoma papilliferum is composed of a papillary epidermis with villous extentions lengthened into cystic spaces (Fig. 10-3). The upper portions of the invaginations are typically lined by squamous epithelial cells. Cystic cavities and their villous projections are lined by columnar cells which may show decapitation secretion. Overlying the columnar cells is a peripheral layer of prominent cuboidal cells. A supporting stroma filled with plasma cells is quite common in this lesion.

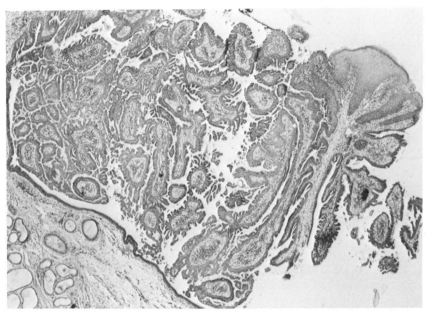

Fig. 10-3 Syringocystadenoma papilliferum. Note papillary epidermis with villous extensions into cystic spaces. (H&E x 150).

DIFFERENTIAL DIAGNOSIS

Hidradenoma papilliferum has microscopic features of cystic papillomatosis, but the lesion is entirely intradermal in its anatomic location, and is almost exclusively a perineal lesion of adult females.

Abrams and Finck[27] have described a salivary gland tumor, *sialadenoma papilliferum*, that is histologically identical to the syringocystadenoma, except for its salivary location.

Syringoma, in its incidence, shows a predisposition of the head and neck area of women. This tumor occurs most often as a collection of small papules or nodules in the periorbital region. Although the lesion is characterized histologically by multiple duct-like and cystic-appearing structures, the tumor differs from the syringocystadenoma in its eccrine origin,[28] and predisposition towards adults. The tumor may occur rarely in children, as crop-like lesions on the face, neck, or chest.

TREATMENT AND PROGNOSIS

Surgical excision is the treatment of choice for the syringo-cystadenoma. Helwig and Hackney[23] reported nine recurrences in their review of 100 patients with syringocystadenoma papilliferum. Follow-up periods ranged from one to nine years. The recurrence rate for the scalp was somewhat higher than the recurrence rate for other sites.

References

1. Moehlenbeck, F.W. "Pilomatrixoma (Calcifying Epithelium)." *Arch. Dermatol.* 108(1973): 532-534.
2. Hauss, H. "Epithelioma Calcificans (Malherbe)." *Dermatologische Wochenshrift* 145 (1962): 209-223.
3. Fust, R. "Bol Liga Contra." *Cancer* 180(1944): 19.
4. Geiser, J.D. "L'epithelioma calcifie de Malherbe." *Annales de Dermatologie et de Syphiligraphie* 86(1950): 259-270, 383-403.
5. Highman, B. and Ogden, G.E. "Calcified epithelioma of Malherbe." *Arch. Pathol.* 37(1944): 169-174.
6. Lever, W.F. and Freisemer, R.D. "Calcifying epithelioma of Malherbe: Report of 15 cases with comments on differentiation from calcified epidermal cyst and on its histogenesis." *Arch. Dermatol.* 59(1949): 506-518.
7. Herzberg, J.J. "Epithelioma calcifie de Malherbe." *Zeitschrift fur Haut und Geschlechtskrankheiten* 22(1957): 78-82.
8. Forbis, R., Jr. and Helwig, E.B. "Pilomatrixoma (calcifying epithelioma)." *Arch. Dermatol.* 83(1961): 606-618.
9. Hashimoto, K.; Nelson, R.G. and Lever, W.F. "Calcifying epithelioma of Malherbe: Histochemical and electron microscopic studies." *J. Invest. Dermatol.* 46(1966): 391-408.
10. McGavran, M.H. "Ultrastructure of pilomatrixoma (calcifying epithelioma)." *Cancer* 18(1965): 1445-1446.
11. Okun, M.R. and Edelstein, L.M. *Gross and Microscopic Pathology of Skin. Dermatopathology.* Boston:Foundation Press, 1976.
12. Lever, W.F. *Histopathology of Skin.* 5th ed. Philadelphia: Lippincott, 1975.
13. Turhan, B. and Krainer, L. "Bemerkungen uber die sogenannten verkalkenden epitheliome der Haut und ihre Genese." *Dermatologica* 85(1942): 73-77.
14. Milstone, E.B. and Helwig, E.B. "Basal cell carcinoma in children." *Arch. Dermatol.* 108(1973): 523-527.

15. Gray, H.R. and Helwig, E.B. "Epithelioma adenoides cysticum and solitary trichoepithelioma." *Arch. Dermatol.* 87(1963): 102-114.
16. Brook, H.G. "Epithelioma adenoides cysticum." *Br. J. Dermatol.* 4(1892): 269-286.
17. Montgomery, H. "Histogenesis of basal cell epithelioma." *Radiology* 25(1935): 8-23.
18. Goldman, H.J. "Multiple benign cystic epithelioma: report of 10 cases in one family." *JAMA* 115(1940): 2253-2257.
19. Werther, L. "Syringoadenoma papilliferum." *Arch. Dermatol.* 116(1913): 865-870.
20. Biberstein, H. "Uber papilliforme syringocystadenome." *Arch. Dermatol.* 152(1926): 602-608.
21. Reuterwall, O. "Naevus syringo-cystadenomatosus papilliferus and its relation to malignancy." *Acta Pathol. Microbiol. Scand.* [A] Supp. 16 (1933): 376-387.
22. Pinkus, H. "Life history of naevus syringoadenomatous papilliferus." *Arch. Dermatol.* 69(1954): 305-322.
23. Helwig, E.B. and Hackney, V.C. "Syringoadenoma papilliferum. Lesions with and without naevus sebaceous and basal carcinoma." *Arch. Dermatol.* 71(1955): 361-372.
24. Jancar, J. "Naevus syringocystadenomatosus papilliferus." *Br. J. Dermatol.* 82(1970): 402-413.
25. Landry, M. and Winkelmann, R.K. "An unusual tubular apocrine adenoma. Histochemical and ultrastructural study." *Arch. Dermatol.* 105(1972): 869-879.
26. Hashimoto, K. "Syringocystadenoma papilliferum. An electron microscopic study." *Archiv fur Dermatologische Forschung* 245(1972): 353-363.
27. Abrams A.N. and Finck, F.M. "Sialadenoma Papilliferum, a previously unreported salivary gland tumor." *Cancer* 24(1969): 1057-1063.
28. Winklemann, R.K. and Gottlieb, B.F. "Syringoma: an enzymatic study." *Cancer* 16(1963): 665-669.

Chapter XI

Leukemia and Lymphoma

LEUKEMIA

INCIDENCE

Leukemias of all types are the most common malignant neoplastic processes of children. Our population-based studies revealed an annual incidence of 3.9 cases per 100,000 children-at-risk per year for children 15 years of age or less; accounting for 39 percent of all malignancies. National data are similar and indicate that about 2500 new cases are diagnosed each year in the United States.

Leukemic presentation as a problem of the head and neck region is extremely rare, but leukemic involvement of the region at some time in the course of diagnosed disease is more common.

AGE AND SEX

The peak incidence of acute leukemia in children is between 3 and 4 years of age. There appears to be no significant difference in occurrence rates between boys and girls.

PATHOGENESIS

Although the cause or causes of leukemias remain(s) unknown, leukemogenic factors and predisposing conditions are clearly recognized. Leukemogenic factors include radiation and chemicals, with anti-cancer chemotherapeutic drugs becoming increasingly more important among this group of agents.

Predisposing conditions, in cases involving twin children, include the incidence, in one of the twins, Down's syndrome, Bloom's syndrome, etc. [1]

Considerable evidence points to a leukemogenic insult on hematopoietic progenitor cells with resultant clonal expansion and uncontrolled proliferation of a leukemic cell population, as the basic pathophysiology in leukemias. [2] There is great heterogeneity, particularly among lymphoid leukemias, as manifested by immunological characteristics. This heterogeneity reflects the scope of differentiation among clones of progenitor cells under leukemogenic influence. [3]

LIGHT MICROSCOPIC FINDINGS

The pathologist is usually presented with material from a "case of leukemia" for determination of the presence or absence of leukemic infiltration. With greater rarity, biopsy material is from a child without a prior diagnosis of leukemia. In either situation, recognition of the presence of leukemia is usually satisfactory to the extent that precise classification of subtype is ordinarily not expected or possible. One can, however, often classify the disease as lymphogenous or "non-lymphogenous" on the grounds of tissue morphology.

Gingival, soft tissue, or mucosal leukemic masses are more likely to be associated with myelocytic or monocytic leukemias, while leukemic lymphadenopathy is usually of lymphogenous derivation.

Tissue patterns of leukemic infiltration are variable, but, the infiltrate is usually deep- to mid-dermis in skin lesions and beneath, rather than in, mucosa of oral lesions. The monotony of cell type in the infiltrate is characteristic. Cells appear individually or free-floating rather than syncytially.

As a rule, lymphoid leukemias feature cells with little or no cytoplasm. Most often, nuclei are round to oval, chromatin is fine-granular, and nucleoli are indistinct (Fig. 11-1). In touch preparations stained with Wright's stain, "lymphoblasts" are readily identified and generally, the morphology is that of the FAB L-1 type[4] (Fig. 11-2).

Myeloid and monocytic leukemias feature cells with readily apparent pink cytoplasm. Nuclei are usually round to irregularly round, have more clumped chromatin, and prominent nucleoli (Fig. 11-3). Distinguishing monocytic from myelocytic morphology is usually impossible in H&E material, although monocytic leukemic cells may show phagocytic activity, but only rarely. Lederer stain, used for chloracetate esterase, favors myelogenous leukemia, while immunoperoxidase demonstration of lysozyme favors monocytic leukemia; although the latter stain may also be positive in myelogenous leukemia with maturation. Wright's stain of touch preparations usually will clarify the type of leukemia, but acute myeloblastic leukemia without Auer rods may be indistinguishable from monoblastic leukemia. Flouride-sensitive alpha naphthol acetate esterase positivity will establish the monocytic cell type of the leukemia.

A tissue diagnosis of leukemia should be made with caution, leading to bone marrow study for confirmation and detailed classification of the process. Myeloid and monocytic leukemias may, on occasion, be present without marrow involvement, which may take months to

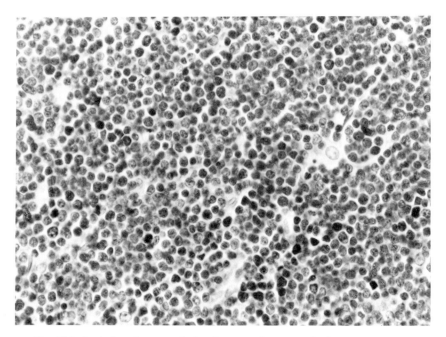

Fig. 11-1 Acute lymphogenous leukemia, appearing as a soft tissue mass, indistinguishable from lymphoblastic lymphoma. (H&E x 250).

evolve. In such cases, it is desirable to have significant evidence for the leukemic cell type before making a definitive diagnosis.

Morphologically, lymphogenous leukemia in lymph node is indistinguishable from lymphoblastic lymphoma; however, immunological features may differ.[5]

The FAB classification of acute leukemias[4] and the refinement of lymphogenous morphology by Miller et al.[6] provided a workable scheme with reasonably well-defined diagnostic criteria. The immunological characterization of acute lymphogenous leukemia is complex and in a state of rapid evolution.[3] Therapeutic relevance of the more sophisticated immunological studies is unproven.

ELECTRON MICROSCOPY

Leukemic cells usually are easily identified upon electron microscopic examination. In contrast to leukemic lymphocytes (Fig. 11-4), those of the granulocytic series contain a rich and varied complement of cytoplasmic organelles. The cells of acute myelogenous leukemia exhibit numerous cytoplasmic granules of varying size and electron density (Fig.

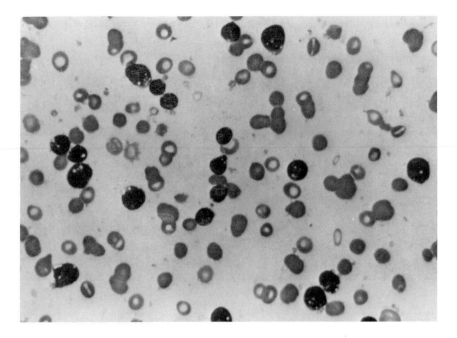

Fig. 11-2 Acute lymphogenous leukemia L1 morphology is demonstrated in this bone marrow smear. (Wright's x 400).

11-5). Leukemic monoblasts, on the other hand, display a monomorphic population of granules, are fewer in number, and are of uniform electron density (Fig. 11-6). Myeloperoxidase and non-specific esterase stains performed at the ultrastructural level[7] can be of value in the identification of poorly-differentiated or atypical leukemic cells in the occasionally problem case.

DIFFERENTIAL DIAGNOSIS

Inflammatory reactions pose the greatest problem in differential diagnosis, although other "small, round cell tumors" may be difficult to distinguish from leukemia. A monotony of cell type is the key point in neoplasm vs. reaction. The free-floating or individuality of cells in leukemia help with this differentiation from the syncytial tumor in the small, round cell group. The value of touch preparations is immeasurable in regard to these differential points.

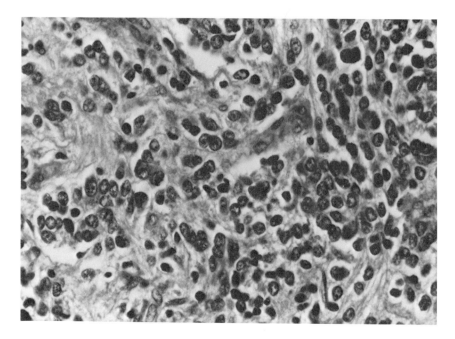

Fig. 11-3 Acute monocytic leukemia. A soft tissue nodular mass features leukemic cells among collagenous tissues. (H&E x 400).

TREATMENT AND PROGNOSIS

Complex and sophisticated chemotherapeutic regimens probably effect a cure rate of over 50 percent in children with acute lymphogenous leukemia who have favorable risk factors.[8]

Monoblastic leukemia in infants probably has a favorable prognosis similar to the lymphogenous type, while monoblastic leukemia in older children and myelogenous leukemia, in general, still have prognoses of less than a 20 percent long-term survival-rate.[8]

Every child with leukemia deserves the type of therapy that can be provided only in a sophisticated pediatric oncology center.

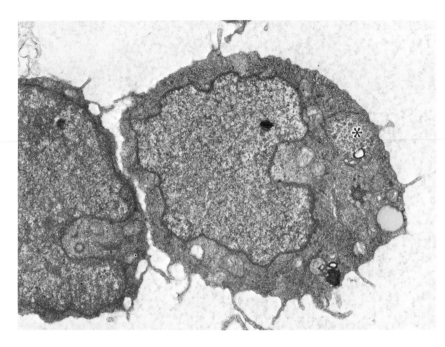

Fig. 11-4 Leukemic lymphocytes exhibit relatively few organelles, with free ribosomes as the dominant cytoplasmic component. Glycogen (asterisk), when present, is focally distributed. (EM x 16,600).

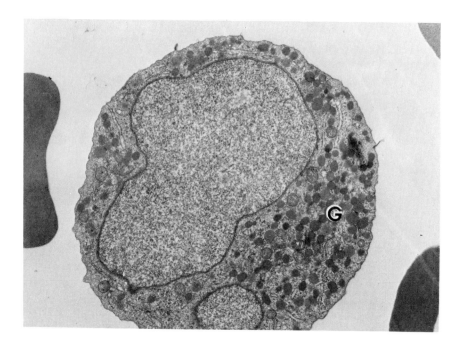

Fig. 11-5 Leukemic myelocytes typically display large numbers of cytoplasmic granules (G), heterogeneous in size and electron density. Glycogen is diffusely distributed through cytoplasm. (EM x 15,700).

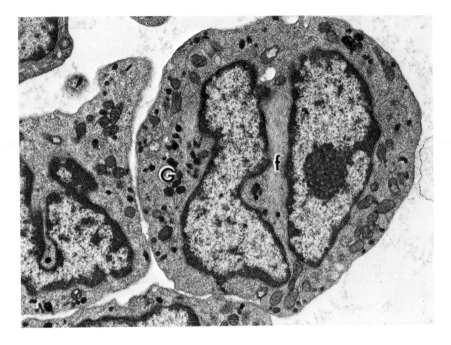

Fig. 11-6 Leukemic monocytes are similar in appearance to myelocytes but exhibit fewer granules (G), all of which are highly electron-dense, and more frequently display bundles of perinuclear cytoplasmic filaments (F). (EM x 15,700).

LYMPHOMA

INCIDENCE

Lymphomatous lymphadenopathy is the most common malignant neoplastic disorder of the head and neck region in children, accounting for nearly 40 percent of such cases. Nearly two-thirds of these children have Hodgkin's disease.[9]

AGE AND SEX

Hodgkin's disease is rare before the age of three, with most cases occurring in children nine- to eleven-years-old. A strong male predominance exists in its incidence (ratios range from 3-to-1 to 11-to-1).[9] Non-Hodgkin's lymphoma shares, with its counterpart, a similar male predominance (a ratio of 4-to-1). About 46 percent of such cases occur in children between the ages of three and ten, 30 percent occurring between the ages of ten and fourteen, 14 percent in those over fourteen years, and 8 percent in those less than three years of age.[10]

PATHOGENESIS

Lymphomas are considered to be malignant processes of the immune system, lacking a clear etiology, and represent problems of lymphocyte differentiation.[11;12] There is a substantial body of evidence for host predisposition in a patient possessing acquired or congenital immunodeficiency,[12] and evidence continues to grow for an etiological role for the Epstein-Barr virus in certain lymphomas.[13] These two factors are exemplified together in the sex-linked immunodeficiency syndrome as described by Purtilo.[14]

The "functional approach to the pathology of malignant lymphomas" espoused by Lukes[12;15] has had tremendous impact upon the discipline of hematopathology and provided the spark for a most exciting era in histopathology.

Hodgkin's disease is classified in children, as in adults, according to the Rye conference modification of the scheme of Lukes et al.[16;17]

Non-Hodgkin's lymphomas of children are rarely nodular and most cases manifest histology of a limited range of tumors: lymphoblastic lymphoma, small non-cleaved follicular center cell lymphomas (Burkitt or Burkitt-like types) and immunoblastic lymphomas. All fall into the so-called "high grade" group of lymphomas as defined by the "working formulation."[18]

Results of lymphoid-marker histology comparative studies suggested that most lymphoblastic lymphomas are of T-cell lineage; the small non-cleaved follicular center cell tumors are of B-cell lineage, and immunoblastic lymphomas may be of either cell line.

CLINICAL FINDINGS

Most lymphomas occur as masses. Lymphadenopathy is, by far, the most common sign of lymphoma, with cervical lymphadenopathy as the initial sign in nearly 90 percent of children manifesting Hodgkin's disease.[17] Involvement of Waldeyer's ring by B-cell tumors may be first manifested as a problem of respiratory obstruction.

About one-third of children with Hodgkin's disease have a fever, weight loss, and other constitutional symptoms at the time of appearance. These symptoms are unusual in non-Hodgkin's lymphomas. In general, symptomatology correlates with extent of lymphomatous disease, but careful and skilled staging procedures are indicated in all cases of lymphoma. Bone marrow evaluation before biopsy is essential.

LIGHT MICROSCOPIC FINDINGS

Criteria for the histological diagnosis of Hodgkin's disease are well-defined.[19] A pattern of lymphoma associated with multinucleated (2 or more nuclei) Reed-Sternberg cells or the presence of the lacunar Reed-Sternberg cell in the histological setting of nodular sclerosis constitutes acceptable histological findings. The latter cells may be difficult to identify in tissues which are fixed in anything other than formalin since that fixative-artifact seems essential for the cytomorphology of the lacunar cell.

Cases of lymphocyte-predominant Hodgkin's disease are often designated to as well-differentiated lymphocytic lymphoma or chronic lymphocytic leukemia. As a result of the extreme rarity of these disorders in children, it is only after careful study of thin sections, that such cases are, in many instances, properly recognized as lymphocyte-predominant Hodgkin's disease.

Tissue lymphoid-marker studies have proven to be of little value in Hodgkin's disease; however, the categorization of cases by the Lukes-Butler scheme has been shown to be relevant to prognosis.

The pathologist should not allow himself to become frustrated by the existing confusion in the literature concerning the classifications of non-Hodgkin's lymphomas. Instead, he should thoroughly familiarize himself with a specific classification for lymphomas based upon morphology, modify it if need be, and then establish a critical understanding with the clinical oncologist in order to co-ordinate the assignment of the appropriate name to each disorder. When inter-institutional relationships exist, the agreement on classification and criteria must necessarily be broader.

Only four types of non-Hodgkin's lymphoma account for nearly all lymphomas affecting children under 16 years of age. Almost all lymphomas of children are essentially diffuse.

There is good evidence favoring selective chemotherapy for lymphoblastic lymphoma. Therefore, the pathologist must be able to distinguish that type of tumor from all others. [10]

LYMPHOBLASTIC LYMPHOMA: [20]

This is the most common type of lymphoma found in children. It has a greater frequency of occurrence in the mediastinum, is rarely found in Waldeyer's ring and the abdomen, but can also occur in cervical nodes. Leukemic conversion is common.

Lymphoblastic lymphoma may feature cells with convoluted or non-convoluted nuclei (the former is the convoluted T-cell lymphoma of Lukes). [21] Generally, the nuclei of lymphoblastic lymphoma are smaller than the nuclei of reactive histocytoses found in the same tissue section. The nuclei may be uniformly round, or they may vary in shape from round to convoluted and clefted. Nuclear chromatin is diffuse and is usually fine and delicate. Nucleoli are generally inconspicuous, although on occasion, they may be somewhat prominent, particularly in the larger cells. The cytoplasm is usually scanty (Figs. 11-7, 11-8). Occasionally, these tumors are PAS positive, and the MGP stain is usually negative. Mitoses may be numerous and a "starry sky" pattern is common. Imprints show cells similar to the L1, and the L2 lymphoblasts of the FAB leukemia classification are occasionally seen as well.

SMALL, NON-CLEAVED CELL LYMPHOMAS:
(Burkitt and Burkitt-like Tumors)

These tumors are most often found in the abdomen. They are extremely rare in the mediastinum and Waldeyer's ring is commonly involved.

BURKITT LYMPHOMA:

The small, non-cleaved cell, Burkitt lymphoma, is diffuse, although a mixed, diffuse, and nodular pattern may be seen. A "starry sky" pattern is common. Nuclei approximate the size of the nuclei of the reactive histiocytes. They may be round to oval, and must be uniform and monotonous in appearance to be called Burkitt (Fig. 11-9). Nucleoli

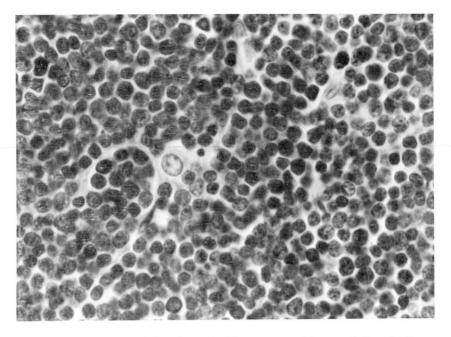

Fig. 11-7 Lymphoblastic lymphoma. A diffuse process, with a population of cells with scanty cytoplasm and indistinct nucleoli. (H&E x 400).

vary from 2-to-5 cm. and are usually prominent. The nuclear chromatin is diffuse or sometimes clumped with clear parachromatin. There is usually a moderate amount of cytoplasm which is amphophilic and pyroninophilic. Cytoplasmic vacuolation can often be seen.

BURKITT-LIKE LYMPHOMA:

The small, non-cleaved cell, Burkitt-like lymphoma, is probably more common than the Burkitt type. Although these tumors occur in the same sites as the Burkitt tumor, they seem to occur in peripheral nodes more frequently than Burkitt tumors. Nuclei approximate the size of, or are larger than, the nuclei of reactive histiocytes, but are larger than the nuclei of the immunoblastic lymphomas. There is considerable variation in nuclear size and shape in contrast to the monotonous and uniform appearance of the Burkitt tumor. Nuclear and cytoplasmic features are otherwise similar to those of the Burkitt tumor (Fig. 11-10).

Imprints of both types of small, non-cleaved cell lymphomas show cells similar to those described as L3 in the FAB classification of

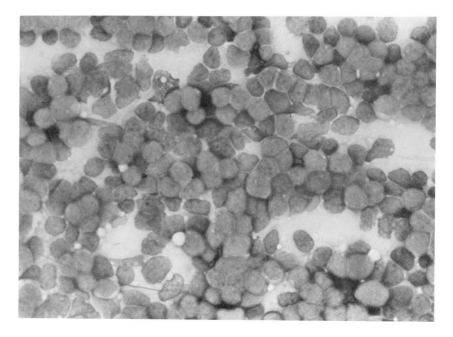

Fig. 11-8 Lymphoblastic lymphoma. A touch-imprint from the lymphoma shown in Fig. 11-7. Indistinguishable from the morphology of leukemia. (Wright's x 400).

leukemias. Cells usually have lipid vacuoles in cytoplasm and are methyl green pyronin positive and PAS negative.

The ability to reliably distinguish Burkitt from Burkitt-like lymphomas is poor even among the best hematopathologists, but it is also likely that the distinction has no therapeutic relevance in children.

IMMUNOBLASTIC LYMPHOMA:

A diffuse pattern without significant "starry sky" effect is the rule in this tumor. Cellularity is usually less dense than in lymphoblastic or small, non-cleaved cell lymphomas. Cells have nuclei which are larger than the nuclei of reactive histiocytes in the tissue section. Cell size is the most important diagnostic element in these tumors as they are large and polymorphous. Nuclei are large, round to oval, with prominent nucleoli and pale chromatin. In some tumors, nuclei are reniform or contorted shapes, chromatin is delicate, and nucleoli are inconspicuous. In some tumors, cells are plasmacytoid and may simulate Reed-Sternberg cells (Fig. 11-11). Other types of non-Hodgkin's lymphoma do occur in children, but are rare.

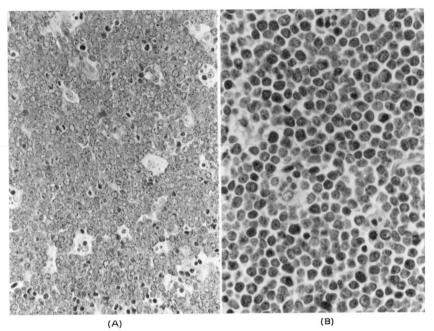

(A)   (B)

Fig. 11-9 Burkitt lymphoma: A. Diffuse lymphoma with prominent "starry sky" pattern. (H&E x 250). B. Monotonous cell pattern with prominent nucleoli and a moderate amount of cytoplasm. (H&E x 400).

Lymphoid-marker studies on cell suspensions prepared from fresh tissue are useful in correlation with morphology and provide additional data that may be clinically relevant at a future date. Our recommendation is to make a diagnosis on morphological grounds and add immunological findings parenthetically; i.e., lymphoblastic lymphoma (cortical thymocytic phenotype).

ELECTRON MICROSCOPY

Although neoplastic lymphocytes display no specific ultrastructural features, the peculiar array of the few cytoplasmic components present is sufficiently characteristic to usually allow easy identification. Polyribosomes occupy most of the cytoplasm. A few scattered clusters of mitochondria and an occasional serpentine profile of rough endoplasmic reticulum are usually the only other organelles present. Centrioles, when observed, are tightly surrounded by the Golgi complex. Cell junctions are not present.

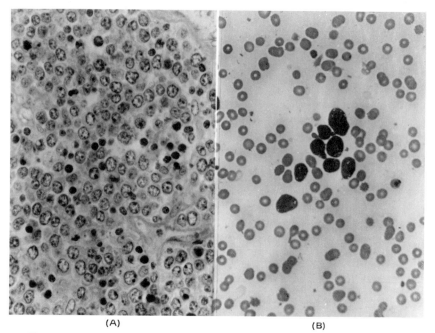

(A)   (B)

Fig. 11-10 Burkitt-like lymphoma: A. A more heterogenous cellular morphology distinguishes the lesion from Burkitt lymphoma. (H&E x 400). B. Cytology of Burkitt and Burkitt-like lymphoma is that of L3 lymphogenous leukemia. (Wright's x 400).

The cells of lymphoblastic lymphoma are indistinguishable from those of acute lymphogenous leukemia (Fig. 11-12). Similar focal deposits of glycogen, although not as commonly observed as in acute lymphogenous leukemia, do occur, and this fact must be taken into account when attempting to distinguish this tumor from Ewing's sarcoma. Electron microscopy can be of value in identifying lymphoblastic lymphoma with convoluted nuclei (Fig. 11-13). The complex folded nuclei which are characteristic of these cells can, at times, be difficult to see by light microscopy, but are easily seen with electron microscopy.

Electron microscopy can be helpful in establishing a diagnosis of Burkitt (or Burkitt-like) lymphoma, especially in cases where the results of conventional histologic stains are equivocal (Fig. 11-14). The classical histochemical triad of pyroninophilia, oil red O or Sudan positivity, and PAS negativity correlates at the ultrastructural level with abundant free ribosomes, numerous lipid inclusions, and the absence of glycogen.

Electron microscopic examination has revealed that the neoplastic cells of nearly all cases of so-called "histiocytic lymphoma" exhibit

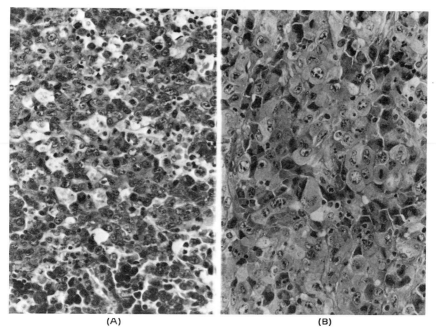

(A)   (B)

Fig. 11-11 Immunoblastic lymphoma: A. A pseudoepithelial pattern is seen in this tumor with B-cell immunological features. (H&E x 250). B. A large cell population manifests bizarre nuclei and highly malignant features. (H&E x 250).

the ultrastructural features of immunoblasts (i.e., transformed lymphocytes), rather than histiocytes or reticulum cells (Fig. 11-15).

Ultrastructural studies can be of great help in distinguishing lymphoma from thymoma, nasopharyngeal carcinoma, or a variety of metastatic epithelial tumors, all of which can be expected to exhibit cell junctions. It must be borne in mind, however, that failure to demonstrate cell junctions does not, in itself, exclude these latter possibilities from consideration.

DIFFERENTIAL DIAGNOSIS

It is absolutely essential that properly fixed tissue be sectioned thinly to render an expert interpretation. Non-neoplastic conditions which must be kept in mind as one examines lymph node histology include: infectious mononucleosis, rheumatoid disease, post-vaccinational adenopathy, toxoplasmosis, herpes zoster adenopathy, angioimmunoblastic lymphadenopathy, and rubella syndrome with immunodeficiency. Comprehensive accurate clinical data is essential for proper

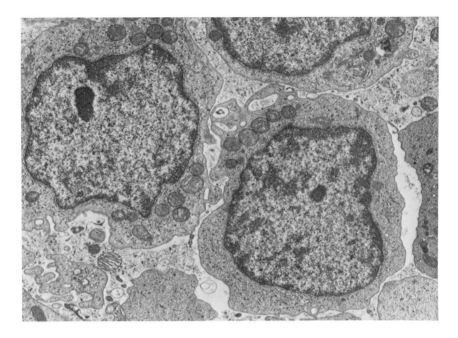

Fig. 11-12 Lymphoblastic lymphomas (without convoluted nuclei) typically display a relatively condensed nuclear chromatin pattern. Abundant polyribosomes impart a stippled appearance to a cytoplasm, otherwise almost devoid of organelles. (EM x 13,000).

interpretation. The fine points of histological differentiation have been published by Hartsock.[22]

Other neoplastic disorders occasionally confused with lymphomas are: metastatic thymoma, nasopharyngeal carcinoma, retinoblastoma, and neuroblastoma.

Cervical thymic tissue must not be confused with lymphomas. The presence of Hassall's bodies is distinctive in such material.

TREATMENT AND PROGNOSIS

Treatment of Hodgkin's disease is stage-dependent, is highly effective in localized disease with a 90 percent or better disease-free survival-rate, and includes radiation and chemotherapy.

Non-Hodgkin's lymphoma therapy is stage-oriented.[10] Localized disease of all histologic types is treated with radiation and chemotherapy. Three-year disease-free survival-data are quoted as approximately 89 percent.

Disseminated disease is treated with chemotherapy. One form of this treatment yields best results with lymphoblastic lymphoma, providing a 73 percent three-year disease-free state, while another form for other types of non-Hodgkin's lymphoma yields a 69 percent disease-free survival-data three years after diagnosis.

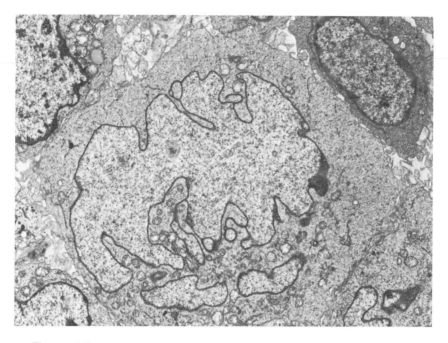

Fig. 11-13 Lymphoblastic lymphomas with convoluted nuclei exhibit, in addition to strikingly irregular nuclear outlines, a charactersitic homogenous electron-lucent nucleoplasm. (EM x 6,600).

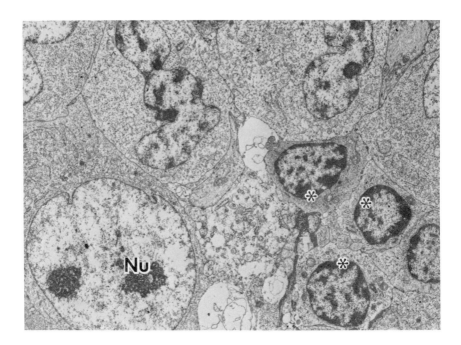

Fig. 11-14 The cells of immunoblastic lymphomas display the ultrastructural features associated with normally transformed lymphocytes. The enlarged nuclei of the neoplastic cells, in comparison to small lymphocytes (asterisks), exhibit prominent nucleoli (Nu) and a less-condensed chromatin pattern. (EM x 15,100).

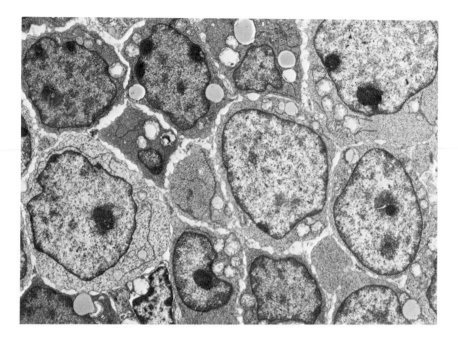

Fig. 11-15 Burkitt and Burkitt-like lymphomas display an especially rich complement of ribosomes and numerous lipid inclusions. (EM x 5,800).

References

1. Baehner, R.L. "Hematologic malignancies: leukemia & lymphoma." In *Smith's Blood Diseases of Infancy & Childhood*, 4th ed., pp. 588-646. St. Louis: C.V. Mosby, 1978.
2. Sallan, S.E. and Weinstein, H.J. "Childhood Leukemia." In *Hematology of Infancy and Childhood*. Vol. II, pp. 979-1022. Philadelphia: W.B. Saunders, 1981.
3. Janossy et al. "Cellular phenotypes of normal & leukemic hemopoietic cells determined by analysis with selected antibody combinations." *Blood* 56(1980): 430-441.
4. Bennett et al. "Proposals for the classification of acute leukemias." *Br. J. Haematol.* 33(1976): 451-458.
5. Callihan, T.R. and Berard, C.W. "Childhood Non-Hodgkin's Lymphomas in Current Histologic Perspective." *Perspect. Pediatr. Pathol.* 7(1982): in press.
6. Miller et al. "Prognostic Importance of Morphology (FAB classification) in Childhood Acute Lymphoblastic Leukemia (ALL)." *Br. J. Haematol.* 48(1981): 199-206.

7. Bozdech, M.J. and Bainton, D.F. "Identification of alpha-naphthyl butyrate esterase as a plasma membrane ectoenzyme of monocytes and as a discrete intracellular membrane-bounded organelle in lymphocytes." *J. Exp. Med.* 153(1981): 182-195.

8. Smithson, W.A.; Gilchrist, G.S. and Burgert, E.O., Jr. "Childhood Acute Lymphocytic Leukemia." *CA* 30(1980): 158-181.

9. Fraumeni, J.F., Jr. and Li, F.P. "Hodgkin's disease in childhood: an epidenologic study." *J. Natl. Cancer Institute* 42(1969): 681-687.

10. Jenkins et al. "Pediatric non-Hodgkin's lymphoma: The Childrens Cancer Study Group Experience — An Interim Report." In *Malignant Lymphomas: Etiology, Immunology, Pathology, Treatment.* pp. 591-601. New York: Academic Press, 1982.

11. Magrath, I.T. "Lymphocyte Differentiation: An essential basis for the comprehension of lymphoid neoplasm." *J. Natl. Cancer Institute* 3(1981): 501-514 (Guest Editorial).

12. Lukes, R.J., "The functional approach to the pathology of malignant lymphomas." In *Malignant Lymphoproliferative Diseases*, pp. 187-211. The Hague: Leiden University Press, 1980.

13. Seemayer, T.A.; Oligny, L.L. and Gartner, J.G. "The Epstein-Barr virus: Historical, Biologic, Pathologic and Oncologic Considerations." *Perspect. Pediatr. Pathol.* 6(1981): 1-34.

14. Purtilo, D.T. "Pathogenesis and phenotypes of an x-linked recessive lymphoproliferative syndrome." *Lancet* 2(1976): 882-886.

15. Lukes, R.J. and Collins, R.D. "Immunologic characterization of human malignant lyphomas." *Cancer* 34(1974): 1488-1503.

16. Lukes et al. "Report of the nomenclature committee." *Cancer Res.* 26(1966): 1131-1139.

17. Schnitzer et al. "Hodgkin's disease in children." *Cancer* 31(1973): 560-564.

18. Dorfman, R.F.; Burke, T.J. and Berard, C.W. "A new working formulation of non-Hodgkin's lymphoma: background, recommendations, histological criteria and relationships to other classifications." In *Advances in Malignant Lymphomas, Proceedings of the Third Annual Bristol-Myers Symposium on Cancer Research.* New York: Academic Press, 1981.

19. Lukes, R.J. "Criteria for involvement of lymph node, bone marrow, spleen and liver in Hodgkin's disease." *Cancer Res.* 31(1971): 1755-1767.

20. Nathwani, B.N.; Kim, H. and Rappaport, H. "Malignant lymphoma; lymphoblastic." *Cancer* 38(1976): 964-983.

21. Barcos, M.P. and Lukes, R.J. "Malignant lymphoma of convoluted lymphocytes: a new entity of possible T-cell type." In *Progress in Clinical and Biological Research*, pp. 147-177. Conflicts in Childhood Cancer, Vol. 4, edited by L.F. Sinks and J.O. Godden. New York: Alan R. Liss, 1975.

22. Hartsock, R.J. "Reactive lesions in lymph nodes." *The Reticuloendothelial System, International Academy of Pathology Monograph*, 16(1975): 152-183.

Chapter XII

Neuroectodermal Tumors and Associated Lesions

MELANOTIC NEUROECTODERMAL TUMOR OF INFANCY

Synonyms

1. Melanotic ameloblastoma
2. Retinal anlage tumor
3. Melanotic progonoma
4. Pigmented congenital epulis
5. Melanotic epithelial odontoma
6. Retinoblastic teratoma

INCIDENCE

The melanotic neuroectodermal tumor of infancy is a rare, benign neoplasm that characteristically appears in the anterior maxilla during the first 12 months of life. The tumor was first described in 1918 as a "congenital melanocarcinoma" by Krompecher.[1] Since then, more than 100 cases have been reported.[2,3] Although 80 percent of the reported cases have occurred in the premaxilla, other documented sites include the mandible, fontanelle, frontal bones, fourth ventricle, scapula, epididymis, cerebellum, and mediastinum.[4,5]

AGE AND SEX

The lesion generally occurs in infants under one year of age; the most common age is from one to three months.[6] There is no apparent sexual predisposition when all sites are considered, although Kerr and Pullon noted a 3-to-2 ratio of sexual predisposition for females in a literature review that excluded tumors not occurring in the maxilla or mandible.[7]

PATHOGENESIS

Four theories of histogenesis have been postulated.[6] Krompecher, in his original description, postulated that the lesion represented a malignant melanocarcinoma derived from pigmented odontogenic or epithelial cells. Studies of the biologic behavior of the tumor have caused this theory to be discounted.

Numerous investigators have proposed a retinal analage theory of histogenesis,[7-9] suggesting that the tumor arose from retinal tissues, which had been misplaced in the course of development. This developmental origin was accepted primarily in view of the tumor's possession of cleft-like alveolar spaces lined by pigmented tumor cells. This morphologic arrangement was considered reminiscent of infoldings resembling the ciliary processes of the eye, but no reported cases describe either a deficiency of retinal or iris tissue.[6] This theory has largely been discarded because entrapment of well-organized retinal tissue by less well-organized maxillary tissue at the time of formation of both tissue components is developmentally incongruous.

An odontogenic origin has been postulated by several investigators.[10-12] Reports which locate the tumor in several extracranial sites seem to discount this theory; in addition, there is little resemblance between tumor cells and either mesenchymal or epithelial portions of the tooth germ.

The theory of neural crest origin enjoys the broadest contemporary acceptance.[6] Embryological evidence of neural crest cell development from ectodermal cords and subsequent migration to the maxilla along with other sites is cited in support of this theory. This lesion presumably represents an overgrowth of these neuroectodermal cells, in either a normal or aberrant location, which usually would be expected to disappear in the normal course of maturation. Dooling and colleagues[13] have suggested, based upon histological similarities between the two tissues, that the fetal pineal may be a normally occuring precursor.

CLINICAL FINDINGS

The most common maxillary manifestation is as a soft tissue mass with intact overlying mucosa (Fig. 12-1). The lesion may contain blue or black areas of pigmentation, and several reported cases document inclusion of rudimentary teeth or displaced tooth germs in the tumor mass.[14]

The lesion may grow large enough to obliterate the labial buccal vestibule which in turn may displace and elevate the lip. Roentgenograms frequently demonstrate a poorly-delineated radiolucency with expansion of the labial or lingual cortices.

Pain and tenderness are seldom symptoms. The rate of tumor growth is variable; in some instances, the lesion may grow quite rapidly, while in others, the growth may be quite slow.[5]

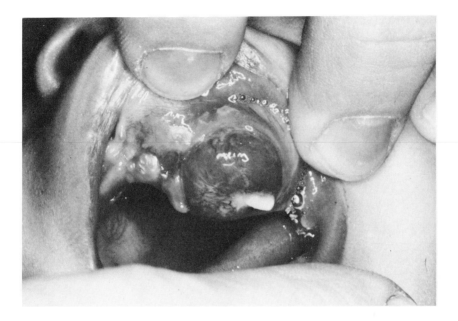

Fig. 12-1 Melanotic neuroectodermal tumor of infancy, involving the anterior maxilla. Courtesy of Drs. Stephen Young, Frederick Rubin, and Michael Rohrer.

LIGHT MICROSCOPY

Histological examination reveals a tumor composed of two cell types (Figs. 12-2, 12-3). The larger of the two cells has large quantities of pale cytoplasm which may contain melanin pigment. Occasionally, these cells are cuboidal or flattened. These larger cells generally line irregular, cleft-like alveolar spaces.

A second, smaller cell is common to the central alveoli. These cells have scant pale cytoplasm and much darker, staining nuclei than the larger cleft-lining cells. The smaller cells are quite basophilic, and generally are tightly packed. Mitotic activity and cellular atypia are uncommon features of either cell. The tumor stroma is composed of well-vascularized interlacing strands of fibrous connective tissue.

ELECTRON MICROSCOPY

Electron microscopy reveals the pigmented cells to be organized into an epithelium, being joined by desmosomes and resting upon a basal lamina. They exhibit abundant organelles, including numerous melanosomes in various stages of development (Fig. 12-4). Found within the

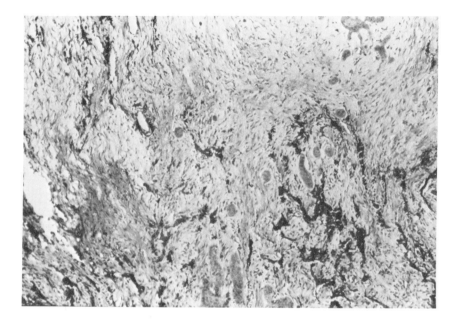

Fig. 12-2 Melanotic neuroectodermal tumor. Note epithelial cell clusters resembling small lymphocytes and scattered melanin. (H&E x 80).

masses of pigmented cells, or separated from them by a fibrocytic stroma, are clusters of the smaller nonpigmented cells (Fig. 12-5), containing relatively few organelles.

Its ultrastructural features support the concept that this tumor represents a neoplastic overgrowth of neuroectodermal cells, which not only maintains its epithelial character and its production of pigment, but includes poorly-differentiated cells resembling "neuroblasts" as well.[13] These poorly-differentiated cells have been described, primarily on the basis of their slender cytoplasmic processes, as resembling the cells of neuroblastoma.[15;16] Interestingly, the occasional patient with this tumor has been reported to exhibit elevated levels of urinary vanillyl-mandelic acid[14;17] —and in one instance, a primary tumor, typical in appearance and occurring with a metastatic lesion, eventually evolved to a point where it closely resembled a conventional neuroblastoma.[18] We hold, nevertheless, to an alternative view[19;20] which claims the nonpigmented cells to be, at least in most instances, simply poorly-differentiated variants of the melanized epithelial cells. This impression is based primarily upon the observation of: occasional premelanosomes within

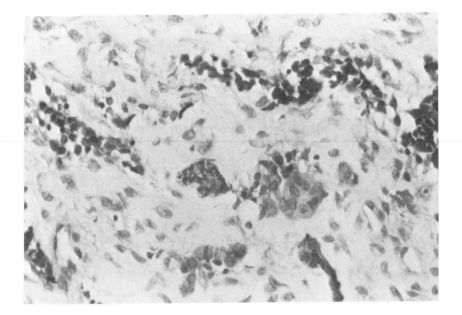

Fig. 12-3 Neoplastic cells displaying larger nuclei and peripheral melanin granules. (H&E x 280).

their cytoplasm, the occurrence of cells appearing to represent transitional forms between the two cell types, and the presence of "neuritic processes" among the well-differentiated pigmented epithelial cells.

DIFFERENTIAL DIAGNOSIS

Several soft tissue lesions can mimic the pigmented neuroectodermal tumor of infancy, including a large eruption cyst, pyogenic granuloma, or peripheral giant cell granuloma. The fact that over 71 percent of pigmented neuroectodermal tumors occur in the premaxilla prior to 12 months of age[21] favors this diagnosis for most pigmented soft tissue lesions in the anterior maxilla of infants.

Radiographs of pigmented neuroectodermal tumors frequently show poorly-marginated borders, thus favoring a roentgenographic diagnosis of malignancy; however, few malignant osseous lesions show a tendency to arise in the premaxilla of infants. Another presumptive diagnostic possibility is central giant cell granuloma, but this lesion is also a distinct rarity in the anterior maxilla of the infant.

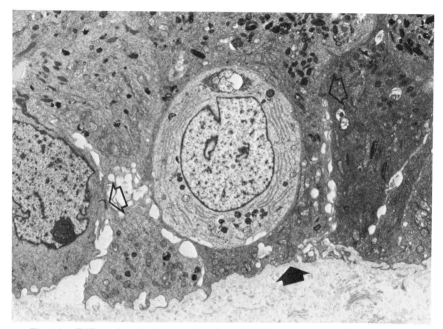

Fig. 12-4 Differentiated (pigmented) cells, exhibiting numerous melanosomes, are joined by desmosomes (open arrows) and rest upon a basal lamina (solid arrow). (EM x 5,300).

On histological grounds, the pigmented neuroectodermal tumor of infancy must be distinguished from other small, round cell tumors including neuroblastoma and lymphoma. The following features should assist in the differentiation of neuroblastoma and lymphoma from the pigmented neuroectodermal tumor. The neuroectodermal tumor of infancy contains tumor cells which: (1) cluster around cleft-like spaces; (2) show a predominance of two cell types; (3) almost invariably show some degree of pigmentation; (4) lack cytologic atypia, and (5) lack a rosette pattern.

TREATMENT AND PROGNOSIS

Most investigators consider the melanotic neuroectodermal tumor of infancy to be a benign neoplasm; the treatment of choice is local surgical excision with vigorous bony curettage. [14;20]

Although the tumor has a prevailing benign behavior, certain cases have shown local aggressive growth. [6;18;22] Local recurrences have

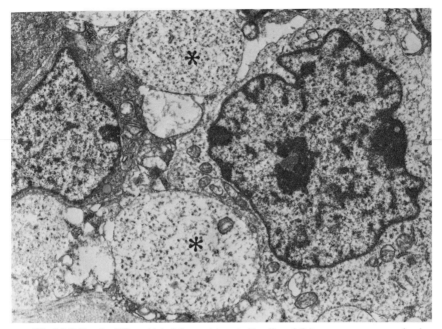

Fig 12-5 Poorly-differentiated (non-pigmented) cells exhibit more numerous, slender cytoplasmic processes (asterisks) than do the pigmented cells, but contain fewer organelles and only rarely exhibit cell junctions, premelanosomes, or basal lamina. (EM x 14,200).

been reported in 15 percent of cases according to the comprehensive review of Stowens and Lin.[23]

Prior to 1979, the only accepted example of malignant melanotic neuroectodermal tumor was reported by Lindahl in a stillborn infant with a maxillary neoplasm and metastases in the liver, adrenal gland, and lymph nodes.[24] Schulz reported a malignant pigmented melanotic tumor of the uterus,[25] but some authorities have suggested that this report is more appropriately a documentation of a malignant teratoma with melanin.[14;24]

Recently, Dehner and associates,[18] Block and co-workers,[22] and Navas and Palacios[26] have reported single cases of malignant melanotic neuroectodermal tumors; however, the final histological manifestation at autopsy in each case was one of a tumor most closely resembling neuroblastoma.

It remains important for the clinician to counsel patients and parents as to the benign yet potentially recurrent nature of the

NEUROBLASTOMA

Synonyms

1. Sympathoblastoma
2. Sympathicoblastoma
3. Sympathogoniona
4. Esthesioneuroblastoma
5. Neuroblastic apudoma

INCIDENCE

Neuroblastoma, the fifth most common malignant neoplasm of the head and neck region of children, is rarely primary in that site. Cervical involvement, usually cervical sympathetic chain or lymph node, occurred in 2.3 percent of neuroblastoma cases of all sites, in several series totaling 1230 cases.[27] The incidence of other soft tissue or bony involvement of the head and neck is extremely low.

AGE AND SEX

The highest incidence of neuroblastoma is in the first three years of life with a slight male predominance, and with whites more often affected than blacks.

PATHOGENESIS

Neuroblastomas are malignant embryonic tumors of neural crest origin and are members of the family of neoplasms of the APUD neuroendocrine system.[28] Tumors with ganglion cell differentiation of varying degrees and amounts (ganglioneuroblastoma), form a continuous spectrum between malignant neuroblastoma and benign ganglioneuroma. Neuroblastoma "maturation" (differentiation) to ganglioneuroma has been well-documented in a significant number of cases.[29]

The sites of involvement and favorable prognosis of widespread (IVs stage) disease in younger infants suggest that IVs neuroblastoma may not be a malignant neoplastic disease at all, but may be a proliferaton of neuroblastic embryonic rests which is destined to develop into either a malignant neoplasm or come under as yet undefined biological controls and undergo spontaneous resolution.[30]

Neuroblastoma of the head and neck should be assumed to be metastatic until proven to be otherwise by thorough tumor staging.

CLINICAL FINDINGS

Most cases manifest, at time of diagnosis, asymptomatic mass or tumor-causing proptosis, nasopharyngeal obstruction, or a tumor associated with a wide array of clinical conditions, some of which are related to catecholamine secretion by the tumor.

VMA (3-methoxy-4-hydroxy mandelic acid) and/or related chemicals can be found in the urine of about 90 percent of children with neuroblastoma [31] and, when present, is a useful marker of tumor activity during follow-up.

Nearly 50 percent of children with neuroblastoma of all sites have metastases at the time of appearance and a tumor can be found in bone marrow in about one half of such cases (25-30 percent of all cases). These data form the indication for pre-operative bone marrow evaluation in all cases of malignant neoplasia in children. A major operative procedure and general anesthesia can be avoided when the tumor is diagnosed from bone marrow studies.

Pre-operative evaluation of the child suspected of having neuroblastoma includes skeletal x-ray survey (or appropriate isotope scan), abdominal and chest x-rays, bone marrow biopsy, and urine catecholamine determinations. Clinical staging of the disease is imperative and forms the basis for management. [32]

GROSS AND LIGHT MICROSCOPIC FINDINGS

Neuroblastoma of the head and neck may occur as a resectable mass but is more often a lesion amenable only to incisional biopsy. The more primitive neuroblastoma is usually a pink to gray cerebroid, friable tissue which may be hemorrhagic and/or focally mineralized. The more differentiated or "mature" tumors are firmer and have a more tan appearance. Such tumors may, when they occur in the sympathetic chain, be associated with intramedullary tumor extension.

The more primitive tumors (neuroblastomas) are composed of cells with small lymphocyte-like nuclei which are round to oval, with fine granular chromatin and indistinct nucleoli. Cytoplasm is ill-defined and nuclei are generally associated with a fine fibrillary matrix or neurophil. Nuclei may form rosettes but usually occur in sheets or compartments formed by delicate connective tissue septae (Figs. 12-6, 12-7). Differentiation is reflected in larger nuclei which are more vesicular and have prominent nucleoli. Cytoplasm is more abundant; cells may be ovoid, polygonal or otherwise ganglion-cell-like. Nissl substance may be present. The occurrence of differentiated ganglion cells

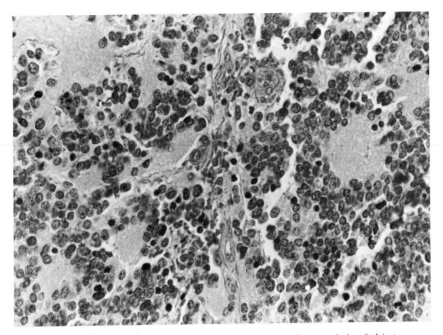

Fig. 12-6 Neuroblastoma. Well-developed rosettes are characteristic of this tumor of the neck. (H&E x 250).

in a distinctive neuro-fibrillary setting is seen in ganglioneuroma. Grading systems based on differentiation are useful.[33]

ELECTRON MICROSCOPY

The most constant and distinguishing ultrastructural feature of neuroblastoma is the presence of long slender "neuritic" processes (Figs. 12-8, 12-9) containing neurosecretory granules, microtubules and fine filaments. These usually can be easily demonstrated even in poorly-differentiated tumors.[34-38] Tumors arising in the olfactory region (esthesioneuroblastomas) are identical to neuroblastomas arising elsewhere. The demonstration of neuritic processes is sufficient to establish a diagnosis of neuroblastoma. Most neuroblastomas exhibit many poorly-formed desmosomes, a feature not present in lymphomas. Small cell carcinomas display well-formed desmosomes and conspicuous tonofilament bundles. Rhabdomyosarcomas rarely possess cell junctions and exhibit myofilaments and external lamina, features not observed in neuroblastoma.[39] We have found, and are in agreement with others, that

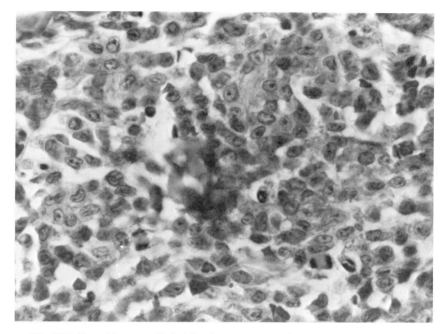

Fig. 12-7 Neuroblastoma. Well-defined rosettes were absent, but neuroblasts, in a neurophile stroma, are shown in this tumor. (H&E x 250).

5-10 percent of neuroblastomas contain cytoplasmic glycogen;[36] therefore, its presence alone cannot be used to distinguish neuroblastomas from tumors such as Ewing's sarcoma. Cell junctions are often difficult to find in Ewing's sarcoma, and when present, are usually not as well-developed as those in neuroblastomas.

DIFFERENTIAL DIAGNOSIS

Electron microscopy is of definite value in distinguishing neuroblastoma from lymphoma, Ewing's tumor, rhabdomyosarcoma, and small cell carcinomas. Special stains such as PAS have limited value and catecholamine autofluoresence is currently an investigative tool. Monoclonal antibodies to neuroblastoma antigen are also being investigated.

TREATMENT AND PROGNOSIS

Prognosis is related to age of the patient and clinical stage of disease at the time of diagnosis. Tumors with ganglion cell differentiation are associated with a better prognosis than those without differentiation. Careful evaluation of the child by surgeon, radiotherapist and pediatric oncologist is essential for proper management, because treatment may embody all three related modalities.

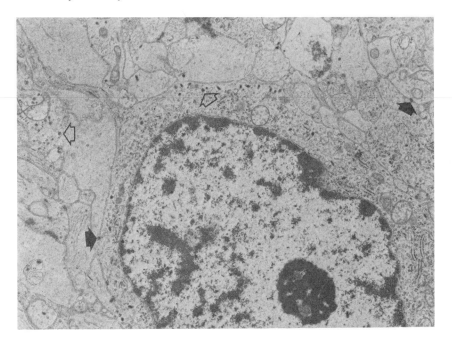

Fig. 12-8 Neuroblastoma cell surrounded by network of characteristic neuritic processes, exhibiting numerous neurosecretory granules (open arrows) and cell junctions (solid arrows). (EM x 13,500).

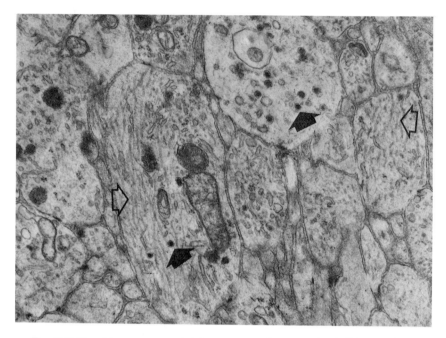

Fig. 12-9 Neuritic processes containing neurosecretory granules (solid arrows), microtubules (open arrows), and fine filaments. (EM x 30,600).

References

1. Krompecher, E. "Sur Histogenese und Morphologie der Adamantinome und Sonstiger Keifergeschwulste." *Beitraege zur Pathologischen Anatomie und Allgemeinen Pathologie* 64(1918): 165.

2. Karma, P.; Rasänen, O. and Karja, J. "Melanotic Neuroectodermal Tumor of Infancy," *J. Laryngol Otol.* 91(1977): 973-979.

3. Lopez, J., Jr. "Melanotic Neuroectodermal Tumor of Infancy: Review of the Literature and Report of a Case." *J. Am. Dent. Assoc.* 93(1976): 1159-1164.

4. Baugh et al. "Melano-Ameloblastoma. Report of a Case." *J. Oral Surg.* 26(1968): 542-545.

5. Batsakis, J.G. *Tumors of the Head and Neck. Clinical and Pathological Considerations* 2nd ed. Baltimore: Williams and Wilkins, 1979.

6. Lucas, R.B. *Pathology of Tumours of the Oral Tissues,* 3rd ed. London: Churchill Livingstone, 1976.

7. Kerr, D.A. and Pullon, P.A. "A Study of the Pigmented Anlage Tumors of Jaws of Infants (Melanotic Ameloblastoma, Retinal Anlage Tumor, Progonoma)." *Oral Surg.* 18(1964): 759-772.

8. Gotcher et al. "Recurrent Melanotic Neuroectodermal Tumor of Infancy: Report of a Case and Tumor Heterotransplantation Studies." *J. Oral Surg.* 38(1980): 702-706.

9. Helpert, B. and Patzer, R. "Maxillary Tumor of Retinal Anlage." *Surgery* 22(1947): 837-841.

10. Clarke, B.E. and Parsons, H. "An Embryological Tumor of Retinal Anlage Involving the Skull." *Cancer* 4(1951): 78-85.

11. Caldwell, J.B., Ernst, K.F. and Thompson, H.C. "Retinal Anlage Tumor of the Maxilla." *Oral Surg.* 8(1955): 796-802.

12. Munmery, J.H. and Pitts, A.T. "Melanotic Epithelial Odontoma in a Child." *Proc. R. Soc. Med.* 19(1926): 11-21

13. Dooling, E.C.; Chi, J.G. and Giles, F.H. "Melanotic neuroectodermal tumor of infancy. Its histological similarities to fetal pineal gland." *Cancer* 39(1977): 1535-1541.

14. Borello, E.D. and Gorlin, R.J. "Melanotic neuroectodermal tumor of infancy. A neoplasm of neural crest origin. Report of a case associated with high urinary excretion of vanillylmandelic acid. *Cancer* 19(1966): 196-206.

15. Nikai et al. "Ultrastructural evidence for neural crest origin of the melanotic neuroectodermal tumor of infancy." *J. Oral Pathol.* 6(1977): 221-232.

16. Taira et al. "Histological and fine structural studies on pigmented neuroectodermal tumor of infancy." *Acta Pathol. Jpn.* 28(1978): 83-98.

17. Brekke, J.B.; Minn, V. and Gorlin, R.J. "Melanotic neuroectodermal tumor of infancy." *J. Oral Surg.* 33(1975): 858-865.

18. Dehner et al. "Malignant melanotic neuroectodermal tumor of infancy. A clinical, pathologic, ultrastructural and tissue culture study." *Cancer* 43(1979): 1389-1410.

19. Neustain, H.B. "Fine structure of a melanotic progonoma or retinal anlage tumor of the anterior fontanel." *Exp. Mol. Pathol.* 6(1967): 131-142.

20. Hayward, A.F., Fickling, B.W. and Lucas, R.B. "An electron microscope study of a pigmented tumour of the jaw of infants." *Br. J. Cancer* 23(1969): 702-708.

21. Greer, R.O. and Mierau, G.W.: In *Tumors of the Oral Mucosa and Jaws in Infants and Children*, pg. 27. Denver: University of Colorado Medical Center Press, 1980.

22. Block et al. "Pigmented Neuroectodermal Tumor of Infancy: An Example of Rarely Expressed Malignant Behavior."*Oral Surg.* 49(1980): 279-285.

23. Stowens, D. and Lin, T.H. "Melanotic Progonoma of the Brain." *Hum. Pathol.* 5(1974): 105-112.

24. Lindahl, F. "Malignant Melanotic Progonoma. One Case." *Acta Pathol. Microbiol. Scand.* (A) 78(1970): 532-536.

25. Schulz, D. "A Malignant Melanotic Neoplasm of the Uterus, Resembling the 'Retinal Anlage' Tumors." *Am. J. Clin. Pathol.* 28(1957): 524-532.

26. Navas, J. and Palacios, J. "Malignant Neuroectodermal Tumor: Light and Electron Microscopic Study." *Cancer* 46(1980): 529-536.

27. Jaffe, B.F. "Pediatric head and neck tumors: A Study of 178 Cases." *Laryngoscope* 83(1973): 1644-1652.

28. Bolande, R.P. "The Neurocristopathies" *Hum. Pathol.* 5(1974): 409.

29. Bolande, R.P. "Benignity of neonatal tumors and the concepts of cancer regression in early life." *Am. J. Dis. Child.* 122(1971): 12-14.

30. Favara, B.E. "Origin of cancer in the neonate", *Am. J. Pediatr. Hematol./Oncol.* 3(1981): 187-191.

31. deGutierrez Moyano, M.B.; Bergada, C. and Becu, L. "Catecholamines in forty children with sympathoblastoma." *J. Pediatr.* 77(1970): 239-244.

32. Evans, A.E.; D'Angio, G.J. and Randolph, J. "A proposed staging for children with neuroblastoma" *Cancer* 27(1971): 374-378.
33. Beckwith, J.B. and Martin, R.F. "Observations on the histopathology of neuroblastoma" *J. Pediatr. Surg.* 3(1968): 106-110.
34. Mackay, B.; Luna, M.A. and Butler, J.J. "Adult neuroblastoma. Electron microscopic observations in nine cases." *Cancer* 37(1976): 1334-1351.
35. Romansky, S.G.; Crocker, D.W. and Shaw, K.N.F. "Ultrastructural studies on neuroblastoma. Evaluation of cytodifferentiation and correlation of morphology and biochemical and survival data." *Cancer* 42(1978): 2392-2398.
36. Yunis et al. "Glycogen in neuroblastoma. A light- and electron-microscopic study of 40 cases." *Am. J. Surg. Pathol.* 3(1979): 313.
37. Taxy, J.B. "Electron microscopy in the diagnosis of neuroblastoma." *Arch. Pathol. Lab. Med.* 104(1980): 355-360.
38. Reynolds et al. "Catecholamine flourescence and tissue culture morphology. Techniques in the diagnosis of neuroblastoma." *Am. J. Clin. Pathol.* 75(1981): 275.
39. Mierau, G.W. and Favara, B.E. "Rhabdomyosarcoma in children: Ultrastructural study of 31 cases." *Cancer* 46(1980): 2035-2040.

Chapter XIII

Peripheral Nerve Tumors

NEUROGENIC TUMORS OF THE HEAD AND NECK

Synonyms

1. *Schwannoma*
   Neurolemmoma
   Neurilemmoma
   Neurinoma
2. *Neurofibroma and Neurofibromatosis*
   Neurofibroma
   Plexiform Neurofibroma
   Solitary Neurofibroma
   Diffuse Neurofibroma
3. *Neurogenic Sarcoma*
   Neurosarcoma
   Malignant Neurilemmoma
   Nerve Sheath Sarcoma
   Malignant Schwannoma
   Neurofibrosarcoma

INTRODUCTION

Peripheral nerve tumors may be categorized either as those of nerve sheath origin or those of sympathetic nervous system origin.[1] The nerve sheath tumors include schwannoma, neurofibroma, and neurogenous sarcoma. *Neurilemmoma* is a solitary and encapsulated tumor usually attached to, or surrounded by, a nerve and is almost never associated with von Recklinghausen's disease or malignant change. Neurites do not traverse the tumor and degenerative changes, such as cystic change or hemorrhagic necrosis, are usually present.

In contrast, neurofibromas are non-encapsulated and usually multiple. They are the harbinger tumors of von Recklinghausen's multiple neurofibromatosis, and in approximately 8 to 10 percent of cases, one of the multiple tumors undergoes a malignant change.[2;3] Neurites pass through this tumor and retrogressive changes are uncommon.

Neurogenous sarcoma is a malignant neoplasm of nerve sheath origin. Although the majority arise from neurofibromas, the noncommittal term, "neurogenous sarcoma" is preferred over "neurofibrosarcoma." These tumors are difficult to remove on primary excision, and tend to recur locally, but are slow to metastasize.

The neoplasms of sympathetic nervous system origin form a spectrum of disease, ranging from neuroblastoma through the mature ganglioneuroma. Neuroblastoma was discussed in Chapter 12. Rare neural tumors and syndromes are discussed under the differential diagnostic headings in the present chapter.

INCIDENCE

The head and neck region is the most common location for benign nerve sheath neoplasms. Das Gupta and colleagues,[4] in reviewing 303 cases of benign nerve sheath tumors seen at Memorial and James Ewing Hospitals in New York from 1926 to 1963, found that 44.8 percent occurred in the head and neck. The vast majority of these lesions occurred in adults; only 12 percent of the lesions were reported to have occurred during childhood or adolescence. Neurogenous malignancies are exceedingly rare. Malignant transformation of neurofibromas in neurofibromatosis occurs in approximately 5.5 to 16 percent of cases.[5;6]

NECK:

The neck is the most common site for neurogenic tumors in the head and neck.[4] Nerve tumors in this location have been subdivided into lesions of the medial and lateral neck by Daly and Raesler,[7] and DiPietro.[8] The medial group arises from the last four cranial nerves and the cervical sympathetic chain; the lateral group arises from the cervical neck trunk, cervical plexus, and brachial plexus.[9] The lateral neck appears to be the site most frequently involved.[9] Rosenfeld and co-workers[10] reviewed 32 primary neurogenic tumors of the lateral neck and found only six tumors in children or adolescents. Five of the six occurred in the first decade of life. One malignancy, a neuroblastoma, was documented in a child 22-months-old.

ORAL CAVITY:

Benign nerve sheath neoplasms of the oral soft tissues are uncommon; the incidence of oral involvement is given as 6.5 percent by Baden and co-workers,[11] and 9 percent by Das Gupta.[4] Wright and Jackson reported that the most common locations are the tongue, buccal or vestibular mucosa, and palate.[12] Malignant change has been reported,[13] but is rare.

INTRAOSSEOUS SITES:

The vast majority of intraosseous head and neck nerve sheath neoplasms occur in the mandible. A 1977 survey of the English-language literature by Ellis, Abrams, and Melrose[14] disclosed 28 acceptable reported cases of primary benign nerve sheath tumors arising in the jaws.[14] Additional single case reports have been added to the literature since then.[15;16] Ellis reported that 11 of 28 cases were in children and adolescents ranging in age from 2 to 18 years.

Malignant central osseous lesions are rare. An extensive review of the literature by Devore and Waldron[17] disclosed only two cases of malignant neurogenous tumors involving the maxilla and seven involving the mandible. Eversole and co-workers[18] reported six additional cases of central osseous neurogenic sarcoma in a 1978 review; one occurred in the mandible of a two-year-old female, the remainder occurred in adults. Nerve sheath neoplasms of the bones of the face and skull have been reported in children, but are rare.

FACIAL NERVE:

Nerve sheath tumors can rarely affect the facial nerve as it transverses the cranium or as it transcends the temporal bone. Sarkor,[19] and Furlow and Walsh[20] have reviewed the subject. Such lesions are exceedingly uncommon in children.

NASAL CAVITY AND PARANASAL SINUSES:

Primary neurogenic tumors arising in the nasal cavity and paranasal sinuses of children are almost curiosities. Kragh and associates reviewed 152 neurilemmomas of the head and neck over a 47-year-period and found that only one involved the paranasal sinuses.[21] Robitaille and associates[22] found only 16 acceptable instances of a peripheral nerve tumor arising in paranasal sinuses directly from opthalmic or maxillary branches of the trigeminal nerve or branches of the autonomic nervous system. All of the tumors they reviewed were benign, and the youngest patient was 19 years of age.

Iwamura and associates[23] reported a case of schwannoma of the nasal cavity in an 18-year-old girl. These authors also reviewed the literature on nasal and maxillary sinus schwannomas and found only 12 reported cases. Nearly three times that number have been reported involving the nose and external sinuses. Batsakis commented that while only 60 total cases of nerve sheath tumors of the nasal cavity and paranasal sinuses are reported in the literature, this figure may be much lower than the true incidence.[9] Neurofibromas and neurogenic sarcomas are exceedingly rare in this area in all age groups.

SALIVARY GLANDS:

Tumors of nerve sheath origin in salivary glands are rare in adults, although neurofibroma, hemangioma, and lymphangioma account for 50 percent of all salivary gland tumors in children.[24] The parotid gland is the favored site for all three lesions.

LARYNX:

Benign neurogenic tumors involving the larynx are uncommon. El-Serafy[25] reported that 89 cases were documented in the literature through 1971. Fourteen of these cases were associated with von Recklinghausen's disease; however, most laryngeal neurogenic tumors are solitary schwannomas.[26] Gibbs, Taylor, and Young[27] and Putney and colleagues[28] have reported benign nerve sheath tumors of the larynx in children. Neurosarcoma in children is exceedingly rare in this anatomic location.

AGE AND SEX

Authors who have reported large series of head and neck *neurilemmomas*[4;10;28] have noted no preponderance of tumors in any age group, but report a sex ratio of approximately six females-to-four males.

As would be anticipated, patients with von Recklinghausen's disease (*multiple neurofibromatosis*) are generally younger than individuals with other peripheral nerve tumors. The mean age of patients with neurofibroma in the head and neck area, regardless of anatomic site, is approximately 15.[3] Manifestations of von Recklinghausen's disease are present in the majority of these patients, including multiplicity of tumors, "cafe au lait" spots, and congenital malformations.[29] It has been generally accepted that any person with more than six "cafe au lait" spots greater than 1.5 cm. in diameter has neurofibromatosis until proven otherwise.[30] Whitehouse[31] has modified this for children to include five or more spots greater than 0.5 cm. Although Oberman and Sullenger[3] reported a greater number of males than females in their review of nerve tumors, it is generally accepted that there is no sexual predisposition for neurofibromas in the head and neck area.

The incidence of sarcomatous change or the development of *neurogenic sarcoma* in association with a pre-existing neurofibroma is reported to range from 5.5 to 13 percent of patients.[5;32] Sarcomatous transformation is more likely to occur in deeply-situated neurofibromas and such change is more frequent in males than females. The peak age incidence is between 2 and 30 years.[33] Although a significant percentage of patients with multiple neurofibromas can be expected to manifest malignant change in one or more of their lesions, malignant alteration is rarely observed in childhood. Oberman and Sullenger[3] reported that none of their patients, first diagnosed as having multiple neurofibromatosis in childhood, developed neurogenous sarcoma after intervals of follow-up extending up to 23 years.

Neurogenous sarcoma unassociated with multiple neurofibromas is primarily a disease of adults, no sexual predisposition has been demonstrated,[3;18] and no correlation between its occurrence and the benign schwannoma has been revealed.[34]

PATHOGENESIS

At present it is generally accepted that peripheral nerve tumors (schwannoma, neurofibroma, neurogenic sarcoma) arise from cells of the sheath of Schwann. Proponents of this theory have produced considerable evidence to support it, based principally on the tissue culture studies of Murray and Stout.[35] Some investigators, however, have maintained that peripheral nerve tumors arise from fibroblasts of the epineurium.[36-38] Their chief objection to the Schwann cell theory lies in the fact that nerve sheath tumors generally contain abundant collagen, a uniquely fibroblastic product. However, recent tissue culture and ultrastructural studies have now shown Schwann cells to be capable of producing collagen,[39] and the Schwann cell origin is, as a result, nearly universally accepted.

CLINICAL FINDINGS

Schwannomas of the head and neck usually occur as solitary well-encapsulated benign tumors characteristically attached to, or running along the course of, a peripheral, cranial, or sympathetic nerve. Small tumors are usually solid, but larger tumors, which may attain a maximum diameter in excess of 10 cm., often exhibit spontaneous degeneration and hemorrhage.[21] Schwannomas are only very rarely associated with von Recklinghausen's disease or malignant change.

Neurofibromas are atypically non-encapsulated and are usually multiple. They are classically associated with von Recklinghausen's disease, with its characteristic skin pigmentation, bony abnormalities, and a tendency to develop neurogenic sarcoma. Since neurites pass through neurofibromas, retrogressive changes such as cystic degeneration, diffuse hemmorhage, and necrosis are not as common as in schwannoma.[9]

Neurofibromas, when seen peripherally, seem to occur in two separate clinical patterns: (1) as multiple discrete nodules, and (2) as great pendulous, often pigmented, masses of tissue[12] (Figs. 13-1A, 13-1B). The radiographic manifestations of neurofibromatosis, especially in children, have been thoroughly reviewed by Holt.[40] These include macrocranium, macroencephaly, cervical kyphosis, and bowing and pseudoarthrosis, especially of the tibia. Acoustic neuromas and optic nerve gliomas have also been associated with neurofibromatosis.[12]

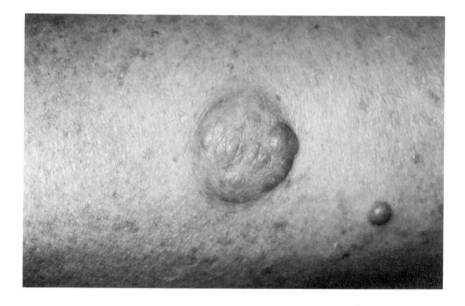

Fig. 13-1A Multiple neurofibromas of the neck. Courtesy of Dr. Loren Golitz.

Ellis, Abrams and Melrose[14] reported that the most commonly manifested symptom of the child with a benign central osseous neurogenic tumor, regardless of histologic type, is swelling or expansion. Pain or paresthesia are less common symptoms. This is in contrast to the clinical symptoms often associated with soft tissue neurofibromas and schwannomas, which dictate that neurofibromas are often reported to be asymptomatic, and schwannomas, painful and tender.

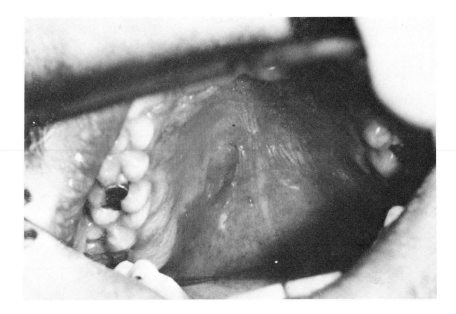

Fig. 13-1B Pendulous solitary neurofibroma of the hard palate.

Roentgenographically, neurilemmomas tend to be well-defined, unilocular radiolucencies, while neurofibromas are more poorly-defined and appear as unilocular as well as multilocular radiolucencies. Cortical perforation is not a common finding with either lesion.

The typical manifestation of the benign neurogenic tumor of the soft tissues of the oral cavity is one of a smooth-surfaced, usually painless, solitary, or multifocal, soft tissue swelling with intact overlying epithelium.[41] Tumors of the medial or lateral neck usually occur as a visible and palpable mass.

In the nose and nasal sinuses, difficulty in breathing may be the principal clinical symptom. Pain is a common symptom of maxillary sinus tumors, and difficulty in swallowing and hoarseness may be associated with pharyngeal and laryngeal lesions respectively. The principal symptomatology of a tumor of the facial nerve is a peripheral facial palsy over a period of months.[9]

Neurogenic sarcoma frequently appears as a rapidly expanding mass which may be quite painful if associated with a large nerve. Most neurogenic sarcomas are firm, lobular, and only roughly circumscribed.[9] Cystic degeneration and tumor necrosis may result in areas that are soft or spongy. Lesions arising centrally within bone usually take the form of multilocular lesions early on, and as "ragged moth-eaten" radiolucencies with ill-defined borders in later stages of development.

LIGHT MICROSCOPY

SCHWANNOMA:

Schwannoma is an encapsulated neoplasm composed of varying quantities of two types of tissue termed Antoni A and Antoni B tissue. Antoni A tissue is characterized by palisading of spindle-shaped Schwann cells around a central acellular area (Fig. 13-2). This whole structure is known as a Verocay body. A second type of tissue (Antoni B) is less cellular and shows microvacuolation of the intercellular substance (Fig. 13-3). The nuclei of the Schwann cells appear less elongated than in Antoni A tissue. In these areas the blood vessels may have thickened walls and mast cells may be found. [12;42]

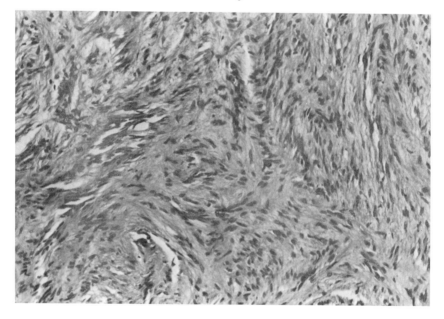

Fig. 13-2 Schwannoma showing distinctive palisading Antoni A type tissue. (H&E x 280).

ANCIENT SCHWANNOMA (ANCIENT NEURILEMMONA):

The ancient schwannoma was first described in the thorax by Ackerman and Taylor in 1951. [43] This lesion is well-encapsulated and

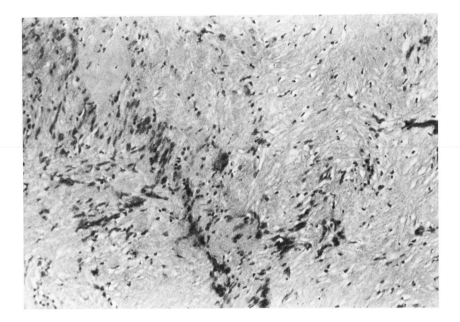

Fig. 13-3 Vacuolated Antoni B tissue is prominent in this medium power photomicrograph of schwannoma. (H&E x 160).

may contain both Antoni A and Antoni B tissue. Inflammatory cells, fibrous areas, and thick-walled blood vessels are usually present, and areas of hemorrhage and hemosiderin may be seen. The tumor also contains many areas with large atypical and pleomorphic nuclei, some of which may be hyperchromatic, although mitoses are not generally a feature of the neoplasm. Three cases from a series reviewed by Wright and Jackson [12] were located in the neck, as were two of eleven cases reported by Dahl. [44] The lesion has also been reported to occur intraorally. [45;46]

NEUROFIBROMA AND NEUROFIBROMATOSIS:

Neurofibromas seem to occur in two forms; solitary and multiple. The distinction is basically a clinical one, because histologically it is often difficult to distinguish a solitary neurofibroma from a manifestation of neurofibromatosis.

The *solitary neurofibroma* is a benign, slowly growing, relatively circumscribed but non-encapsulated neoplasm, originating in a nerve and consisting of Schwann cells, perineural cells, and varying amounts of mature collagen (Fig. 13-4). Microscopic examination usually reveals a lesion well-demarcated from surrounding tissue, in contrast to many neurofibromas seen in association with neurofibromatosis.

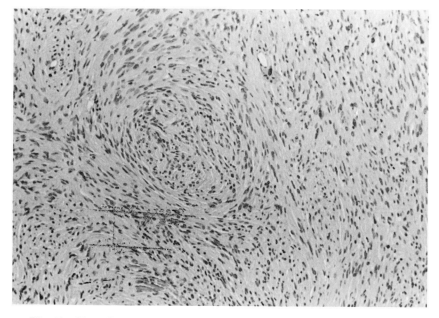

Fig. 13-4 Neurofibroma. Note the course of nerve sheath cells concentrically around nerve. (H&E x 180).

Tumor cells are elongated, fusiform, and often have "comma-shaped" nuclei (Fig. 13-5). These cells are set in a myxomatous, microvacuolated matrix of wavy collagen fibers, and mast cells (said to be more numerous than in the Antoni B tissue of the schwannoma), are common, and may constitute a useful diagnostic feature.[42]

Histologically, the lesions of neurofibromatosis show the same features as those described in solitary neurofibroma, —excepting the usual absence of a distinct margin found between the neurofibroma and the surrounding tissue. Lesions are often plexiform in character, containing distorted masses of myxomatous peripheral nerve still contained within perineurium and surrounded by neurofibroma. Harkin and Reed[47] suggested that the plexiform neurofibroma seems to occur only with neurofibromatosis.

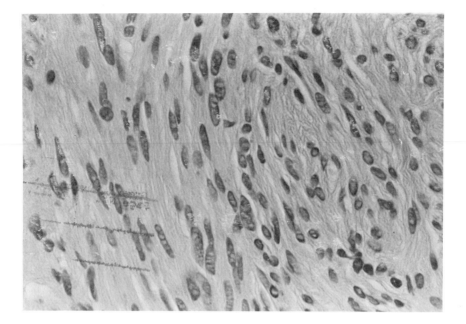

Fig. 13-5 Higher power, showing elongated fusiform cells of neurofibroma. (H&E x 360).

NEUROGENIC SARCOMA:

Neurogenic sarcoma can be divided into two relatively broad categories. The first is a malignant change in lesions of neurofibromatosis, designated by Harkin and Reed[47] as neurofibrosarcoma. The second is either a malignant neural tumor, diagnosed, in the absence of neurofibromatosis, on the basis of surgical or radiographic evidence of origin from a nerve trunk, or, those malignant neoplasms which, on histologic examination, show (as does malignant epithelioid schwannoma) a recognizable neural pattern. Neurogenic sarcoma is not a common diagnosis if the preceding criteria are used.[12]

Histologically, neurogenic sarcoma is a highly cellular neoplasm composed of plump spindle-shaped cells, usually with elongated cytoplasmic processes (Fig. 13-6). The cells are often arranged in characteristic streaming or swirling patterns,[12] and the stroma ranges from collagenous to myxomatous. There may be varying degrees of nuclear pleomorphism, and mitoses are often numerous. Atypical cellular areas in neurofibromas, especially in patients with neurofibromatosis, may be suggestive of malignant change. One histological type of malignant tumor shows round to polyhedral cells which are sometimes arranged in nests reminiscent of melanoma. This pattern has tentatively been classified as *malignant epithelioid schwannoma* by Harkin and Reed.[47]

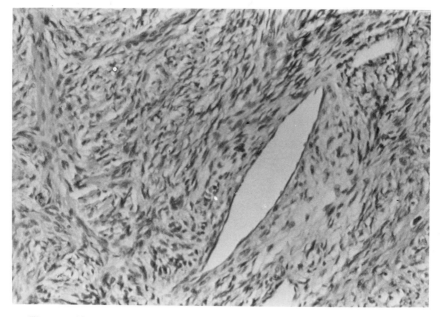

Fig. 13-6 Neurogenic sarcoma composed of a highly cellular proliferation of plump, often hyperchromatic, spindle-shaped cells. (H&E x 160).

ELECTRON MICROSCOPY

The neoplastic Schwann cells of benign nerve sheath tumors are easily identified using electron microscopy. Like their normal counterparts, they display a cytoplasm relatively poor in organelles (Fig. 13-7). Most conspicuous are scattered mitochondria, variable numbers of lysosomes, and numerous delicate, randomly-oriented cytoplasmic filaments. The cytoplasmic filaments of Schwann cells are neither as densely-packed nor as well-organized as are those of smooth muscle cells or myofibroblasts, and are not associatd with fusiform bodies or peripheral condensation plaques. It is also noteworthy that Schwann cells do not exhibit the prominent rough endoplasmic reticulum characteristic of fibroblasts. They typically possess long, slender cytoplasmic processes which, in the absence of nerve fibers, often appear to express their aborted potential for forming myelin sheaths by attempting to envelop each other. The cells frequently exhibit pinocytotic activity, and characteristically, are surrounded by an external lamina. Modified desmosomal-type attachment sites occur between adjacent cells. "Luse" bodies,[48] cross-banded bundles of collagen with a periodicity of 100-120 nm., were at one time considered pathognomonic of schwannoma but have since been demonstrated in a number of other neoplastic and non-neoplastic conditions. Although nonspecific, their frequency of occurrence in Schwann cell tumors makes them of some diagnostic value.

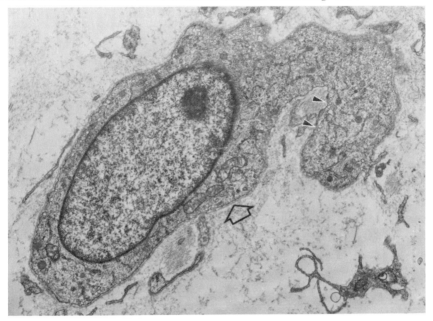

Fig. 13-7 Schwann cells, characteristically, are enveloped by an external lamina (arrow) and typically display numerous pinocytotic vesicles (arrowheads) and delicate cytoplasmic filaments, but only a modest amount of rough endoplasmic reticulum. (EM x 13,100).

Electron microscopic studies have thus far done more to fuel than to resolve the controversy surrounding the histogenesis of *neurofibroma*. Current thoughts regarding whether these tumors derive from Schwann cells, fibroblasts, or a common progenitor cell have been summarized by Ghadially.[49] Whatever their derivation, neurofibromas are found to display, usually in abundance, both Schwann cells and fibroblasts (Fig. 13-8) within a collagenous matrix, which will also often contain unmyelinated (Fig. 13-9) and/or myelinated nerve fibers.

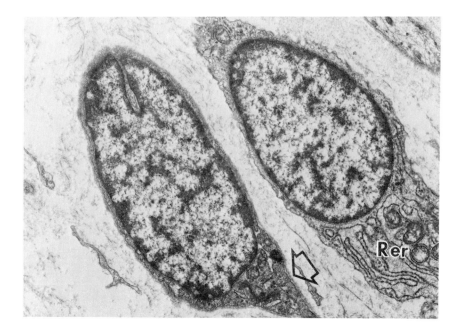

Fig. 13-8 The Schwann cells of neurofibromas (cell on the left) are easily distinguished from associated fibroblasts (cell on the right) by their well-developed external lamina (arrow) and relative paucity of rough endoplasmic reticulum (Rer). (EM x 13,500).

By enabling positive identification of Schwann cells, electron microscopy can prove of value in the occasional troublesome case. It should be recognized, however, that the proportion of Schwann cells present in these tumors is quite variable and that, in some instances, even with careful attention to sampling, ultrastructural studies may fail to establish the diagnosis.

Malignant Schwann cells tend to be less well-differentiated than their benign counterparts, but often retain sufficient features to enable identification. In some instances, their characteristic external lamina is lost altogether, but it commonly persists in an attenuated and/ or interrupted form or as a less clearly-defined flocculent coating along the plasma membranes (Fig. 13-10). The slender intertwining cell processes and intercellular junctional complexes also seen in benign schwannomas, are variably present. We have not observed "Luse" bodies in malignant Schwann cell tumors. Although the cells may appear plumper than those of non-neoplastic Schwann cells, in general they

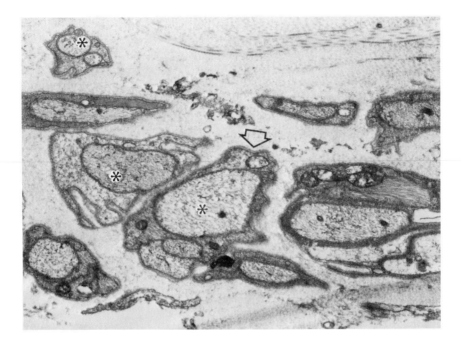

Fig. 13-9 Frequently observed in neurofibromas are unmyelinated axons (asterisks), ensheathed by Schwann cells and their associated external lamina (arrow). (EM x 16,500).

display a similar organelle-poor cytoplasm containing numerous randomly-oriented delicate filaments.

Our experience with presumed malignant schwannomas has been similar to that of Taxy and associates,[50] who reported electron microscopic studies to have been helpful in establishing a diagnosis in 8 of 15 cases examined.

DIFFERENTIAL DIAGNOSIS

Benign nerve sheath neoplasms may be clinically indistinguishable from other mesenchymal neoplasms. Microscopically, since this group of tumors is composed of benign-appearing spindle cells associated with varying amounts of collagen, they must frequently be distinguished from leiomyoma, spindle cell nevus, nodular fasciitis, central odontogenic fibroma, and the group of benign fibrous histiocytomas occurring on sun-exposed surfaces. The characteristic histological features of each of these lesions are discussed under their specific heading in this text and the reader is referred to those sections.

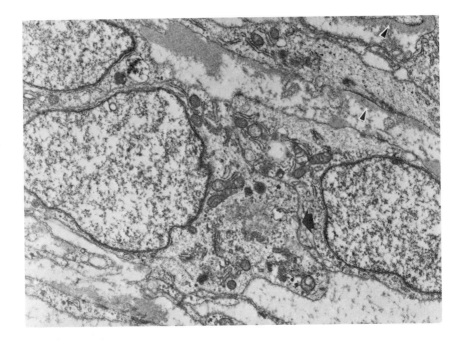

Fig. 13-10 The neoplastic cells of this neurogenic sarcoma are recognizable as being of Schwann cell lineage by the presence of basal lamina-like material (arrowheads), surrounding slender cytoplasmic processes, junctional complexes (arrow), and numerous fine cytoplasmic filaments. (EM x 13,600).

Distinction of neurogenic sarcoma from fibrosarcoma has been a long-standing dilemma for the surgical pathologist. Stout[51] has proposed the use of special stains to demonstrate so-called "straight-line" reticulin fibers parallel to the axis of the cells to assist in distinguishing neurogenic sarcoma from fibrosarcoma. Batsakis[9] reported that he had not found this to be a reliable aid, and we concur.

It is perhaps much more important to be able to distinguish schwannoma, neurofibroma, and neurogenic sarcoma from other neural tumors and nerve-associated syndromes in the head and neck, specifically: traumatic neuroma, nerve sheath myxoma, ganglioneuroma, multiple endocrine neoplasia syndrome, and acoustic neuroma.

Traumatic or *amputation neuroma* is a non-neoplastic proliferation of nerve fibers, Schwann cells and fibrous tissue occurring at the proximal end of a severed peripheral nerve. Lesions arise following trans-section or crushing injury to a peripheral nerve. Axons, in their myelin sheaths, proliferate and, being unable to penetrate the scar tissue, grow laterally or collapse upon themselves. This produces a tangled mass of axons and Schwann cells in dense scar tissue.[12]

Clinically, the traumatic neuroma most often appears as a small soft tissue nodule that may be quite painful on palpation. Rarely may the traumatic neuroma be seen centrally within bone. The mandible is the most common intraosseous site, according to Eversole.[52] Histologically, the lesion consists of dense masses of fibrous connective tissue, throughout which there are bundles of nerve fibers, axons, and Schwann cells. A trichrome stain may be useful in identifying collagen. Wright and Jackson reported that an alcian blue stain may prove helpful in staining perineural mucins which are present in the scar tissue.[12]

Simple surgical excision is the treatment of choice. Presumably because the scar tissue is eliminated, there is little tendency for recurrence.[12]

Nerve sheath myxoma was first described by Harkin and Reed,[32] although reports of similar lesions prior to that time used the descriptive term pacinian neurofibroma.[53] Too few cases of nerve sheath myxoma have been reported to permit any conclusions as to its definitive clinical manifestation, although tumors have occurred in children, especially in the palatal mucosa.[12] Histologically, the tumor consists of well-defined lobules of myxomatous tissue separated by fibrous septa. The cellularity varies, but stellate or hyperchromatic bipolar cells are usually present. Multinucleated cells appearing as a syncytium may also be seen along with palisading of nuclei. In addition, structures resembling pressure receptors have been reported.[12] The tumor stains intensely with alcian blue. Webb[54] found ultrastructural features which suggested that the cell of origin for this neoplasm is the perineural cell. The lesion has a benign behavior pattern and simple surgical excision effects cure.

Ganglioneurofibroma generally occurs in children and young adults in the posterior mediastinum. The tumor is thought to arise by differentiation of immature neuroblasts.[55] Occasionally, lesions which histologically resemble ganglioneurofibromas are found in the floor of the mouth and in the neck. In the neck, these lesions are thought to represent non-neoplastic sympathetic ganglia or perhaps involvement of a sympathetic ganglion by neurofibroma.[47;55] Thoma and Goldman[56] have reported a very unusual case with numerous ganglion cells arising centrally within the mandible following avulsion of the mandibular nerve.

There are no absolute histological criteria to distinguish a ganglioneurofibroma from a non-neoplastic ganglion or involvement of a ganglion by neurofibroma.[12] The presence of binucleate or multinucleate ganglion cells favors a diagnosis of ganglioneuroma.

Multiple endocrine neoplasia III, an autosomal dominantly inherited syndrome, is characterized by multiple mucosal neuromas, medullary carcinoma of the thyroid, pheochromocytoma, and marfanoid habitus. It was apparently first described in 1922-1923[57] and more recently amplified by Williams and Pollack,[58] Gorlin and Mirkin,[59] and Khairi and associates.[60] The basic defect appears to be hyperplasia and neoplasia of neural crest derivatives. Oral mucosal, palpebral conjunctiva, or eyelid lesions precede the development of thyroid carcinoma and pheochromocytoma, thus early diagnosis of skin and oral lesions may prove life-saving.

The *acoustic neuroma* is, in reality, most often a schwannoma arising from the sheath of the vestibular portion of the eighth nerve within the auditory canal. Acoustic neuromas are extremely uncommon in children, but occasionally they have been reported.[61]

TREATMENT AND PROGNOSIS

Most benign neurogenic tumors in the head and neck can be treated by surgical excision, although laryngeal lesions may require sequential excision.[9]

Because as many as 16 percent of all patients with neurofibromatosis may ultimately develop an associated sarcomatous lesion, close follow-up and excision of individual tumors in such patients may be necessary.

GRANULAR CELL TUMOR

Synonyms

1. Granular cell myoblastoma
2. Myoblastic myoma
3. Granular cell schwannoma
4. Embryonal rhabdomyoblastoma
5. Uniform myoblastoma

INCIDENCE

Since Abrikossoff's classic description of the granular cell tumor in 1926,[62] over 1,200 cases have been reported in the literature.[63] Although the lesion has been reported in virtually every organ and tissue in the human body, the incidence of subcutaneous lesions and lesions of the oral cavity and larynx have accounted for over 67 percent of all its reported cases.[63] The oral cavity is, by far, the most common anatomic location in the head and neck region.[64] Some reports stated that as many as 50 percent of all granular cell tumors occur in the oral cavity.[64] However, the comprehensive survey of Peterson[63] showed that only 28 percent occurred in the oral cavity.

AGE AND SEX

Although the lesion has been reported in all age groups, most cases have occurred in the third, fourth, or fifth decades of life. Miller and associates[65] reviewed 25 cases of granular cell tumor in a comprehensive 1977 study and found that 72 percent of the lesions observed occurred in patients between twenty-one and fifty years of age. Only two tumors were reported in children, and both patients were 10-years-old. Some investigators[9;66] have considered the *congenital epulis of the newborn* and the granular cell tumor to be identical lesions, but, because of the age specificity and unusual location of patients with congenital epulis, we favor the view of Custer and Fust,[66] which separates the two entities. Discussion of the latter lesion will be covered in depth under the differential diagnosis heading of this section.

Many authors have suggested there is no difference in incidence between males and females with granular cell tumors;[64;67;68] however, the recent investigations of Peterson,[63] Miller and colleagues,[65] and Thawley and co-workers[69] suggested that females are affected almost twice as often as males.

PATHOGENESIS

Although its unique microscopic morphology permits easy diagnosis, the histogenesis of this unusual tumor has not been satisfactorily delineated. Originally, the tumor was thought to arise, in response to trauma or inflammation,[62] from a myoblastic precursor, hence the appellation *granular cell myoblastoma* was applied. This theory could not be supported with ultrastructural observations and, as a result, a host of histogenetic proposals ensued, including a histiocytic theory (histiocytes storing metabolites),[70] a fibroblastic theory,[71] and a neurogenic theory.[72]

The neurogenic theory maintains that the cell of origin is the Schwann cell, and that the lesion should therefore be called granular cell schwannoma rather than granular cell myoblastoma. Support for this name and theory of origin has become quite strong.[70;72-74] Recently, Eversole and Sabes[73] have postulated that no single cell type is responsible for this tumor and that perhaps various sheath cells with histiocytic-like potential are the cells of origin; therefore, the name *granular sheath cell lesion* was proposed. In light of the sustained taxonomic controversy, the World Health Organization has proposed the noncommittal name, granular cell tumor.

CLINICAL FINDINGS

The tongue is the most frequent site of granular cell tumor, followed by the lip, buccal mucosa, the floor of the mouth, and palate.[63] Tongue lesions usually manifest as clinically asymptomatic, firm lumps, measuring less than 2 cm. in greatest dimension[74] (Fig. 13-11). Lesions of the lateral border, tip, and tongue dorsum are most common. Lesions involving other oral sites have been reported to be nodular, flat, or button-like.[9] Multiple granular cell tumors have been reported, primarily involving the skin and subcutaneum.[69;75]

LIGHT MICROSCOPY

Histologically, the granular cell tumor is a non-encapsulated, circumscribed nodule covered by skin or mucous membrane. The overlying epithelium is reported to show pseudoepitheliomatous hyperplasia in 50 to 65 percent of cases[9] (Fig. 13-12). Our experience with 13 granular cell tumors observed over a 10-year-period has been one where 10 of the 13 showed peudoepitheliomatous hyperplasia.

The supporting connective tissue is largely replaced by granular cells which are uniform in size and may collectively vary from 20-to-50μ

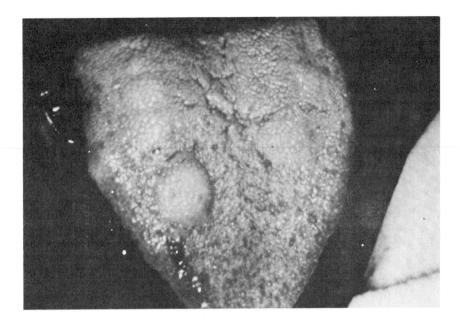

Fig. 13-11 Granular cell tumor of the tongue. Courtesy of Dr. Doran Ryan.

in diameter and vary collectively from distinctly polyhedral to spindle-shaped (Fig. 13-13). The cytoplasm is usually heavily granulated. In sections stained with hematoxylin and eosin, the concentration and distribution of granules is generally not uniform within the cytoplasm. In methylene blue-stained sections, this variation in size, distribution, and concentration of granules is more apparent.

Tumor cell nuclei are ovoid, of uniform size, are relatively small, as compared to overall cell size, and a prominent nuclear membrane and nucleolus are present. Nuclei of adjacent striated muscle are also ovoid and stain deeply.

Clusters of granular cells are generally separated from each other by bundles of collagen. Specimens obtained from the tongue will usually show intermingling of granular cells and muscle fibers. In areas of pseudoepitheliomatous hyperplasia of the covering epithelium, granular cells are generally intimately associated with epithelial cells, with no separation by collagen fibers. Cytoplasmic processes of basal cells of the epithelium may protrude into the granular cell region without an apparent connective tissue condensation.

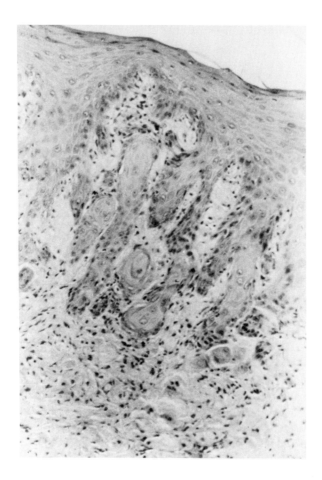

Fig. 13-12 Granular cell tumor, showing pseudoepitheliomatous hyperplasia overlying a lamina propria, filled with granular cells. (H&E x 160).

Batsakis[9] reported a frequent pattern of the tongue granular cell tumor is one where tumor cells are concentrically arranged around a myelinated nerve. Our experience with 13 of these lesions has been one where multiple level sections of oral tumors demonstrated nerve bundles or fibers in every case.

Granular cell tumors have a special histochemistry quite different from that of muscle.[9] Granular cells are reported to contain no glycogen, and reported to stain Periodic-Acid-Schiff positive.[76] They also react positively with Sudan Black B.[76]

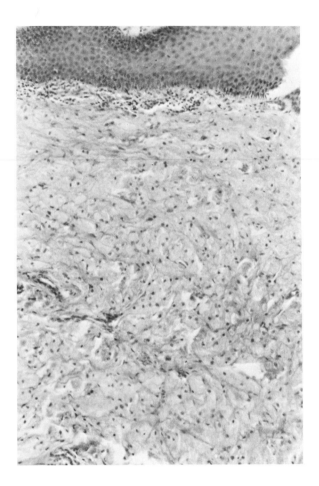

Fig. 13-13 Granular cell tumor in a child, showing cells with a prominent granular cytoplasm. (H&E x 220). Courtesy of Dr. Bruce Jafek.

ELECTRON MICROSCOPY

Granular cell tumors present a striking ultrastructure, and are characterized by cells displaying numerous large pleomorphic lysosomal granules. The granular cells are loosely organized into clusters, which are surrounded by a well-developed basal lamina (Fig. 13-14). Junctional complexes between the cells have not been demonstrated convincingly. Found between the clusters of granular cells is another unusual cell type; a spindle-shaped cell, containing membrane-bounded fibrillar structures known as "angulate bodies" (Fig. 13-15). The angulate body cells occur singly, are not surrounded by basal lamina-like material, and often display pinocytotic activity.

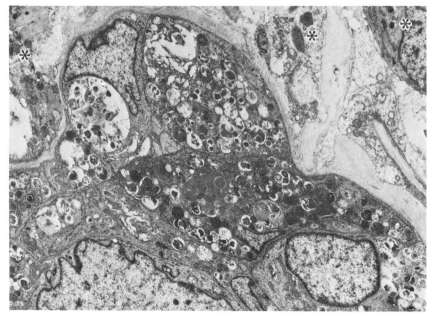

Fig. 13-14 Granular cell tumors display nests of granular cells, between which lie spindle-shaped angulate body cells (asterisks). (EM x 6,000).

In dealing with tumors displaying an abundant eosinophilic granular cytoplasm, electron microscopy can be of value in establishing whether the cytoplasmic granularity is due to lysosomal granules, or some other organelle (e.g. mitochondria). Identification of the characteristic granules is not sufficient evidence in itself, to establish a diagnosis of granular cell tumor, as similar granules may be found in a variety of other neoplastic and reactive lesions. Demonstration of the associated angulate body cells is important as these are not present in the other lesions (e.g. congenital epulis, granular cell ameloblastoma, ameloblastic fibroma) featuring morphologically similar granular cells.

DIFFERENTIAL DIAGNOSIS

The granular cell tumor has to be distinguished from other granular cell lesions, the most significant of which is the *congenital epulis of the newborn*. While the histogenesis of the congenital epulis is

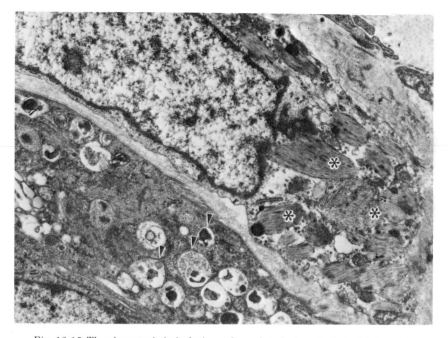

Fig. 13-15 The characteristic inclusions of angulate body cells (asterisks) contain densely packed fibrils, while those of the granular cells (arrowheads) contain a heterogenous assortment of myelin figures, small vesicles and dense bodies. (EM x 15,200).

unknown, odontogenic,[77] undifferentiated mesenchymal,[78] and hamartomatous origins have been proposed.[66] The lesion was first described by Neumann[79] as a peculiar maxillary tumor in a newborn. Since that time, only 81 additional cases have been documented in the English literature.[78] The most comprehensive recent review is by Lack and associates,[78] who reviewed 21 cases.

The congenital epulis, usually quite apparent at birth, occurs almost exclusively in females (an 8-to-1 predominance) as a localized nodular excrescence of the anterior maxillary alveolar gingiva (Fig. 13-16). The most frequent location appears to be within the area overlying future canine or lateral incisor teeth,[78] and lesions are generally in the range of 0.4 to 2 cm. in diameter, when discovered.

The histopathology of the congenital epulis is quite similar, if not identical, to that of the granular cell myoblastoma. However, Batsakis[9] has noted several practically applicable histological features separating the two entities: (1) the congenital epulis shows a greater

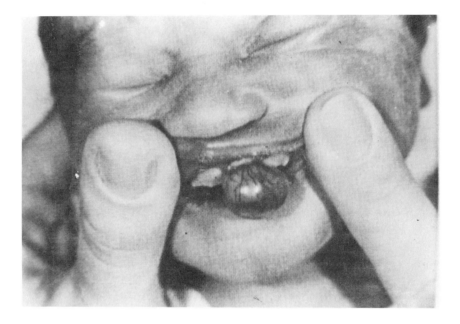

Fig. 13-16 Congenital epulis of the anterior maxilla. Courtesy of Dr. Al Leider.

frequency of entrapped odontogenic epithelial rests and osseous metaplasia than the granular cell myoblastoma; (2) there is characteristically no pseudoepitheliomatous hyperplasia of overlying epithelium in the congenital epulis, and (3) there appears to be a greater degree of vascularity of the supporting stroma present in the congenital epulis.

The ultrastructure of congenital epulis has not been adequately characterized, having been commented upon in only six reported cases. In four of the cases, tissue for electron microscopic examination had been retrieved from paraffin blocks,[78] and in the remaining two cases,[74;80] the tissues had initially been fixed in formalin. We have had the opportunity to examine one optimally preserved specimen (courtesy of Dr. Peter J. Philpott).

In general, the cells of congenital epulis bear a close resemblance to those of granular cell tumors, but differ in several respects. The cells of congenital epulis tend to be individually compartmentalized within a fibrous stroma and are not invested by a well-formed external lamina, whereas the cells of granular cell tumors are organized into cell clusters, surrounded by a well-developed basal lamina (Fig. 13-17). Moreover,

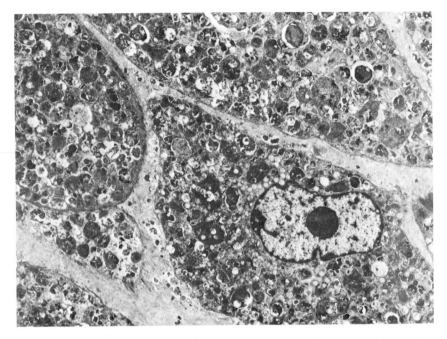

Fig. 13-17 The cells of congenital epulis resemble those of granular cell tumors, but are not organized into nests surrounded by basal lamina. Angulate body cells are not present. (EM x 6,000).

where adjacent cells of congenital epulis are in intimate contact, poorly-developed attachment sites are occasionally seen. Pinocytotic vesicles are commonly observed.

While the cytoplasmic granules of congenital epulis are strikingly similar to those found in granular cell tumors, this need not imply that the two tumors are histogenetically related. It is worth noting in this regard that similar granules are known also to occur in a variety of other neoplasms of differing histogenesis. They have been found, for example, in granular cell ameloblastomas[81;82] (which exhibit the well-formed desmosomes, characteristic of epithelial cells), oligodendrogliomas,[83] a Wilms' tumor,[84] and schwannomas, and may be present in a number of non-neoplastic conditions as well. It seems probable that these divergent lesions share only a common pathway to the production of such granules.

The congenital epulis of the newborn must be distinguished from the rare, well-differentiated rhabdomyoma, that has been described by Misch.[85] Histochemically, the lesion can be distinguished from the rhabdomyoma, in that the intercellular granules seen in the congenital epulis are not composed of glycogen and glycoproteins, as they are in rhabdomyoma.[86]

The preferred treatment for congenital epulis is surgical resection with care not to interfere with the unerupted dentition. There has been no documented instance of recurrence even if the congenital epulis is incompletely removed, and malignant behavior is unknown.

TREATMENT AND PROGNOSIS

The granular cell tumor is a benign lesion that is amenable to conservative local excision with adequate peripheral normal tissue because of the sometimes ill-defined borders. A recurrence rate of approximately eight percent can be expected.[78]

Multiple or multicentric granular cell tumors, reportedly accounting for 5-to-16 percent of all granular cell tumors,[78] may prove somewhat more locally aggressive than solitary growths and thus be more difficult to eradicate surgically.

Although development of malignant granular cell tumor from an existing benign granular cell tumor has been reported,[78;87] Batsakis[9] concluded that many of the reported malignancies are, in reality, soft-part sarcomas, histiocytomas, or rhabdomyosarcomas.

References

1. Oberman, H.A. and Abell, M.R. "Neurogenous Neoplasms of the Mediastinum." *Cancer* 13(1960): 882-898.
2. Saxen, E. "Tumors of Sheaths of Peripheral Nerves—Studies of Their Structure, Histogenesis and Symptomatology." *Acta Pathologica et Microbiologica Scandinavica* 79(1948): 1-135.
3. Oberman, H.A. and Sullenger, G. "Neurogenous Tumors of the Head and Neck." *Cancer* 11(1967): 1192-2001.
4. Das Gupta et al. "Benign Solitary Schwannomas (Neurilemmomas)." *Cancer* 24(1969): 355-366.
5. Preston, F.W.; Walsh, W.S. and Clark, T.H. "Cutaneous Neurofibromatosis (von Recklinghausen's Disease). Clinical Manifestations and Incidence of Sarcoma in 61 Male Patients." *Arch. Surg.* 64(1952): 813-827.
6. Holt, J.F. and Wright, E.M. "Radiologic Features of Neurofibromatosis." *Radiology* 58(1948): 647-664.
7. Daly, J.F. and Raesler, H.K. "Neurilemmoma of the Cervical Sympathetic Chain." *Arch. Otolaryngol.* 77(1963): 262-267.
8. DiPietro, J. "Tumors of Peripheral Nerves." *Tumori* 46(1960): 430-466.
9. Batsakis, J.G. *Tumors of the Head and Neck. Clinical and Pathological Considerations*, 2nd ed. Baltimore: Williams and Wilkins, 1979.
10. Rosenfeld, L.; Graves, H. and Lawrence, R. "Primary Neurogenic Tumors of the Lateral Neck." *Ann. Surg.* 167(1968): 847-855.

11. Baden, E.; Pierce, H.E. and Jackson, W.F. "Multiple Neurofibromatosis with Oral Lesions." *Oral Surg.* 8(1955): 263-280.

12. Wright, B.A. and Jackson, D. "Neural Tumors of the Oral Cavity: A Review of the Spectrum of Benign and Malignant Oral Tumors of the Oral Cavity and Jaws." *Oral Surg.* 49(1980): 509-522.

13. Carstens, P.H.B. and Schrodt, G.R. "Malignant Transformation of a Benign Encapsulated Neurilemmoma." *Am. J. Clin. Pathol.* 51(1969): 144-149.

14. Ellis, G.L.; Abrams, A. and Melrose, R. "Intraosseous Benign Neural Sheath Neoplasms. Report of 7 New Cases and Review of the Literature." *Oral Surg.* 44(1977): 731-743.

15. Satterfield, S.D.; Elzay, R.P. and Mecuri, L. "Mandibular Schwannoma. Report of Case." *J. Oral Surg.* 39(1981): 776-777.

16. Rengaswamy, V. "Central Neurilemmoma of the Jaws." *Int. J. Oral Surg.* 7(1978): 300-304.

17. Devore, D.T. and Waldron, C.A. "Malignant Peripheral Nerve Tumors of the Oral Cavity." *Oral Surg.* 14(1961): 56-68.

18. Eversole, L.R.; Schwartz, W.D. and Sabes, W.R. "Central and Peripheral Fibrogenic and Neurogenic Sarcoma of the Oral Regions." *Oral Surg.* 36(1973): 49-62.

19. Sarkor, S. "Neurinoma of the Facial Nerve." *J. Laryngol. Otol.* 73(1959): 129-132.

20. Furlow, L.T. and Walsh, T.E. "Neurilemmoma of the Facial Nerve." *Laryngoscope* 69(1959): 1075-1984.

21. Kragh, L.V.; Soule, E.H. and Masson, J.K. "Benign and Malignant Neurilemmomas of the Head and Neck. " *Surg. Gynecol. Obstet.* 111(1960): 211-218.

22. Robitaille, Y.; Seemayer, T.A. and Deiry, A.E. "Peripheral Nerve Tumors Involving Paranasal Sinuses: A Case Report and Review of the Literature." *Cancer* 35(1975): 1254-1258.

23. Iwamura, S.; Sugiura, S. and Nomura, Y. "Schwannoma of the Nasal Cavity." *Arch. Otolaryngol.* 96(1972): 176-177.

24. Thackray, A.C. and Lucas, R.B. *Tumors of the Major Salivary Glands. Atlas of Tumor Pathology*, 2nd series, fascicle 10. Washington, D.C.: Armed Forces Institute of Pathology, 1964.

25. El-Serafy, S. "Rare Benign Tumors of the Larynx." *J. Laryngol. Otol.* 85(1971): 837-851.

26. Chang-Lo. "Laryngeal Involvement in von Recklinghausen's Disease. A Case Report and Review of the Literature." *Laryngoscope* 87(1977): 435-442.

27. Gibbs, N.M.; Taylor, M. and Young, A. "von Recklinghausen's Disease in the Larynx and Trachea of an Infant." *J. Laryngol. Otol.* 71(1957): 626-630.

28. Putney, F.J.; Moran, J.J. and Thomas, G.K. "Neurogenic Tumors of the Head and Neck." *Laryngoscope* 74(1964): 1037-1059.

29. Crowe, F.W. "Axillary Freckling as a Diagnostic Aid in Neurofibromatosis." *Ann. Intern. Med.* 61(1964): 1142-1143.

30. Wright, B.A. and Jackson, D. "Neural Tumors of the Oral Cavity." *Oral Surg.* 49(1980): 509-522.

31. Whitehouse, D. "Diagnostic Value of the Cafe au-Lait Spot in Children." *Arch. Dis. Child.* 41(1966): 316-319.

32. Harkin, J.C. and Reed, R.J. *Tumors of the Peripheral Nervous System. Atlas of Tumor Pathology,* 2nd series, fascicle 3, pg. 94. Washington, D.C.: Armed Forces Institute of Pathology, 1969.

33. Heard, G. "Nerve Sheath Tumors and von Recklinghausen's Disease of the Nervous System." *Ann. R. Coll. Surg. Engl.* 31(1962): 229-248.

34. D'Agostino, A.N.; Soule, E.H. and Miller, R.H. "Primary Malignant Neoplasms of Nerves (Malignant Neurilemmoma) in Patients Without Manifestations of Multiple Neurofibromatosis (von Recklinghausen's Disease)." *Cancer* 16(1963): 1003-1014.

35. Murray, M. and Stout, A.P. "Schwann Cell Versus Fibroblast in Origin of Specific Nerve Sheath Tumor, Observations Upon Normal Nerve Sheath and Neurilemmomas *in vitro.*" *Am. J. Pathol.* 16(1940): 41-60.

36. Mallory, F.B. "The Type of Cell of the So-Called Dural Endothelioma." *J. Med. Res.* 41(1920): 349-364.

37. Tarlov, I.M. "Origin of Perineural Fibroblastoma." *Am. J. Pathol.* 16(1940): 33-40

38. Penfield, W. "Encapsulated Tumors of the Nervous System." *Surg. Gynec. Obstet.* 45(1927): 178-188.

39. Fisher, E.R. and Vezuvski, V.D. "Cytogenesis of Schwannoma (Neurilemmoma) Neurofibroma, Dermatofibroma and Dermatofibrosarcoma, As Revealed by Electron Microscopy." *Am. J. Clin. Pathol.* 49(1968): 141-154.

40. Holt, J.F. "Neurofibromatosis in Children." *Am. J. Roentgenol.* 130(1978): 615-639.

41. Chen, S.Y. and Miller, A.S. "Neurofibroma and Schwannoma of the Oral Cavity." *Oral Surg.* 47(1979): 522-528.

42. Isaacson, P. "Mast Cells in Benign Nerve Sheath Tumors." *J. Pathol.* 119 (1976): 193-196.

43. Ackerman, L.V. and Taylor, F.H. "Neurogenous Tumors Within the Thorax." *Cancer* 4(1951): 669-691.

44. Dahl, I. "Ancient Neurilemmoma (Schwannoma)." *Acta. Pathol. Microbiol. Scand.* [*A*] 85(1977): 912-818.

45. Eversole, L.R. and Howell, R.M. "Ancient Neurilemmoma of the Oral Cavity." *Oral Surg.* 32(1971): 440-443.

46. Marks, R.B.; Carr, R.F. and Kreller, A.J. "Ancient Neurilemmoma of the Floor of the Mouth. Report of Case." *J. Oral Surg.* 34(1976): 731-735.

47. Harkin, J.C. and Reed, R.J. *Tumors of the Peripheral Nervous System. Atlas of Tumor Pathology,* 2nd series, fascicle 3, pp. 29, 51, 60-64, 148, 149. Washington, D.C.: Armed Forces Institute of Pathology, 1969.

48. Luse, S.A. "Electron Microscopic Studies of Brain Tumors." *Neurology (Minneap.)* 10(1960): 881-905.

49. Ghadially, F.N. *Diagnostic Electron Microscopy of Tumors.* London: Butterworth, 1980.

50. Taxy et al. "Electron Microscopy in the Diagnosis of Malignant Schwannoma." *Cancer* 49(1981): 1381-1391.

51. Stout, A.P. *Tumors of the Peripheral Nervous System. Atlas of Tumor Pathology,* section 2, fascicle 6. Washington, D.C.: Armed Forces Institute of Pathology, 1949

52. Eversole, L.R. "Central Benign and Malignant Neural Neoplasms of the Jaws. A Review." *J. Oral Surg.* 27(1969): 716-721.

53. Pritchard, R.W. and Custer, R.P. "Pacinian Neurofibroma." *Cancer* 5(1952): 297-301.

54. Webb, J.N. "The Histogenesis of Nerve Sheath Myxoma: Report of a Case with Electron Microscopy." *J. Pathol.* 127(1979): 35-37.

55. Abell, M.R.; Hart, W.R. and Olsen, J.R. "Tumors of the Peripheral Nervous System." *Hum. Pathol.* 1(1970): 503-551.

56. Thoma, K.H. and Goldman, H.M. *Oral Pathology*, 5th ed., p. 1307. St. Louis: C.V. Mosby, 1960.

57. Gorlin, R.J.; Pindborg, J.J. and Cohen, M.M., Jr. *Syndromes of the Head and Neck*, 2nd ed., pp. 513-519. New York: McGraw-Hill, 1967.

58. Williams, E.D. and Pollack, D.J. "Multiple Mucosal Neuromata: A Syndrome Allied with von Recklinghausen's Disease." *J. Pathol. Bacteriol.* 91(1966): 71-80.

59. Gorlin, R.J. and Mirkin, L.B. "Multiple Mucosal Neuromas, Medullary Carcinoma of the Thyroid, Pheochromocytoma and Marfanoid Body with Muscle Wasting." *J. Kinderheilkd* 113(1972): 313-325.

60. Khairi et al. "Mucosal Neurofibroma, Pheochromocytoma and Medullary Thyroid Carcinoma. Multiple Endocrine Neoplasia Type 3." *Medicine* 54(1975): 89-112.

61. Anderson, M.S. and Bentinck, B.R. "Intracranial Schwannoma in a Child." *Cancer* 29(1972): 231-234.

62. Abrikossoff, A.I. "Uber myome, ausgehend von der guesgestreiften Willkurlicken muskylatur." *Virchows Arch. [Pathol. Anat.]* 260(1926): 215.

63. Peterson, L.J. "Granular Cell Tumor, Review of the Literature and Report of a Case." *Oral Surg.* 37(1974): 728-735.

64. Day, R.C.B. "Granular Cell Myoblastoma." *Br. J. Oral Surg.* 2(1964): 65-70.

65. Miller et al. "Oral Granular Cell Tumors. Report of Twenty-Five Cases with Electron Microscopy." *Oral Surg.* 44(1977): 227-237.

66. Custer, R.P. and Fust, J.A. "Congenital Epulis." *Am. J. Clin. Pathol.* 22(1953): 1044-1053.

67. Herschfus, L. and Walter, J.G. "Granular Cell Myoblastoma of the Oral Cavity." *Oral Surg.* 29(1970): 341-352.

68. Syers, C.S. and Keen, R.R. "Granular Cell Myoblastoma Occurring in the Upper Lip." *J. Oral Surg.* 27(1969): 143-144.

69. Thawley, S.E. and Ogura, J.H. "Granular Cell Myoblastoma of the Head and Neck." *South. Med. J.* 67(1974): 1020-1024.

70. Aparicio, S.R. and Lumsden, C.E. "Light and Electron Microscope Studies on the Granular Cell Myoblastoma of the Tongue." *J. Pathol.* 97(1969): 339-355.

71. Garancis, J.C.; Komorowski, R.A. and Kuzma, J.F. "Granular Cell Myoblastoma." *Cancer* 25(1970): 542-550.

72. Sobel et al. "Granular Cell Myoblastoma: An Electron Microscopic and Cytochemical Study Illustrating the Genesis of Granules and Aging of Myoblastoma Cells." *Am. J. Pathol.* 65(1971): 59-71.

73. Eversole, L.R. and Sabes, W.R. "Granular Sheath Cell Lesions." *J. Oral Surg.* 29(1971): 867-871.

74. Regezi, J.A.; Batsakis, J.G. and Courtney, R.M. "Granular Cell Tumors of the Head and Neck." *J. Oral Surg.* 37(1979): 402-409.

75. Moscovic, E.A. and Azar, H.A. "Multiple Granular Cell Tumors (Myoblastoma)." *Cancer* 20(1967): 2032-2047.

76. Allek, D.S.; Johnson, W.C. and Grahman, J.H. "Granular Cell Myoblastoma: A Histological and Enzymatic Study." *Arch. Dermatol.* 98(1968): 532-547.

77. Kaempfer, L.G. "Congenital Epulides (Odontoblastomata). A Clinical and Pathologic Study." *Surg. Gynecol. Obstet.* 12(1911): 357-366.

78. Lack et al. "Gingival Granular Cell Tumors of the Newborn (Congenital Epulis). A Clinicopathologic Study of 21 Patients." *Am. J. Surg. Pathol.* 5(1981): 37-45.

79. Neumann, E. "Ein Fall von Congenitaler Epulis." *Arch. Heilk.* 12(1871): 189-190.

80. Kay, S.; Elzay, R.P. and Willson, M.A. "Ultrastructural observations on a gingival granular cell tumor (congenital epulis)." *Cancer* 27(1971): 674.

81. Navarrete, A.R. and Smith, M. "Ultrastructure of granular cell ameloblastoma." *Cancer* 27(1971): 948.

82. Tandler, B. and Rossi, E.P. "Granular cell ameloblastoma: Electron microscopic observation." *J. Oral Pathol.* 6(1971): 401.

83. Takei, V.; Mirra, S.S. and Miles, M.L. "Eosinophilic granular cells in oligodendrogliomas." *Cancer* 38(1976): 1968.

84. Kurtz, S.M. "A unique ultrastructural variant of Wilms' tumor. Its possible histogenetic implications." *Am. J. Surg. Pathol.* 3(1979): 257.

85. Misch, K.A. "Rhabdomyoma purum: A benign rhabdomyoma of tongue." *Journal of Pathology and Bacteriology* 75(1958): 105.

86. Cherrick, H.M. "The Jaws and Teeth." In *Surgical Pathology*, edited by W.F. Coulson, pg. 36. Philadelphia: J.B. Lippincott, 1978.

87. Cadotte, M. "Malignant granular—cell Myoblastoma." *Cancer* 33(1974):1417-1421.

Chapter XIV

Tumors of Muscle
RHABDOMYOSARCOMA

Synonyms

Myosarcoma

INCIDENCE
Rhabdomyosarcoma is the second most common tumor of the head and neck region in children; lymphoma is the most common.

AGE AND SEX
Nearly one-third of rhabdomyosarcomas in children occur in the head and neck region with peak incidence at around four years of age. There is no significant predisposition of sex or race.

PATHOGENESIS
Rhabdomyosarcomas are tumors of primitive mesenchyme with varying degrees of myogenous differentiation. They arise most often in the nasopharynx, orbit, middle ear, or soft tissues of the neck when the head and neck region is involved. Tumors need not arise in skeletal muscle.

CLINICAL FINDINGS
Patients may manifest symptoms directly related to mass, such as nasopharyngeal obstruction, proptosis, ear pain, or pain due to pressure on sensitive facial tissues (Fig. 14-1). There is more often subtle clinical manifestation of nerve involvement, otitis media, sinusitis, or, either reactive or metastatic lymphadenopathy without obvious tumor mass.

Definition of tumors may be greatly augmented by use of computerized tomography. Tumors in parameningeal sites such as nasopharynx, paranasal sinuses, and middle ear (orbital tumors are not included in this group), are associated with a high frequency of meningeal extension and high mortality rate.[1]

Clinical staging of the extent of disease forms the basis for therapy and prognostication. Preoperative evaluation of bone marrow and cerebrospinal fluid for tumor involvement is essential.

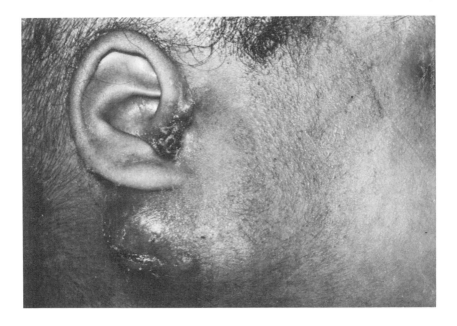

Fig. 14-1 Preauriclular hard mass with ulceration—rhabdomyosarcoma.

GROSS AND LIGHT MICROSCOPIC FINDINGS

Rhabdomyosarcomas of the head and neck are usually amenable to no more than incisional biopsy because they are usually not resectable. The lesion is generally fleshy, gray, and without distinct margins; however, tumors adjoining nasal or sinus cavities may have the "botryoid" configuration featuring polypoid, edematous, or gelatinous masses.

Histological patterns are heterogeneous in a given tumor and in different tumors. "Problems of morphologic classification" and histological diagnostic criteria for rhabdomyosarcoma were summarized by Gonzales-Crussi and Black-Schaffer.[2] In general these tumors feature primitive mesenchymal cells with spindle shapes, myxoid appearance, and/or alveolar patterns in the presence of variable signs of rhabdomyogenic differentiation such as fibrillary eosinophilic cytoplasm, cross-striations, or tandem multinucleation (Figs. 14-2, 14-3).

Features of differentiation are often more evident on ultrastructural study, and immunohistological identification of myglobin or creatine kinase in the tumor cell population may be very helpful.

Subclassification of rhabdomyosarcoma based on histology has not proven to be of clinical relevance.

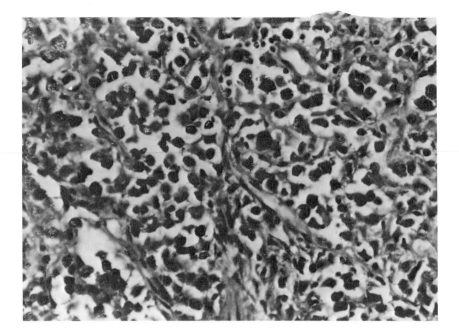

Fig. 14-2 Rhabdomyosarcoma. An alveolar pattern is seen in this tumor from the nasopharynx. (H&E x 250).

ELECTRON MICROSCOPY

Ultrastructural diagnosis of rhabdomyosarcoma rests upon detection of specific thin (actin) and thick (myosin) cytoplasmic filaments and/or Z-band material. Other, less specific, features of myoblasts include pinocytotic vesicles, monoparticulate glycogen, and "basement membrane"[3] (Fig. 14-4).

Electron microscopic examination may provide conclusive evidence for a diagnosis of rhabdomyosarcoma. However, in about one-half of the cases with a light microscopic diagnosis of rhabdomyosarcoma, this cannot be verified by electron microscopy.

The differential diagnostic ultrastructural features of malignant fibrous histiocytoma, granular cell tumor (myoblastoma), Ewing's sarcoma and neuroblastoma (tumors which may occur in the head and neck and present differential diagnostic problems) are discussed elsewhere. Tumors morphologically similar to the renal "rhabdoid" tumor can arise in extra-renal sites. These tumors, which resemble rhabdomyosarcoma histologically, show distinctive ultrastructural features including cell junctions and dense whorls of nonspecific cytoplasmic filaments.[4]

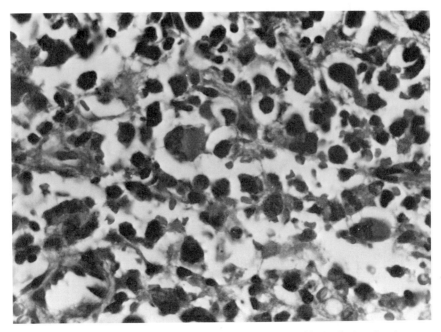

Fig. 14-3 Rhabdomyosarcoma. The large cells mimic myoblasts. Such cells often stain for myoglobin by immunological techniques. (H&E x 400).

Alveolar soft part sarcoma can be easily identified by the presence of characteristic crystalline cytoplasmic inclusions.[5]

TREATMENT AND PROGNOSIS

Prognosis and therapy are based on the clinical stage of disease at the time of diagnosis. The national collaborative Intergroup Rhabdomyosarcoma Study uses clinical groupings of cases as defined by the surgeon at operation and confirmed by the pathologist. Lymph node dissection is not recommended as a rule. Comments on therapy and prognosis as shown below are from Intergroup Rhabdomyosarcoma Study data.

Group I — Localized disease, completely resected. Chemotherapy is recommended and over 90 percent of patients should be cured.

Group II — Grossly resected tumor with microscopic residual disease. Chemotherapy and radiation are recommended and the tumor-free survival-rate may be as high as 70 percent.

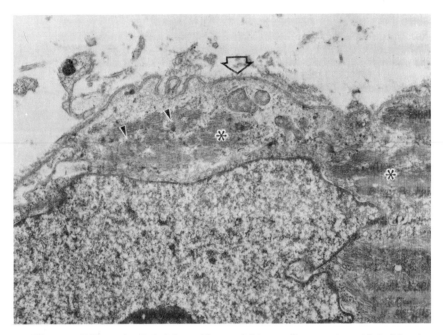

Fig. 14-4 Differentiated rhabdomyoblasts exhibit myofilaments (asterisks), Z-band material (arrow heads), monoparticulate glycogen, and pinocytotic vesicles, and are enveloped by "basement membrane" (arrow). (EM X 16,000).

Group III — Incomplete resection or biopsy with gross residual disease. Chemotherapy and radiation are recommended and the tumor-free survival-rate may be as high as 50 percent.

Group IV — Metastatic disease present. Chemotherapy may be expected to result in a disease-free survival-rate of about 12 percent.

Parameningeal tumors are associated with extremely high mortality rate and represent a special management challenge. Orbital tumors are not included in this group.

References

1. Berry, P. and Jenkin, R.D. "Parameningeal rhabdomyosarcoma in the young." *Cancer* 48,2nd suppl.(1981): 281-288.
2. Gonzales-Crussi, F. and Black-Schaffer, S. "Rhabdomyosarcoma of infancy and childhood." *Am. J. Surg. Pathol.* 3(1979): 157-171.
3. Mierau, G.W. and Favara, B.E. "Rhabdomyosarcoma in children: ultrastructural study of 31 cases" *Cancer* 46(1980): 2035-2040.

4. Haas et al. "Ultrastructure of malignant rhabdoid tumor of the kidney." *Hum. Pathol.* 12(1981): 646-657.

5. Shipkey et al. "Ultrastructure of alveolar soft part sarcoma" *Cancer* 17(1964): 821-830.

Chapter XV

Vascular Tumors
HEMANGIOMA

Synonyms

1. Hemangioendothelioma
2. Juvenile hemangioma
3. Juvenile angioma
4. Plexiform angioma

INCIDENCE

Hemangiomas are developmental vascular abnormalities common in the head and neck regions of children. Many well-documented case reports and literature reviews have been assembled concerning these tumors, but probably there have been none as impressive or comprehensive as the study of Watson and McCarthy.[1] These investigators reviewed 1,363 blood and lymph node tumors over an eight-year-period and found vascular tumors to account for five percent of all hospital admissions at their institution.

Over 50 percent of all hemangiomas occur in the head and neck area,[2,3] even though this area constitutes less than one-seventh of the body surface. The incidence of hemangiomas of the head and neck is considerably higher in children than in adults. Shklar and Meyer suggested that hemangiomas are 7 to 8 times as frequent in children as compared to adults.[4] Multiple vascular lesions are also much more common in children. Multiple lesions were found in 16 percent of the patients reviewed by Watson and McCarthy.[1]

AGE AND SEX

Hemangiomas are generally considered to occur far more commonly in males than females,[5] although there exist a few large series in the literature reporting a male predominance.[6] In most instances hemangiomas occur very early in life. Of the 1,363 cases reviewed by Watson and McCarthy,[1] 73 percent were present at birth and 85 percent had developed by the end of the first year of life. Margileth and Museles reported that the majority of the 336 patients with hemangiomas they reviewed over a seven-year-period at U.S. Naval hospitals were also under one year of age.[6]

PATHOGENESIS

Hemangiomas were initially described and reported as soft tissue tumors in the early part of the nineteeth century;[7] nonetheless, some degree of controversy continues to surround their histogenesis. Ribbert[8] and Bowman[9] supported the theory that hemangiomas resulted from a primary failure of developing embryonic rudiments which affected the angioblastic vessel anlage. The most widely accepted current theory is that the hemangioma is a consequential development of mesenchymal rests that undergo endothelial differentiation and proliferation as blood vessels,[4;10;11] —thus the lesion is most commonly regarded as a developmental hamartoma. This histogenesis of osseous hemangiomas has been reviewed by Jacobs and Kimmelstiel,[12] who suggested that the increase in bone dimension with osseous hemangiomas is not the result of cellular growth as one would expect with a true neoplasm, but a secondary change due to variation in intersinusoidal pressure, in turn leading to increased metalaxis of bone tissue.

CLINICAL FINDINGS

SKIN:

Hemangiomas of skin surfaces of the head and neck are common in children. Margileth and Museles reported that 38 percent of the 36 hemangiomas they reviewed in a study of cutaneous hemagiomas in children were in the head and neck area.[6] They delineated four distinctive types of cutaneous lesions.

    I. Strawberry Mark — The strawberry mark (hemangioma simplex), a capillary hemangioma, is the most common (Fig. 15-1). It is usually bright or purplish-red with well-defined borders and consists of a myriad of minute capillaries protruding from the skin surface. When pressure is applied, the strawberry lesion blanches incompletely; on palpation, it is a solid, firm mass which compresses only slightly in most instances, if at all.

    II. Cavernous — The cavernous hemangioma usually has poorly-defined borders and is subsurface. It may also be well-circumscribed and occur as a (dermal) elevation. The lesion is composed primarily of large venous channels which impart a red-blue discoloration to the overlying skin. It frequently feels like a bag of worms. These tumors may compress easily to half the original size and then, upon release of pressure, quickly revert to their former size. They become larger upon straining and may darken when the child cries.

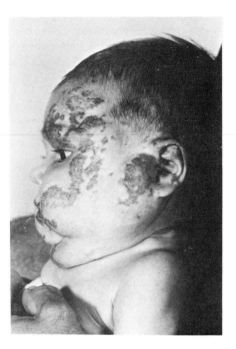

Fig. 15-1 Large capillary hemangioma of the face. Courtesy of Dr. Loren Golitz.

III. Mixed — The mixed (combined) hemangioma consists of the cavernous type with an overlying capillary (strawberry or port wine) component.

IV. Others — The port wine mark, spider nevus, and erythema nuchae are rare in children.

ORAL MUCOUS MEMBRANES:

Hemangioma is a common lesion of the oral mucosa. It is less commonly found in the deeper connective tissue and muscle, and is rarely a bone lesion of the maxilla and mandible. Oral angiomas are now generally considered to be developmental malformations or hamartomatous lesions rather than true neoplasms. Oral hemangiomas may exist as small superficial lesions, as larger superficial lesions, extending with some depth, into the underlying connective tissue, or as extensive lesions involving large areas of underlying connective tissue and musculature, which results in gross deformity of the oral tissues. The small superficial hemangiomas may be rounded, pedunculated, or flattened, with a broad base. Larger superficial lesions have less distinct boundaries and may appear as lobulated, somewhat raised configurations. Superficial lesions have a red-purple or deep red color. Deeper lesions are surrounded or "encapsulated" by connective tissue and are covered with epithelium, so that their color is a light red or pink rather than purple. The surface may be raised if the lesion is sufficiently large. Extensive hemangiomas of the lips and tongue may cause gross deformity, resulting in macrocheilia or macroglossia[4] (Fig. 15-2). Patients manifesting deep hemangiomas are usually less than five years of age.[4] Cavernous hemangiomas of the oral cavity and hypopharynx are rare, with only ten cases reported between 1887 and 1961,[13] and only an additional 20 cases reported since then.[5]

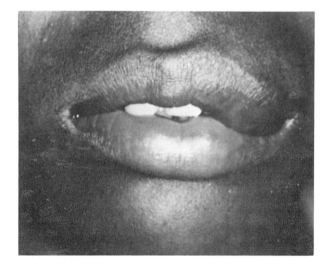

Fig. 15-2 Hemangioma of the lip and oral mucosa, resulting in macrocheilia.

Hemangiomas often develop as multicentric lesions, so that there may be a grouping of several hemangiomas in a given area. As the lesions develop and increase in size, they often blend into one large lesion; these extensive surface lesions may manifest a pebbled surface suggestive of a confluence of many small individual lesions.

Hemangiomas can occur in any area of the oral cavity, but the tongue, buccal mucosa, and lower lip are the two regions most commonly involved.[4]

An important fact to be remembered by the surgical pathologist is that many oral angiomatous proliferations are found in association with syndromes having a systemic vascular counterpart. Important syndromes include hereditary hemorrhagic telangiectasia, Sturge-Weber syndrome, and Maffuci's syndrome. The pyogenic granuloma may also resemble hemangioma both clinically and microscopically.

MUSCLE:

Intramuscular hemangioma was first reported by Liston in 1843 when he reported an erectile tumor of the popliteal space. More recently, Scott,[14] in a study of 393 cases of intramuscular hemangioma, found the lower limbs to be the most common site for occurrence. Thirteen-and-one-half percent of Scott's cases were found in the head and neck region, with the masseter and trapezius muscles most frequently involved. The lesions occurred between birth and 30 years of age in almost 95 percent of the cases, supporting the theory that they are congenital. There is no reported sexual predisposition for intramuscular hemangiomas. Since Scott's review, numerous reports have described the intramuscular hemangioma; the most recently reported case involved the obicularis oris muscle.[15] The most common initial symptom for the muscular hemangioma, regardless of site, is swelling.

The lesion is usually described as a smooth-surfaced, rubbery mass with distinct margins. Frequently it is mobile and can be moved across the line of the muscle but not along its length. Pulsations, bruits and thrills are rarely found. In most cases, the tumor is not compressible. The overlying skin is usually of normal coloration, and pain is reported in many cases, probably produced by compression of adjacent tissues. Loss of function of the involved muscle may occur as the lesion enlarges, with deformity as an end result. Radiographic examination occasionally discloses phleboliths in the muscle or surrounding soft tissue. Because of its usual clinical manifestation, the muscular angioma is rarely diagnosed preoperatively.[15]

Lesions described a *"invasive" hemangiomas* are most often deep muscular lesions that are, upon treatment, refractory in behavior. Children exceed adults 10-to-1 in the acquisition of deeply "invasive" benign hemangiomas.

OSSEOUS:

Hemangiomas of bone occur most frequently in the vertebrae and skull. The cavernous type is the most common subtype encountered. In a comprehensive review of 6,221 bone tumors, Dahlin reported a total of 69 hemangiomas of bone.[16] Forty-four of these lesions were in the head and neck area. The skull and maxilla were the two most susceptible sites.

Central hemangioma of the jaws is rare. In a comprehensive review by Piercell and others[17] in 1975, only 53 cases were found in the literature. Lund,[18] in a review of 35 cases in 1970, found a ratio of 2-to-1 towards an incidence in females and also observed that, for unknown reasons, the mandible is affected twice as frequently as the maxilla. The peak incidence is in the second decade of life.[19;20]

The initial signs and symptoms of central hemangioma of the jaws are highly variable and frequently of no diagnostic value. In many cases of maxillary hemangioma, the initial symptoms are either a swollen cheek or a severe nosebleed, whereas in cases of mandibular hemangioma, the usual symptom is mucosal bleeding from the gingiva, often nocturnal, or unexpected hemmorrhage after tooth extraction. The lesion may also be asymptomatic, in which case it will only be discovered as a result of change from routine dental radiography or when uncontrollable hemorrhage necessitates emergency surgery. Jaw lesions often have a "soap-bubble" radiographic appearance.

The most common finding during an examination is a firm, nonpainful, bony swelling associated with a subjective pulsating sensation or throbbing discomfort. Severe, clinically evident pain is uncommon. There may be paresthesia of affected nerves as well as derangement of the normal arch and occlusion. The soft tissues can be hyperthermic or show venous dilation, and the overlying gingiva is sometimes discolored or congested with blood.

Although skull lesions were common in Dahlin's review, he reported that many of the hemangiomas of the calvarium in his series were asymptomatic and were discovered during roentgenographic study conducted for other reasons.[16]

SALIVARY GLANDS:

The juvenile hemangioma is by far the most common salivary gland tumor of infancy. The parotid gland is most often affected, although the submandibular gland may occasionally be involved. Howard and co-workers,[21] in a thorough review of the literature, discovered the vast majority of all reported lesions to occur during the first year of life. There is an apparent slight female predisposition and a common denominator in the physical findings is a painless swelling during the first few months of life. Lesions may become evident as a bluish discoloration, or they can have a cystic quality, or spongy texture. Anterior extension of the lesion over the mandibular ramus with displacement of the ear lobe outward, upwards, or backwards may be noted on clinical inspection.

LIGHT MICROSCOPY

The microscopic features of juvenile hemangioma are varied. Classically, they show a prominent proliferation of endothelial cells. The endothelial cells form vascular spaces ranging from small capillary configurations to large cyst-like spaces filled with erythrocytes. In some cases, the endothelial proliferation results in sheets and cords of cells with few patent vascular spaces. The connective tissue component of hemangioma may consist of a minimal amount of loose myxomatous tissue, or it may consist of extremely dense hyalin-like material.

The classification of hemangiomas on a histologic basis is interesting, but of little value in relation to prognosis of the lesions. Shklar[4] found no correlation between histological type and clinical behavior of oral hemangiomas. The majority of the small superficial pedunculated lesions tend to be of the capillary type. The larger superficial lesions and the deeper lesions tend to be cavernous, or represent a mixture of capillary and cavernous patterns. Solid cellular lesions are uncommon.

CAPILLARY TYPE:

This type of hemangioma is composed of large numbers of small blood vessels, predominately of capillary size (Fig. 15-3). Stromal infiltration of inflammatory cells is usually minimal; however, it must be remembered that some raised pedunculated lesions in the head and neck area, especially those of oral mucosa, are easily traumatized, and thus varying degrees of inflammatory infiltration should not be considered unusual. Surface ulceration may also occur occasionally. The distinction of capillary hemangioma from granuloma pyogenicum is often difficult to make when inflammatory infiltration is dense.

CAVERNOUS TYPE:

In this type of hemangioma, the vascular spaces are quite large; an entire small lesion may be composed of one or two "cyst-like" spaces lined with endothelial cells and filled with erythrocytes. Generally, these

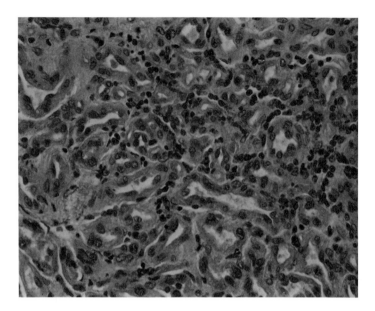

Fig. 15-3 Prominent capillary network and rich endothelial cell proliferation are seen in this high-power photomicrograph of juvenile capillary hemangioma. (H&E x 425).

lesions are diffuse, more deeply-seated than the capillary type, and composed of numerous, large, irregular vascular spaces separated by dense connective tissue.

MIXED TYPE:

Many hemangiomas are actually mixtures of capillary and cavernous types. In such types, small and large vascular spaces may be interspersed or may exist in different areas of a large lesion.

CELLULAR TYPE:

Some lesions present a pattern of solid sheets and cords of endothelial cells with occasional vascular spaces. This type of hemangioma has often been thought to be composed of more primitive cell types, although there is little rationale for this concept. The term *hemangioendothelioma* has been used to describe such lesions. This terminology is now considered outmoded.

SCLEROSING TYPE:

This type of lesion is usually found in deeper structures and is composed of vascular spaces separated by extremely dense fibrous connective tissue. The connective tissue component comprises a large portion of the lesion and often presents an amorphous hyalin-like appearance.[4]

Allen and Enzinger[22] recently classified the intramuscular hemangioma according to vessel size, namely: small vessel, large vessel, and mixed type. They reported that small vessel hemangiomas (capillary) were found most frequently in the trunk (30 percent in the head and neck regions) and had a recurrence rate of 20 percent after treatment. Large vessel hemangiomas were found most frequently in the lower limbs (19 percent in the head and neck) with a 9 percent recurrence rate. Mixed type hemangiomas were encountered most frequently in the trunk (5 percent in the head and neck) and were seen to possess a relatively high recurrence rate of 28 percent.

ELECTRON MICROSCOPY

Electron microscopy can be helpful in demonstrating the vascular nature of tumors of uncertain origin and for the purpose of identifying the cell type undergoing proliferation. An excellent recent review of the ultrastructure of vascular neoplasms, with an assessment of the role of electron microscopy in the diagnosis of these tumors, has been presented by Waldo and others.[23] Hemangiomas typically display normal-appearing small vessels, surrounded by multilayered basement membranes (Fig. 15-4).

DIFFERENTIAL DIAGNOSIS

Inflammatory lesions with a vascular component may easily be confused with a true hemangioma. The most significant of these lesions is the *pyogenic granuloma*. The pyogenic granuloma is a hemorrhagic, elevated benign growth which can be found in universal distribution throughout the body, but is most common on the skin and oral mucous membranes (Figs. 15-5A, 15-5B). The oral mucosa is by far the most common anatomic site for its incidence in the head and neck. Moreover, pyogenic granulomas have been reported on the tonsils and laryngeal mucosa, usually following intubation.[24]

Oral lesions occur most frequently on the gingiva; other oral sites in descending order of frequency are: the lips, tongue, and cheek.[25] From a study of a group of 30 cases of pyogenic granuloma in children, Standish and Shafer[26] concluded that the incidence of the lesion

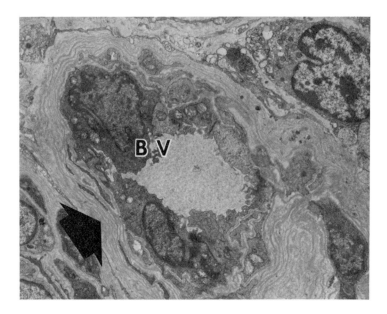

Fig. 15-4 The blood vessels (BV) of hemangiomas are lined by a single layer of normal-appearing endothelial cells and, typically, are surrounded by a multi-layered basement membrane (arrow). (EM x 5,700).

indicates no sexual predisposition; —however, large reviews of patients in all age groups suggest that females are more susceptible.[25] While infection and hormonal influences have been suggested as possible etiological factors, the pathogenesis of pyogenic granuloma is considered, by most authorities, to center around trauma.[27]

Microscopic examination of pyogenic granuloma will reveal a circumscribed mass of granulation tissue usually covered at least partially by an epithelial surface. The granulation tissue usually manifests extreme vascularity, with extensive endothelial proliferation, and often, larger vascular channels engorged with erythrocytes (Fig. 15-6). A mixed inflammatory infiltrate is common in the supporting connective tissue. Some lesions ultimately mature and become totally fibrous. The pyogenic granuloma may be microscopically indistinguishable from hemangioma, particularly if the hemangioma has been traumatized or secondarily infected. Conservative local surgical excision is the preferred treatment; a 10-to-16 percent recurrence rate has been reported.[25]

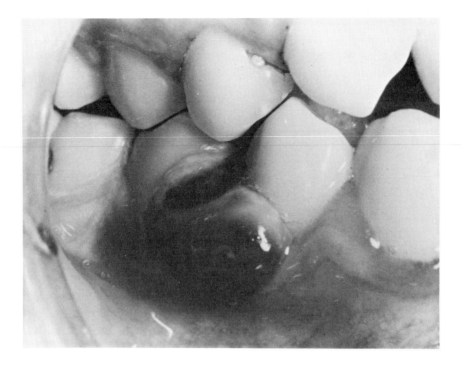

Fig. 15-5A Gingival pyogenic granuloma. Note the hemorrhage color of the extremely vascular lesion seen in this figure and that of Fig. 15-5B. Courtesy of Dr. Paul Casamassimo.

THE ARTERIOVENOUS FISTULA:

Arteriovenous fistulas may be congenital or acquired. Either type may be accompanied by a swelling, a mass, or by spontaneous bleeding. Lesions of the oral soft tissues, face, and scalp are much more frequently encountered than bony lesions. Acquired lesions are usually the result of trauma, while congenital lesions are thought to be the result of persistence of embryonic channels.[24] The head, neck, and the extremities are the most common sites of incidence of arteriovenous fistulas. Although both subsets of the lesion represent an abnormal connection between arterial or venous channels, the following points of difference exist: (1) In the congenital type, there may be multiple links between arteries and veins as opposed to single links in the acquired type, and (2) Congenital fistulas produce less marked systemic effects such as cardiac hypertrophy or decompensation. Batsakis noted that the

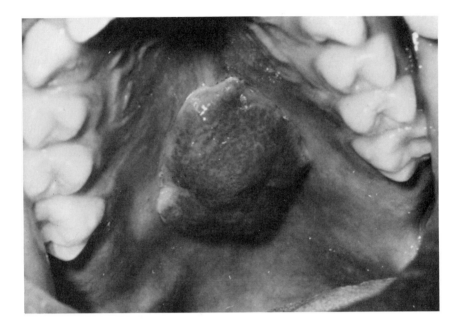

Fig. 15-5B Palatal pyogenic granuloma.

prognosis of untreated fistulas in the head and neck region is uncertain, although he reported the head and neck lesions are better tolerated than lesions of the extremities.[24]

STRAWBERRY NEVUS:

The strawberry nevus was definitively classified as a hypertrophic capillary hemangioma by Batsakis in 1974.[24] The lesion typically appears as a small red area involving subcutaneous areas of the head and neck shortly after birth. A rapid growth rate may follow, to the extent that the lesion often appears quite aggressive. The strawberry nevus rarely reaches a size greater than 1 cm. before undergoing regressive involution during early childhood. The histopathology is quite dynamic and dependent upon the growth phase of the lesion. Both capillary and cavernous elements may be seen in this disorder.

OSLER-RENDU-WEBER SYNDROME:

Hereditary hemorrhagic telangiectasia or angiomatosis is a familial disorder characterized by angiomas appearing at puberty or later in life. The most susceptible sites are the labial, oral and nasal mucosa, pharynx, conjunctiva, and face.[28-31] Individual lesions are small

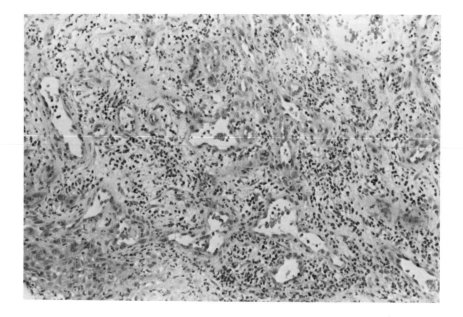

Fig. 15-6 Capillary proliferation in a reactive stroma, filled with acute and chronic inflammatory cells is characteristic of pyogenic granuloma. (H&E x 130).

and appear as minute, deep-red papules. Hemorrhages from the mucosal lesions are a common problem and treatment with electrocoagulation is often necessary. Microscopically, the lesions are hemangiomas of the capillary variety, with occasional larger cavernous spaces. Neurofibromatosis, elliptocytosis, and arteriovenous aneurysm of the lung have also been found in association with this syndrome.

STURGE-WEBER SYNDROME:

This disorder is a neurocutaneous syndrome consisting of angiomatosis of the skin, mucosa, and leptomeninges of the brain.[32-34] Cutaneous hemangiomas tend to be unilateral and usually appear on the face. Both cutaneous and mucosal hemangiomas tend to be of the capillary type.[34] Oral lesions are usually localized to the gingiva and appear as diffuse gingival enlargements. Hemangiomatous lesions of the leptomeninges most often occur over the occipital lobes of the brain, and meningeal lesions often contain calcified laminated concretions.

Symptoms related to the brain are rare, and intracranial pressure is not appreciably increased, even by relatively large lesions. Epilepsy, mental retardation, and hemiplegia may occur in certain cases.

MAFFUCCI'S SYNDROME:

This extremely rare syndrome consists of dyschondroplasia in association with hemangiomas of the skin and oral mucous membrane. The syndrome first appears at puberty or during childhood, and affects boys more frequently than girls. The dyschondroplasia is seen in the long bones and may result in deformity and a tendency to spontaneous fractures. Chondrosarcoma is very often a grave complication of the osseous lesions.[35]

HEMANGIOPERICYTOMA:

The hemangiopericytoma of children is a distinct entity with a biologic behavior pattern that is unique to this age group. Commonly referred to as infantile or congenital hemangiopericytomas, these lesions were first described by Stout and Murray[36] in 1942, and later by Kauffman and Stout[37] who described a series of 31 cases. Recently, Enzinger and Smith have thoroughly delineated the pathology of infantile hemangiopericytoma as separate and distinct from the adult variety.[38] These authors reported that in contrast to the adult form of hemangiopericytoma, the childhood tumors are benign, affect the newborn through the very young, and occur primarily in the subcutis.

Infantile hemangiopericytoma can be found in a variety of anatomic locations. Eleven of the 31 tumors reviewed by Kauffman and Stout occurred in the head and neck region. The tongue was the only head and neck location in which more than one tumor was identified. Thirteen of the tumors they observed were congenital, and seven of these were in the head and neck area. A male predominance has most often been reported.

The histopathology of the tumor is characterized by a pronounced collagen matrix, a rather irregular distribution of the vascular pattern, and most significantly, according to the studies of Enzinger and Smith, features suggesting a transition between hemangiopericytoma and hemangioendothelioma[37] (Fig. 15-7). This tumor may concurrently show areas of necrosis, atypical mitotic activity, and perivascular extension by tumor cells beyond the main tumor mass, —and still remain biologically benign.

The juvenile hemangiopericytoma is grossly similar to other mesenchymal neoplasms and, upon inspection at the surgical bench, it

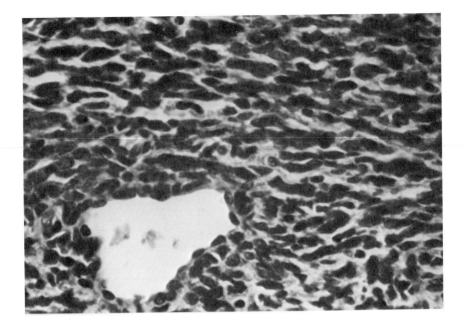

Fig. 15-7 Hemangiopericytoma showing an irregular arrangement of neoplastic cells in a perithelial location. (H&E x 220). Courtesy of Dr. Bruce Jafek.

has no observable uniqueness. Histologically, it must be distinguished from several other mesenchymal neoplasms. Upon staining with hematoxylin and eosin preparations, juvenile hemangioma can imitate the hemangioperocytoma because the lining endothelial cells are often flattened while the surrounding endothelial cells are rounded. In juvenile hemangioma, a reticulin stain should show a reticulin vascular sheath enclosing both flattened lining cells and rounded surrounding cells, an indication that all of them are endothelial cells.[38] However, using the same stain with hemangiopericytoma, the surrounding rounded or elongated cells will be outside the vascular reticulin sheath.[38] In most instances, with the exception of some malignant examples, each pericyte will be surrounded by reticulin fibers, which is not the case with the endothelial cells of a simple juvenile hemangioma.

Another tumor which may be confused with the hemangiopericytoma is the *vascular leiomyoma*, especially since pericytes may be closely related to smooth muscle cells.[38] If no myofibrils and no special acidophile tendency in the tumor cells can be demonstrated, one should suspect that the cells are pericytes. Neurilemmoma has sometimes been confused with hemangiopericytoma, perhaps because of its propensity for containing groups of vessels with thick collagen collars.[38] However, neurilemmoma has distinctive features not seen in hemangiopericytoma, such as: division of Antoni A and B tissue; dominent nuclear palisading, and finally, the distribution of reticulin fibers paralleling the long axes of the Schwann cells instead of being wrapped about them.

Sclerosing hemangioma (fibrous xanthoma) may be confused with hemangiopericytoma, but the former tumor almost always has histiocytes containing lipid and/or hemosiderin. It also most commonly involves the skin, while hemangiopericytoma is generally subcutaneous or deeper.

A hemangiopericytoma that shows prominent spindling and collagen formation may mimic a fibrous histiocytoma histologically, but the latter usually shows a storiform or cartwheel pattern and a less well pronounced, less intricate vascular network.[38]

The ultrastructure of juvenile hemangiopericytoma has recently been reviewed by Eimoto.[39] The versatility of the primitive pericyte was discussed and the author noted that some tumor cells showed the characteristic ultrastructural features of fibroblasts, endothelial cells, and smooth muscle cells.

The infantile hemangiopericytoma is most often managed by wide surgical excision. All of the cases discussed by Enzinger and Smith[38] followed a benign clinical course. Batsakis reported a greater "malignant potential" for patients in the pre-adolescent and adolescent age groups.

ANGIOSARCOMA:

Malignant vascular tumors occur at all ages but are almost curiosities in children. Southwich collected only three angiosarcomas out of 70 malignant tumors of the head and neck in children.[40] Nonetheless, Girard[41] reported that angiosarcoma tends to occur more frequently in children than adults.

In an analysis of 28 cutaneous angiosarcomas, Girard and others[41] discovered the face and the scalp to be the most common locations for angiosarcoma. Bundens and Brighton[42] reviewed the world literature and reported 32 cases of this lesion in the bone, adding two cases of their own. They found that angiosarcoma occurred almost twice as often in males as females; the femur was involved most frequently, and there were eleven lesions of multifocal origin. Only one case occurred in the mandible. Shklar and Meyer,[4] in a review of 694 oral vascular tumors and tumor-like proliferations, reported only three angiosarcomas. More recently, Wesley and others[43] reviewed 20 primary oral malignant hemangioendotheliomas from the literature and added a case of their own. Of their 20 cases, 11 appeared in females and 8 in males (the sex of one patient was not specified). The age span ranged from 1 day to 67 years. Ten lesions involved the mandible, one involved the maxilla, three were in the gingiva, two in the maxillary sinus, one in the tongue, one in the lower lip, one in the floor of the mouth, and one in the palate.

Zachariades and associates[44] reviewed the world literature on angiosarcoma of the maxilla and mandible and reported a case of their own. Quite interestingly, they found that 14 of a total of 46 lesions occurred in children.

The histogenesis of angiosarcoma is obscure. The outstanding chief complaint is usually the presence of a rapidly growing mass, with rapid onset and minimal symptoms.

Stout[45] established the following criteria for the diagnosis of angiosarcoma: (1) the presence of atypical endothelial cells in a number greater than required to line a vessel (Fig. 15-8), and (2) the formation of vascular tubes, the lamina of which have a distinct tendency to anastomose with a delicate framework of reticulin fibers. In extreme anaplasia, it may be difficult to distinguish this lesion from leiomyosarcoma, or fibrosarcoma.

A problem often arising when the tumor is viewed using light microscopy is one of differentiation between a tumor of pericyte origin and a tumor arising from the endothelium.[46] To solve the problem, a silver reticulin stain may prove helpful. When the tumor cells are located outside the reticulin sheath, pericytes are considered to be the cells of origin.[43;47]

Ultrastructurally, the principal difference between hemangiopericytoma and hemangioendothelioma is the spacing of tumor cells in relation to the surrounding extracellular material. Extracellular material is relatively thin in the former, whereas it is much more abundant with the latter.

Batsakis reported that, when feasible, the treatment of choice for an angiosarcoma is complete excision controlled by frozen sections for adequacy of margins.[24] The five-year survival-rate is frequently less than 25 percent.[44]

KAPOSI'S SARCOMA:

Kaposi's sarcoma is rare in childhood. Dutz and Stablet reviewed 1,256 cases and reported that only 40 (3.2 percent) occurred in

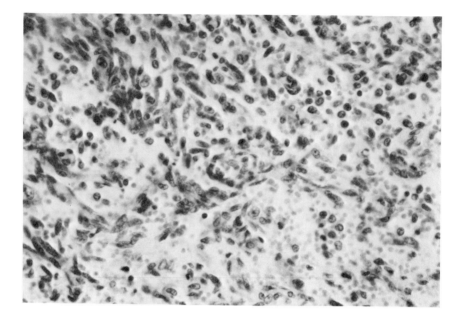

Fig. 15-8 Poorly-differentiated angiosarcoma, showing abundant proliferation of atypical endothelial cells. (H&E x 180). Courtesy of Dr. Bruce Jafek.

patients under six years of age. Interestingly, 18 of their 40 cases were from Africa.

Olweny and others[48] reviewed 12 cases of childhood Kaposi's sarcoma seen at the Uganda Cancer Institute over a seven-year-period. The disease usually manifested as generalized lymphadenopathy, with sparsely distributed cutaneous nodules. Females outnumbered males among children with the disease, whereas males outumbered females in its incidence among adults to a proportion as great as 13-to-1. Primary disease in the head and neck area appeared in very few patients. The histology is usually of mixed cell type. If not treated, childhood Kaposi's sarcoma runs a fulminating course, but disease control with chemotherapy is associated with prolonged survival.

ANGIOFIBROMA

Synonyms

1. Juvenile angiofibroma
2. Nasopharyngeal angiofibroma
3. Juvenile nasopharyngeal angiofibroma
4. Juvenile fibroangioma

INCIDENCE

Angiofibroma is reported to account for 0.5 percent of all head and neck neoplasms.[24] Hora and Brown reported that the tumor accounts for approximately one in five-to-six thousand otolaryngological admissions to hospital clinics.[49] Apostol and Frazell reviewed the total clinical experience of the head and neck service at the Sloan-Kettering Memorial Cancer Center over a 30-year-period and documented 40 cases.[50]

AGE AND SEX

The incidence of angiofibroma shows a marked male predominance. The predisposition of males is so great that, until recently, some authorities thought the tumor occurred exclusively in males. However, Batsakis, Osborn and Sokolovski, and Svoboda and Kirschner[24;51;52] have reported cases with all the clinical and histological hallmarks of angiofibroma in females.

Most angiofibromas occur during adolescence. In a review of 29 cases, Martin and associates[53] found that the age of the onset of symptoms varies from 7 to 19 years, with an average age of 14.

In a review of 26 cases of angiofibroma, which had all occurred in male caucasians, Hubbard[54] found an age range from 9 to 50 years. He excluded one case found in a 50-year-old man, and reported the average age to be 16 years. The duration of symptoms prior to initial examination ranged from 3 months to 5 years in Hubbard's review, with an average of about 15 months.

Apostol and Frazell[50] reviewed 40 cases, including 25 previously reported by Sternberg.[55] All patients were white males. Although Apostol and Frazell reported an onset age that ranged from 8-to-27 years, the ages in the majority of cases ranged from 10-to-17 years with a median age of 17.

Batsakis[24] reported the incidence of this tumor in the United States and Europe to be much lower than its incidence in Egypt, India, Southeast Asia, and Kenya.

PATHOGENESIS

The pathogenesis of the nasopharyngeal angiofibroma has not yet been fully explained. Hall and Wilkins[56] cited four theories of origin that have been popularized:

1. In 1878, Verneuil theorized that the tumor originated from the periochondrium of the cartilage uniting the basioccipital bone to the sphenoid. It was his belief that during the second decade of life, the cartilage underwent ossification, destroying the site of origin of the tumor. This supports the idea of "spontaneous regression" but not sexual predisposition.
2. Bunner postulated that nasopharyngeal fibroma originated from the basilar fascia or pharyngeal aponeurosis of the superior constrictor muscle covering the posterior wall and roof of the nasopharynx.
3. Schiff believed that the angiofibroma is "pituitary bound" and is a sexually stimulated cavernous connective tissue, probably of the inferior turbinate type. He was of the opinion that the tumor developed from the nasopharyngeal periosteum.
4. Willis suggested that the angiofibroma developed from an inflammatory allergic state, much as a polyp does, and is not a true tumor.

Hubbard postulated that the tumor is a distinctive and destructive type of hemangioma.[54]

A more detailed and still popular theory is that of a sex-endocrine relationship as proposed by Martin and associates.[57] Their observations suggested that the angiofibroma may result from a deficiency of androgen activity or from increased production of estrogens. This theory lends itself to the question of regressive sexual maturity in patients afflicted with the juvenile nasopharyngeal angiofibroma. Although a number of cases have been reported in which the patient did show signs of sexual underdevelopment, there does not appear to be a constant relationship.[58]

CLINICAL FINDINGS

Unquestionably the most common symptoms of manifestation are epistaxis and nasal obstruction. Repeated episodes of epistaxis may result in anemia.[58] Obstruction of nasal airways is usually unilateral, although it can be bilateral.[54] Kerwin,[59] stated that obstruction is usually the earliest manifesting sign and that it occurs when the tumor has reached a size of roughly 3 cm. He further mentioned that many young boys fail to pay much attention to such minor complaints and the nasal obstruction goes unnoticed. As a result, the most apparent complaint is usually nasal bleeding, and the previous history of obstruction is elicited only upon questioning. Oral breathing is often a manifestation of the nasal obstruction.

The angiofibroma commonly grows in a foward direction from its origin in the nasopharynx[58] (Fig. 15-9). Depending upon the size the mass attains and its path of extension, a number of clinical manifestations may be noted. These signs include orbital involvement with exophthalmos, maxillary involvement with resultant facial deformity, palatal bulging, sinusitis, otitis media, mastoiditis, headache, and speech difficulty.[50;60;61] Bhatia and associates[62] have reported four cases of juvenile nasopharyngeal angiofibroma with intracranial extensions. Occasionally, one may find a tumor growing in a downward direction, causing anterior displacement of the soft palate. In such an instance, the mass occurs in the oropharynx.

Direct clinical visualization of the tumor is best accomplished by posterior rhinoscopy, facilitated by use of a topical anesthetic and retraction of the palate. Occasionally, the mass may be seen through one of the nares. Angiographic techniques may be employed to reveal a blood supply usually originating from the internal maxillary and the ascending pharyngeal arteries.[59]

According to Holman and Miller,[63] there are distinctive roentgenographic characteristics providing aid in the diagnosis of juvenile nasopharyngeal angiofibroma. These features include: (1) anterior bowing of the posterior maxillary wall adjacent to an expanding tumor; (2) erosion through the floor of the sphenoid bone with a resultant radiolucency, surrounded by a sclerotic border, and (3) in some cases, enlargement of the superior orbital fissure when the lower margin is eroded by expansion of the tumor. In addition, Sternberg[55] noted deviation of the nasal septum away from the involved side in 6 of 25 cases he reviewed.

GROSS AND LIGHT MICROSCOPIC FINDINGS

Grossly, the tumors are rounded or nodular masses, exhibiting a sessile or slightly pedunculated base (Fig. 15-10). The erythematous mucosal covering may show ulceration. Sectioning reveals resilient, pliable tissues.

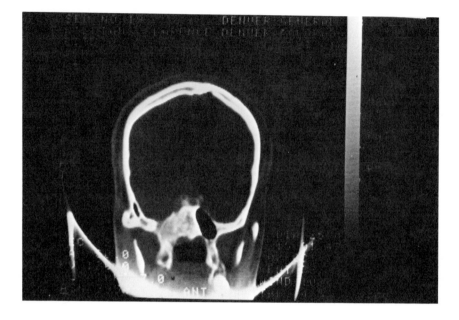

Fig. 15-9 Computerized tomographic view of nasopharyngeal angiofibroma with extension into the paranasal and maxillary sinuses. Courtesy of Dr. Bruce Jafek.

Histologically, the tumor is composed of a nonencapsulated admixture of spindle and stellate fibroblasts in a varying amount of collagenous matrix. Overlying respiratory surface epithelium may show a degree of squamous metaplasia, but the basic histological pattern is derived from the tumor's vascular component and its connective tissue stroma. The vascular network consists of simple endothelially-lined vessels of irregular shape and varied caliber (Fig. 15-11). Characteristically, the advancing edge of an enlarging angiofibroma exhibits the most prominent vascular proliferation. This region can be seen to blend gradually with the deeper portions of the tumor, where larger, anastomosing vascular channels are found. On occasion, the large, deep vessels may individually resemble those seen in a cavernous hemangioma. Thick-walled vessels may represent pre-existing vascular channels. Secondary changes of vascular occlusion and thrombosis may be noted in tumors exhibiting evidence of regression. Focal obliteration of vessels by stromal compression results in double rows of endothelial cells in some parts of the tumor. Degenerative changes in the vessel walls may occasionally be noted, and include diffuse or focal hyalinization, and

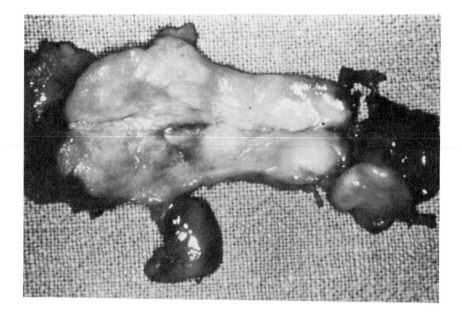

Fig. 15-10 Firm nodular mass with glistening cut surface, characteristic of angiofibroma. Courtesy of Dr. Bruce Jafek.

areas of myxomatous degeneration. An apparent fibrinoid necrosis is rarely seen. The fibrous connective tissue stroma consists of interwoven fine and coarse collagen fibers, imparting a streaming fascicle-like appearance.

ELECTRON MICROSCOPY

Taxy[64] postulated from ultrastructural findings that the tumor cells in the juvenile angiofibroma are, in fact, a hybridized mesenchymal cell, most likely a myofibroblast.

DIFFERENTIAL DIAGNOSIS

Clinically, one must rule out a variety of inflammatory conditions, as well as other neoplastic growths. Nasal polyps present the most frequent difficulty in clinical differentiation from angiofibroma. Nevertheless, histological differences are usually sufficient to avoid confusion.[58]

The *glomus jugular tumor* may resemble juvenile nasopharyngeal angiofibroma histologically, but, the former is, typically, quite a bit

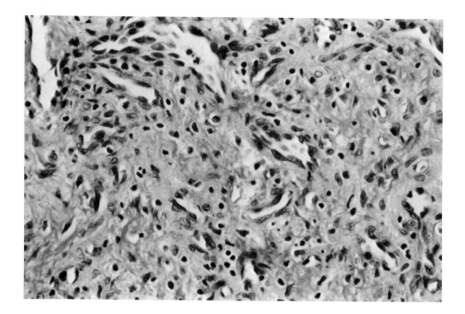

Fig. 15-11 Angiofibroma showing a vascular component, composed of channels lined by endothelial cells. The vascular network is supported by a relatively mature connective tissue stroma. (H&E x 240). Courtesy of Dr. Bruce Jafek.

more vascular than the latter, and the stromal desmoplastic reaction is less prominent.

It is probably most important to distinguish angiofibroma from the more common capillary hemangioma because of the somewhat greater destructive biological potential of the latter. Rosai[65] commented that hemangiomas are accompanied by a sparser amount of fibrous tissue, and their vessels do not have the so-called erectile tissue appearance characteristic of nasopharyngeal angiofibroma.

Although odontogenic myxoma (fibromyxoma) may resemble angiofibroma, myxomas lack the vascularity of angiofibroma. Myxoma also shows a dominant stellate fibroblastic histopathological pattern often accompanied by entrapped epithelial odontogenic rests. Such rests have not been reported in angiofibroma.

TREATMENT AND PROGNOSIS

The primary treatment of angiofibroma remains surgical excision. Apostol and Frazell,[50] in their review, documented five common modes of management including local surgery, external radiation therapy, seed implants, testosterone therapy, and external carotid artery ligation. Radiation therapy is now considered to be contraindicated and testosterone is not successful as a primary or adjunctive management tool.

Stilbestrol has been used with varying degrees of success but its side effects often negate its use.

Surgical management ranges from conservative to radical. Batsakis[24] maintained that regardless of the surgical technique employed, the approach must be tailored to provide adequate exposure and to allow a controlled removal of the tumor.

Hora[49] reported a mortality rate of three percent for the tumor. The prognosis for the young juvenile with this disease is nonetheless quite good, although recurrences may pose a problem of morbidity, along with a depressed psychological condition. Smith and co-workers[66] reported a recurrence rate of 2.5 in 19 of 40 patients they treated; in one patient, they documented 12 recurrences.

LYMPHANGIOMA

Synonyms

1. Simple lymphangioma
2. Cavernous lymphangioma

INCIDENCE, AGE AND SEX

The vast majority of lymphangiomas are noted at birth. Sixty-seven percent of 27 patients reviewed at the Johns Hopkins Hospital over a 28-year-period by Harkins and Sabiston[67] had congenital lesions. Batsakis[24] reported that 80 to 90 percent of the lesions are detected by the end of the second year of life.

The head and neck area is the most frequently affected anatomic site followed by the lower extremities, arms, axilla, and trunk. Bhaskar reported that along with hemangiomas, lymphangiomas account for 27 percent of all oral tumors in children. The incidence of lymphangiomas indicates no apparent sexual predisposition.

PATHOGENESIS

Lymphangiomas are best characterized as hamartomas rather than true neoplasms; —as such they probably arise as developmental malformations characterized by large endothelially-lined spaces forming small plexuses which develop into lymph sacs. Sabin[68] has shown that all lymphatics begin as capillaries, and that their method of growth is by the sprouting of the cellular material and by nuclear division of the capillary wall endothelium. Subsequently, there is a continuous growth and invasion of the body by lymphatic channels from the primary sprouts emerging from the veins and ultimately forming the peripheral lymphatic capillaries. Lymphangiomas are often regarded as the enlargement of lymphatic spaces; a process secondary to failure of the lymphatics' normal drainage into the venous system.[68]

CLINICAL FINDINGS

The most common sites for the occurrence of lymphangiomas are the neck, tongue, cheek, and floor of the mouth. Lesions of the neck usually become manifest as *cystic hygromas* (Fig. 15-12). These hygroma colli are predominately found in the posterior triangle of the neck beneath the platysma. Kreller and colleagues[69] reported that larger hygromas may extend beyond the sternocleidomastoid muscle into the anterior compartment of the neck and often across the midline. Lesions that arise towards the anterior tend to invade the floor of the mouth and base of the tongue. Large lesions may result in respiratory stridor, spontaneous hemorrhage, or pain. Small lesions are usually unilocular while large lesions tend to be multilocular. Both types of lesions may ordinarily be seen with transillumination. Multilocular lesions tend to intercommunicate and are usually filled with watery or straw-colored fluid.[69]

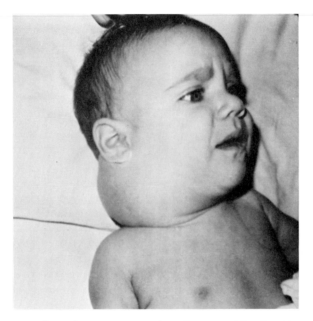

Fig. 15-12 Cystic hygroma in an infant. Courtesy of Dr. Ray Wood.

Lesions of the oral mucosa occur as superficial small papillary masses or as deeper lesions of the submucosa (Fig. 15-13). Deep lesions tend to show elevation of the overlying mucosa and generally have a rubbery consistency. Large lesions may result in macrocheilia or macroglossia.

LIGHT MICROSCOPY

Lymphangioma is composed of a mass of lymph vessels characterized by a thin, delicate endothelium and absence of erythrocytes within the lymph spaces. The size of these lymph spaces varies considerably, and the terms *simple* or *cavernous* may be used to highlight their size differences.

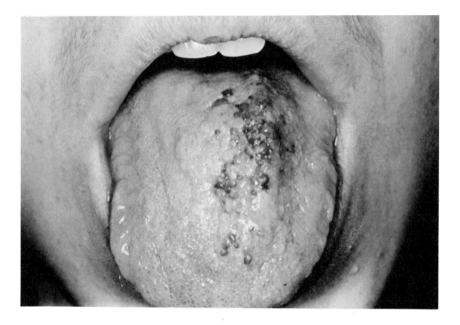

Fig. 15-13 Lymphangioma of the tongue. Courtesy of Dr. Roy Eversole.

The cavernous type of lymphangioma, with large, obvious spaces, is by far the most common (Fig. 15-14). Its walls are extremely thin, and this often offers a means of distinguishing the lesion from hemangioma. The vessels are separated by varying amounts of fibrous connective tissue, and covered by stratified squamous epithelium.

The simple lymphangioma is usually small, superficial, and composed histologically of small dilations of subepithelial lymphatic channels. In contrast, *cystic hygroma* is composed of multiple dilated and collapsed lymphatic channels lined by a single layer of flattened endothelium. Focal lymphocytic infiltrations as well as small sprouts or buds of lymphangiomatous tissue may extend into adjacent normal tissue.

DIFFERENTIAL DIAGNOSIS

Watson and McCarthy[1] have emphasized the necessity for differentiation between cystic hygroma and cavernous lymphangioma. Both lesions tend to occur in infants and in specific anatomic sites. The diagnosis depends on the appearance of the lesion upon operation as well as its microscopic characteristics. Cystic hygroma is composed of large,

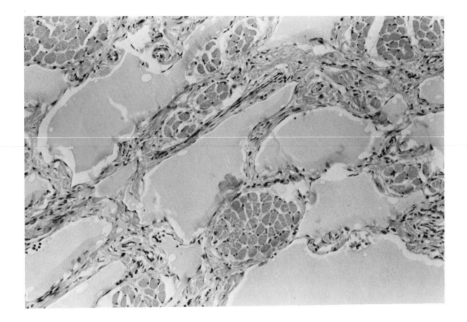

Fig. 15-14 Lymphangioma of the tongue, showing marked lymphangectasia in the lamina propria and muscular submucosa. (H&E x 240).

multiloculated cysts which are more or less clearly delineated. More solid, small to microscopic cysts are common to cavernous lymphangioma. Histologically, the endothelium in cystic hygroma tends to be more flattened, with less fibrous stroma, than that in cavernous lymphangioma.

In some instances, it is impossible to state categorically whether the vascular elements in a lymphangioma are lymphangiomatous channels into which bleeding has occurred or whether a hemangioma is present as well. If lymphangiomatous tissue is strongly the predominant type, the lesion is usually classified as cavernous lymphangioma.

The differentiation between lymphangioma and lymphangiosarcoma may be difficult to make. Lymphangiosarcoma is rare and this diagnosis is generally reserved for lesions showing either rapid growth or cytological evidence of malignancy. It represents a type of tumor which is highly invasive and rarely seen in children. Stewart and Treves,[70] as well as Stout,[71] have reported several cases of this type occurring in the upper extremities following radical mastectomy, but head and neck tumors are rare.

TREATMENT AND PROGNOSIS

The preferred treatment for oral lymphangiomas is usually surgical; although cryosurgery, radiotherapy, and injection of sclerosing substances have all been employed.

Batsakis reported that the optimum age for surgical management of a cystic hygroma is 18 months to 2 years. Observation of the lesion until adolescence, along with aspiration, cryosurgery, and radiation therapy, have all been employed as management modalities for the cystic hygroma. None, except the modality first cited, is considered to be a reasonable alternative to a thorough surgical removal.[24]

Harkins and associates[67] reported a high rate of recurrence associated with lymphangiomas regardless of their anatomic location in the head and neck area. This high incidence of local recurrence is illustrated by the fact that a total of 88 surgical procedures were performed in a group of only 27 patients studied by Harkins. Although high mortality rates are uncommon, such cases have only been reported in association with extensive cystic hygromas of the perinatal child where cellulitis, repiratory obstruction, and hemorrhage have occurred.

References

1. Watson, W.L. and McCarthy, W.D. "Blood and lymph vessel tumors. Report of 1,056 cases." *Surg. Gynecol. Obstet.* 71(1940): 569-588.
2. Friedman et al. "Cavernous hemangioma of the oral cavity — review of the literature and report of case." *J. Oral Surg.* 31(1973): 617-619.
3. Herarg et al. "The use of cryotherapy in the management of intraoral hemangioma." *South Med. J.* 65(1972): 1123-1127.
4. Shklar, G. and Meyer, I. "Vascular tumors of the mouth and jaws." *Oral Surg.* 19(1965): 335-358.
5. Saunders, B. *Pediatric Oral and Maxillofacial Surgery.* St. Louis: C.V. Mosby, 1979.
6. Margileth, A.M. and Museles, M. "Cutaneous hemangiomas of children. Diagnosis and conservative management." *JAMA* 194(1965): 523-526.
7. Johnson, E.W., Jr. "Hemangiomas of the extremities." Thesis, University of Minnesota, 1950.
8. Ribbert. "Uber bau, wachsthum und genese der angiome." *Virchows Archiv: Abteilung A: Pathologische Anatomie* 151(1898): 381-401.
9. Bowman, K. "A clinico-histologic investigation on hemangioma." *Acta Chir. Scand.* 83(1940): 185-224.
10. Hartley, J.H. and Schatten, W.E. "Cavernous hemangioma of the mandible" *Plast. Reconstr. Surg.* 50(1972): 287-290.
11. Shira, R.B. and Guemsey, L.H. "Central cavernous hemangioma of the mandible: report of a case." *J. Oral Surg.* 23(1965): 636-642.
12. Jacobs, J.E. and Kimmelstiel, P. "Cystic angiomatosis of the skeletal system." *J. Bone Joint Surg.* 35A(1953): 409-420.

13. Cocke, E.W., Jr. "Cavernous hemangioma of the oral cavity and hypopharynges." *Am. J. Surg.* 102(1961): 798-802.
14. Scott, J.E. "Hemangiomata in skeletal muscle." *Br. J. Surg.* 44(1957): 496-501.
15. Kinni, J.E.; Webb, R.I. and Christensen, R.E. "Intramuscular hemangioma of the obicularis oris muscle: report of case." *J. Oral Surg.* 39(1981): 780-782.
16. Dahlin, D.C. *Bone Tumors. General Aspects of and Data on 6,221 Cases*, 3rd ed. Springfield: Charles C. Thomas, 1978.
17. Piercell, M.P.; Waite, D.E. and Nelson, R.L. "Central hemangioma of the mandible." *J. Oral Surg.* 33(1975): 225-232.
18. Lund, B.A. "Hemangiomas of the mandible and maxilla." *J. Oral Surg.* 22(1964): 234-242.
19. Schnidel et al. "Central cavernous hemangioma of the jaws." *J. Oral Surg.* 36(1981): 803-807.
20. Martis, C. and Karakasn, D. "Central hemangioma of the mandible: report of case." *J. Oral Surg.* 31(9173): 613-616.
21. Howard et al. "Parotid tumors in children." *Surg. Gynecol. Obstet.* 90(1950): 307-319.
22. Allen, P.W. and Enzinger, R.M. "Hemangioma of skeletal muscle." *Cancer* 29(1972): 8-22.
23. Waldo, E.D.; Vuletin, J.C. and Kaye, G.I. "The ultrastructure of vascular tumors: additional observations and a review of the literature." *Pathol. Annu.* 12(1977): 279.
24. Batsakis, J.G. *Tumors of the Head and Neck. Clinical and Pathological Considerations*, 2nd ed. Baltimore: Williams and Wilkins, 1979.
25. Bhaskar, S.N. and Jacoway, J.R. "Pyogenic granuloma—clinical features, incidence, histology and result of treatment: report of 242 cases." *J. Oral Surg.* 24(1966): 391-398.
26. Standish, S.M. and Shafer, W.G. "Gingival reparative granulomas in children." *J. Oral Surg.* 19(1961): 367-375.
27. Kerr, D.A. "Granuloma pyogenicum." *Oral Surg.* 4(1951): 158-176.
28. Osler, W. "On a family form of recurring epistaxis associated with multiple telangiectases of the skin and mucous membranes." *Bulletin of the Johns Hopkins Hospital* 12(1901): 333-337.
29. Garland, H.G. and Anning, S.T. "Hereditary hemorrhagic telangiectasia: a genetic and bibliographical study." *Br. J. Dermatol.* 62(1950): 289-310.
30. Goldstein, H.I. "Goldstein's heredofamilial angiomatosis with recurring familial hemorrhages (Rendu-Olser-Weber's disease)." *Arch. Intern. Med.* 49(1931): 836-865.
31. Stock, M.F. "Hereditary hemorrhagic telangiectasia (Osler's disease)." *Arch. Otolaryngol.* 40(1944): 108-114.
32. Weber, F.P. "Multiple hereditary developmental angiomata (telangiectases) of the skin and mucous membranes associated with recurring hemorrhages." *Lancet* 2(1907): 160-162.
33. Weber, F.P. "A note on association of extensive hemangiomatous naevus of the skin with cerebral (meningeal) hemangioma, especially, cases of facial vascular naevus with contralateral hemiplegia." *Proc. R. Soc. Med.* 22(1929): 431-442.
34. Peterman et al. "Encephalotrigeminal angiomatosis (Sturge-Weber disease): clinical study of thirty-five cases." *JAMA* 167(1958): 2169-2176.

35. Lewis R.J. and Ketcham, A.S. "Maffucci's syndrome: functional and neoplastic significance. Case report and review of the literature. *J. Bone Joint Surg.* 55(1973): 1465-1479.

36. Stout, A.P. and Murray, M.R. "Hemangiopericytoma — a vascular tumor featuring Zimmerman's pericytes." *Ann. Surg.* 116(1942): 26-33.

37. Kauffman, S.L. and Stout, A.P. "Hemangiopericytoma in children." *Cancer* 13(1960): 695-710.

38. Enzinger, F.M. and Smith, B.H. "Hemangiopericytoma. An analysis of 106 cases." *Hum. Pathol.* 7(1976): 61-82.

39. Eimoto, T. "Ultrastructure of an infantile hemangiopericytoma." *Cancer* 40(1977): 2161-2170.

40. Southwick, H.W.; Slaughter D.P. and Majarakis, J.D. "Malignant disease of the head and neck in childhood." *Arch. Surg.* 78(1959): 678-681.

41. Girard, C.; Waine, C.J. and Graham, J.H. "Cutaneous angiosarcoma." *Cancer* 23(1970): 868-883.

42. Bundens, W.D. and Brighton. C.T. "Malignant hemangioendothelioma of bone." *J. Bone Joint Surg.* 47A(1965): 762-772.

43. Wesley, R.K.; Mintz, S.M. and Wertheimer, F.W. "Primary malignant hemangioendothelioma of the gingiva." *Oral Surg.* 39(1975): 103-112.

44. Zachariades et al. "Primary hemangioendotheliosarcoma of the mandible. Review of the literature and report of case." *J. Oral Surg.* 39(1980):288-296.

45. Stout, A.P. "Hemangioendothelioma: a tumor of blood vessels featuring vascular endothelial cells." *Ann. Surg.* 118(1943): 445-464.

46. Orlian, A.I. "Benign hemangiopericytoma of the tongue." *J. Oral Surg.* 31(1973): 936-938.

47. Phillips, H.; Brown, S. and Ball, M. "Hemangioendothelioma: report of case." *J. Oral Surg.* 27(1969): 286-288.

48. Olweny et al. "Childhood Kaposi's sarcoma: clinical features and therapy." *Br. J. Cancer* 33(1976): 555-560.

49. Hora, J.F. and Brown, A.K. "Paranasal juvenile angiofibroma." *Arch. Otolaryngol.* 76(1962): 457-459.

50. Apostol, J.V. and Frazell, E.L. "Juvenile nasopharyngeal angiofibroma." *Cancer* 18(1965): 869-878.

51. Osborn, D.A. and Sokolovski, A. "Juvenile nasopharyngeal angiofibroma in a female." *Arch. Otolaryngol.* 82(1965): 629-632.

52. Svoboda, D.J. and Kirschner, F. "Ultrastructure of nasopharyngeal angiofibroma." *Cancer* 19(1966): 1949-1962.

53. Martin, H.; Erlich, H.E. and Abels, J.E. "Juvenile nasopharyngeal angiofibroma." *Ann. Surg.* 127(1948): 513-536.

54. Hubbard, E.M. "Nasopharyngeal angiofibromas." *Arch. Pathol.* 65(1958): 192-204.

55. Sternberg, S.S. "Pathology of the juvenile nasopharyngeal angiofibroma. A lesion of adolescent males." *Cancer* 7(1954): 15-28.

56. Hall, L.J. and Wilkins, S.A. "Nasopharyngeal fibroma." *Am. J. Surg.* 116(1968): 530-537.

57. Martin, H.; Erlich, H.E. and Abels, J.E. "Juvenile nasopharyngeal angiofibroma." *Ann. Surg.* 127(1948): 513-536.

58. Hicks, J.L. and Nelson, J.F. "Juvenile nasopharyngeal angiofibroma." *Oral Surg.* 35(1973): 807-817.

59. Kerwin, R.W. "Juvenile nasopharyngeal angiofibroma." *Arch. Otolaryngol.* 53(1951): 397-405.

60. Conley et al. "Nasopharyngeal angiofibroma in the juvenile." *Surg. Gynecol. Obstet.* 126(1968): 825-837.

61. Chhangani, D.L.; Sharma, S.D. and Popli, S.P. "Intracranial extensions in nasopharyngeal fibroma." *J. Laryngol. Otol.* 82(1968): 1137-1144.

62. Bhatia, M.L; Mishra, S.C. and Prakash, J. "Intracranial extensions of the juvenile angiofibroma of the nasopharynx." *J. Laryngol. Otol.* 81(1967): 1395-1403.

63. Holman, C.B. and Miller, W.E. "Juvenile nasopharyngeal angiofibroma." *Amer. J. Roentgen.* 94(1965): 292-298.

64. Taxy, J. "Juvenile angiofibroma, an ultrastructural study." *Cancer* 39(1977): 1044-1053.

65. Rosai, J. *Ackerman's Surgical Pathology,* 6th ed. St. Louis: C.V. Mosby, 1981.

66. Smith, M.F.W.; Boles, R. and Work, W.P. "Cryosurgical techniques in removal of angiofibromas." *Laryngoscope* 74(1964): 1071-1080.

67. Harkins, G.A. and Sabiston, D.C. "Lymphangioma in infancy and childhood." *Surgery* 47(1960): 811-822.

68. Sabin, F.R. "The origin and development of the lymphatic system." *Johns Hopkins Med. J.* 17(1916): 347.

69. Kreller, J.S.; Carr, R.F. and Quinn, J.H. "Cystic hygroma in a 17-year-old patient: report of case." *J. Oral Surg.* 36(1978): 808-813.

70. Stewart, F.W. and Treves, N. "Lymphangiosarcoma in postmastectomy lymphedema. A report of six cases in elephantiasis chirurgica." *Cancer* 1(1948): 64-81.

71. Stout, A.P. *Tumors of the Soft Tissues. Atlas of Tumor Pathology,* section 2, fascicle 5. Washington, D.C.: Armed Forces Institute of Pathology, 1953.

Chapter XVI

Metastatic and Miscellaneous Tumors

INCIDENCE

The most common metastatic tumors in the head and neck region of children are, in our experience, neuroblastoma, retinoblastoma, and Wilm's tumor or nephroblastoma.

Primary tumors of the head and neck other than thyroid tumors and those covered in previous chapters of this text are exceedingly rare but include: chordoma, mesenchymoma, paraganglioma, meningioma, leiomyosarcoma, alveolar soft parts sarcoma, and synovial sarcoma.

GENERAL COMMENT

Neuroblastoma may on occasion manifest as a metastatic orbital tumor with "black eyes" and proptosis. Most patients in whom the disease occurs in this fashion have bone marrow metastases as well, and a diagnosis can be made through biopsy of that tissue (Fig. 16-1). Nearly one third of neuroblastomas are said to eventually involve the orbit through metastatic disease.[1] Cervical nodal and skull metastases are also not uncommon in patients with neuroblastoma of abdominal or thoracic primary sites.

Retinoblastoma rarely appears with evidence of metastatic disease at the time of diagnosis and, in those rare situations, central nervous system or bone marrow metastases are more often seen. In recent years we have seen late (8-10 years after primary tumor removal) cervical node involvement by retinoblastoma (Fig. 16-2). Wilm's tumor (nephroblastoma) may on rare occasions metastasize to cervical lymph nodes or, more commonly, the base of the skull.

References

1. Dehner, L.P. In *Pediatric Surgical Pathology*, p.175. St. Louis: C.V. Mosby, 1975.

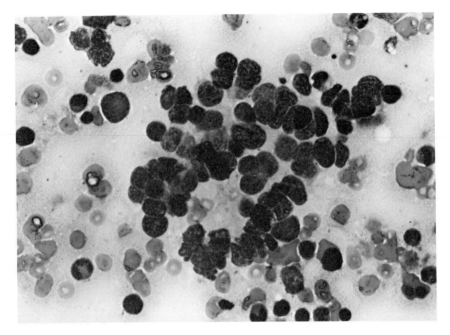

Fig. 16-1 Neuroblastoma metastatic to bone marrow. Clusters of cells suggest a rosette configuration. Electron microscopy of such cellular aggregates is often definitively diagnostic. (Wright's x 400).

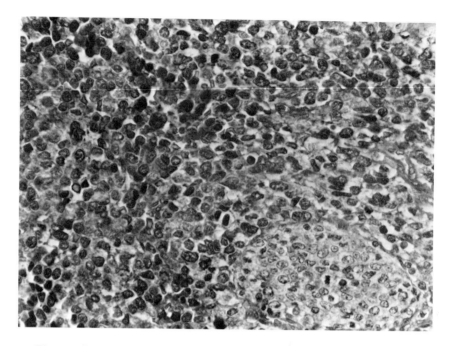

Fig. 16-2 Retinoblastoma in a cervical node with a follicular center cell aggregate. Poor-differentiation is characteristic of such metastatic disease. (H&E x 250).

Index

ABOUT THE AUTHORS

ROBERT O. GREER, JR., D.D.S., Sc.D.

Dr. Greer received his undergraduate education at Miami University, Oxford, Ohio, graduating with an A.B. in Zoology in 1965. His dental education and D.D.S. were obtained at Howard University College of Dentistry in 1969.

Dr. Greer completed Anatomic and Oral Pathology residencies at Boston University Hospital and the Boston University School of Graduate Dentistry. He received a Sc.D. in Pathology in 1974 from Boston University.

In 1974 he joined the University of Colorado Health Sciences Center and presently holds the rank of Professor and Chairman of the Oral Pathology and Oncology Division.

Dr. Greer is also Director of the Western States Regional Pathology Laboratory in Denver.

GARY W. MIERAU, PH.D.

Undergraduate studies leading to a Bachelor of Arts degree (in education) with a major in Biology, were completed by Dr. Gary Mierau at Kearney State College (Nebraska) in 1967. His graduate studies in Wildlife Ecology at Colorado State University earned Dr. Mierau a Master of Science degree in 1968, and a Doctor of Philosophy degree in 1974.

The position he currently holds, that of Electron Microscopist in the Department of Pathology at The Children's Hospital, Denver, was taken in 1969.

Dr. Mierau's principle special interests currently lie in the application of electron microscopy to diagnostic human pathology, particularly neoplastic diseases of childhood. His many research activities, however, continue to range well outside the realm of medicine, including such areas as environmental pollution and wildlife ecology.

BLAISE E. FAVARA, M.D.

Dr. Favara's undergraduate education was obtained at the University of Arizona with a major in Chemistry and Zoology, concluding with a B.S. degree granted in 1954. His medical education and M.D. were obtained at St. Louis University School of Medicine, St. Louis, Missouri, in 1958. He served his internship at City of Memphis Hospital, University of Tennessee, while subsequent active duty in public health service at Louisville University, Kentucky, provided Dr. Favara with experience in Pediatric Cardiology.

Residency in Pediatrics and Pediatric Pathology was served by Dr. Favara at St. Louis University Hospital System, Boston Children's Hospital, and Boston Lying-In Hospital. Upon completion of training, Dr. Favara held the position of Pathologist and Director of Laboratories at LaBonner Children's Hospital, Memphis, Tennessee, and was an assistant Professor of Pediatrics and Pathology at the University of Tennessee.

In 1968, Dr. Favara took the position which he currently holds: Chairman of the Department of Pathology at The Children's Hospital, Denver, Colorado. His special areas of interest within the field of Pediatric Pathology revolve about oncologic pathology with special interest in hematopathology.

Dr. Favara is a member of the editorial boards of the Journal of Pediatric Pathology and the American Journal of Clinical Pathology.

His research interests are dominated by studies in histiocytic diseases of children with emphasis on morphologic and immunologic features.